The Year book of sports
medicine

2000
YEAR BOOK OF
SPORTS MEDICINE®

Statement of Purpose

The YEAR BOOK Service

The YEAR BOOK series was devised in 1901 by health professionals who observed that the literature of medicine and related disciplines had become so voluminous that no one individual could read and place in perspective every potential advance in a major specialty. That has never been more true than it is today.

More than merely a series of books, YEAR BOOK volumes are the tangible results of a unique service designed to accomplish the following:

- to *survey* a wide range of journals
- to *select* from those journals papers representing significant advances and statements of important clinical principles
- to provide *abstracts* of those articles that are readable, convenient summaries of their key points
- to provide *informed commentary* about their relevance

These publications grow out of a unique process that draws on the talents of outstanding authorities in clinical and fundamental disciplines, trained literature specialists, and professional writers—all supported by the resources of Mosby, the world's preeminent publisher for the health professions.

The Literature Base

Mosby and its editors survey approximately 500 journals published worldwide, covering the full range of the health professions. On an annual basis, the publisher examines usage patterns and polls its expert authorities to add new journals to the literature base and to delete journals that are no longer useful as potential YEAR BOOK sources.

The Literature Survey

More than 250,000 peer-reviewed articles per year are scanned systematically—including title, text, illustrations, tables, and references—by the publisher's team of literature specialists. Each scan is compared, article by article, to the search strategies that the publisher has developed in consultation with the nearly 200 outside experts who form the pool of YEAR BOOK editors. A given article with broad scientific or clinical implications may be reviewed by any number of YEAR BOOK editors, from one to a dozen or more, regardless of the discipline for which the paper was originally published. In turn, each editor who receives the article reviews it to determine whether it should be included in his or her volume. This decision is based on the article's inherent quality, its relevance to readers of that YEAR BOOK, and the editor's goal to represent a comprehensive picture of a given field in each volume of the YEAR BOOK. In addition, the editor indicates when to include figures and tables from the article to help the YEAR BOOK reader better understand the information.

Of the quarter million articles scanned each year, only 5% are selected for publication within the YEAR BOOK series, thereby assuring readers of the high value of every selection.

The Abstract

The publisher's abstracting staff is headed by a seasoned medical editing professional and includes individuals with extensive experience in writing for the health professions. When an article is selected for inclusion in a YEAR BOOK, it is assigned to a member of the abstracting staff. The abstractor, guided in many cases by notations supplied by the physician editor, writes a structured, condensed summary designed to rapidly communicate to the reader the essential information contained in the article.

The Commentary

The YEAR BOOK editorial boards, sometimes assisted by guest contributors, write comments that place each article in perspective. This provides the reader with insights from authorities in each discipline that point out the value of the article and that often reflect the authority's thought processes in assessing the article.

Additional Editorial Features

The editorial boards of each YEAR BOOK organize the abstracts and comments to provide a logical and satisfying sequence of information. To enhance the organization, editors also provide introductions to sections or individual chapters, comments linking a number of abstracts, citations to additional literature, and other features.

The published YEAR BOOK contains enhanced bibliographic citations for each selected article, including extended listings of multiple authors and identification of author affiliations. Each YEAR BOOK contains a Table of Contents specific to that year's volume. From year to year, the Table of Contents for a given YEAR BOOK may vary, depending on developments within the field.

Every YEAR BOOK contains a list of the journals from which articles have been selected. This list represents a subset of approximately 500 journals surveyed by the publisher and occasionally reflects a particularly pertinent article from a journal that is not surveyed routinely.

Finally, each volume contains a comprehensive subject index and an index to authors of each selected article.

The 2000 Year Book Series

Year Book of Allergy, Asthma, and Clinical Immunology™: Drs Rosenwasser, Boguniewicz, Milgrom, Routes, and Spahn

Year Book of Anesthesiology and Pain Management™: Drs Tinker, Abram, Chestnut, Roizen, Rothenberg, and Wood

Year Book of Cardiology®: Drs Schlant, Collins, Gersh, Graham, Kaplan, and Waldo

Year Book of Chiropractic®: Dr Lawrence

Year Book of Critical Care Medicine®: Drs Parrillo, Balk, Calvin, Franklin, and Shapiro

Year Book of Dentistry®: Drs Zakariasen, Boghosian, Dederich, Hatcher, Horswell, and McIntyre

Year Book of Dermatology and Dermatologic Surgery™: Drs Thiers and Lang

Year Book of Diagnostic Radiology®: Drs Osborn, Birdwell, Dalinka, Groskin, Maynard, Oestreich, Pentecost, Ros, Smirniotopoulos, and Young

Year Book of Emergency Medicine®: Drs Burdick, Cydulka, Cone, Hamilton, Loiselle, and Niemann

Year Book of Endocrinology®: Drs Mazzaferri, Fitzpatrick, Horton, Kannan, Kreisberg, Meikle, Molitch, Morley, Osei, Poehlman, and Rogol

Year Book of Family Practice®: Drs Berg, Bowman, Davidson, Dexter, Morrison, and Scherger

Year Book of Gastroenterology™: Drs Lichtenstein, Dempsey, Ginsberg, Katzka, Kochman, Morris, Nunes, Rosato, and Stein

Year Book of Hand Surgery®: Drs Amadio and Hentz

Year Book of Medicine®: Drs Barkin, Frishman, Jett, Klahr, Loehrer, Malawista, Mandell, and Mazzaferri

Year Book of Neonatal and Perinatal Medicine®: Drs Fanaroff, Maisels, and Stevenson

Year Book of Nephrology, Hypertension, and Mineral Metabolism: Drs Schwab, Bennett, Emmett, Moe, and Textor

Year Book of Neurology and Neurosurgery®: Drs Bradley and Gibbs

Year Book of Nuclear Medicine®: Drs Gottschalk, Blaufox, Coleman, Strauss, and Zubal

Year Book of Obstetrics, Gynecology, and Women's Health®: Drs Mishell, Herbst, and Kirschbaum

Year Book of Oncology®: Drs Loehrer, Eisenberg, Glatstein, Gordon, Johnson, Pratt, and Thigpen

Year Book of Ophthalmology®: Drs Wilson, Cohen, Eagle, Grossman, Laibson, Maguire, Nelson, Penne, Rapuano, Sergott, Shields, Spaeth, Tipperman, Ms Gosfield, and Ms Salmon

Year Book of Orthopedics®: Drs Morrey, Beauchamp, Currier, Swiontkowski, Tolo, and Trigg

Year Book of Otolaryngology–Head and Neck Surgery®: Drs Paparella, Holt, and Otto

Year Book of Pathology and Laboratory Medicine®: Drs Raab, Dabbs, Olson, Silverman, and Stanley

Year Book of Pediatrics®: Dr Stockman

Year Book of Plastic, Reconstructive, and Aesthetic Surgery®: Drs Miller, Bartlett, Garner, McKinney, Ruberg, Salisbury, and Smith

Year Book of Psychiatry and Applied Mental Health®: Drs Talbott, Ballenger, Frances, Jensen, Meltzer, Simpson, and Tasman

Year Book of Pulmonary Disease®: Drs Jett, Castro, Maurer, Peters, Phillips, and Ryu

Year Book of Rheumatology, Arthritis, and Musculoskeletal Disease™: Drs Panush, Hadler, Hellmann, LeRoy, Pisetsky, and Simon

Year Book of Sports Medicine®: Drs Shephard, Alexander, Kohrt, Nieman, Torg, and Mr George

Year Book of Surgery®: Drs Copeland, Bland, Deitch, Eberlein, Howard, Luce, Seeger, Souba, and Sugarbaker

Year Book of Urology®: Drs Andriole and Coplen

Year Book of Vascular Surgery®: Dr Porter

2000

The Year Book of SPORTS MEDICINE®

Editor-in-Chief
Roy J. Shephard, MD, PhD, DPE, FACSM
Professor Emeritus of Applied Physiology; Faculty of Physical Education and Health, University of Toronto

Editors
Marion J.L. Alexander, PhD
Professor, Faculty of Physical Education and Recreation Studies; Research Affiliate, Health, Leisure and Human Performance Research Institute, University of Manitoba, Winnipeg, Manitoba

Francis J. George, ATC, PT
Director of Sports Medicine, Brown University, Providence, Rhode Island

Wendy M. Kohrt, PhD
Professor of Medicine, Division of Geriatric Medicine, University of Colorado Health Sciences Center, Denver

David C. Nieman, PhD
Professor of Health and Exercise Science, Appalachian State University, Boone, North Carolina

Joseph S. Torg, MD
Professor of Orthopedic Surgery, MCP-Hahnemann School of Medicine; Interim Chairman, Hahnemann University Hospital, Philadelphia, Pennsylvania

American College of Sports Medicine Liaison Representative
Robert E. Sallis, MD, FACSM
Kaiser Permanente Medical Center, Alta Loma, California

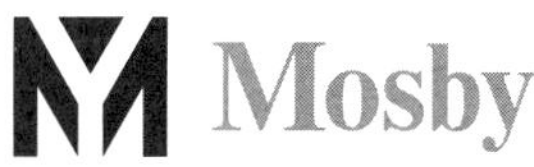 Mosby

St. Louis   Baltimore   Boston   Carlsbad   Naples   New York   Philadelphia   Portland   London
Madrid   Mexico City   Singapore   Sydney   Tokyo   Toronto   Wiesbaden

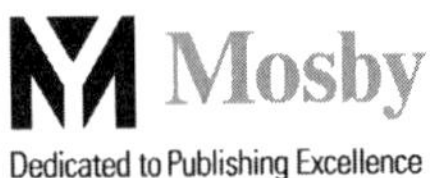

Publisher: Susan Patterson
Developmental Editor: Karen Moehlman
Manager, Periodical Editing: Kirk Swearingen
Production Editor: Amanda Maguire
Project Supervisor, Production: Joy Moore
Project Assistant, Production: Betty Dockins
Manager, Literature Services: Idelle L. Winer
Illustrations and Permissions Specialist: Steve Ramay

Printed in the United States of America
Composition by Thomas Technology Solutions, Inc.
Printing/binding by Maple-Vail

Mosby, Inc.
11830 Westline Industrial Drive
St. Louis, MO 63146

International Standard Serial Number: 0162-0908
International Standard Book Number: 0-323-00730-9

Table of Contents

Journals Represented

Mosby and its editors survey approximately 500 journals for its abstract and commentary publications. From these journals, the editors select the articles to be abstracted. Journals represented in this YEAR BOOK are listed below.

Age and Ageing
American Journal of Cardiology
American Journal of Clinical Nutrition
American Journal of Emergency Medicine
American Journal of Epidemiology
American Journal of Gastroenterology
American Journal of Medicine
American Journal of Physiology
American Journal of Public Health
American Journal of Respiratory and Critical Care Medicine
American Journal of Roentgenology
American Journal of Sports Medicine
Annals of Internal Medicine
Archives of Family Medicine
Archives of Ophthalmology
Archives of Pediatrics and Adolescent Medicine
Arthroscopy
British Journal of Sports Medicine
British Medical Journal
Chest
Circulation
Clinical Biomechanics
Clinical Orthopaedics and Related Research
Cutis
Diabete et Metabolisme
Diabetes Care
Epilepsia
Foot & Ankle International
Heart
Injury
International Journal of Epidemiology
International Journal of Sports Medicine
Journal of Allergy and Clinical Immunology
Journal of Applied Physiology: Respiratory, Environmental and Exercise
    Physiology
Journal of Athletic Training
Journal of Bone and Joint Surgery (American Volume)
Journal of Bone and Joint Surgery (British Volume)
Journal of Bone and Mineral Research
Journal of Clinical Endocrinology and Metabolism
Journal of Clinical Epidemiology
Journal of Clinical Pathology
Journal of Computer Assisted Tomography
Journal of Gerontology. Series A Biological Sciences and Medical Sciences
Journal of Internal Medicine
Journal of Orthopaedic Research
Journal of Orthopaedic and Sports Physical Therapy

Journal of Pediatrics
Journal of Rheumatology
Journal of Sports Medicine and Physical Fitness
Journal of Sports Sciences
Journal of Trauma: Injury, Infection, and Critical Care
Journal of the American Academy of Orthopaedic Surgeons
Journal of the American Board of Family Practice
Journal of the American College of Cardiology
Journal of the American Geriatrics Society
Journal of the American Medical Association
Journal of the Royal College of Surgeons of Edinburgh
Lancet
Mayo Clinic Proceedings
Medical Journal of Australia
Medical Problems of Performing Artists
Medicine and Science in Sports and Exercise
Metabolism: Clinical and Experimental
New England Journal of Medicine
Ophthalmology
PACE - Pacing and Clinical Electrophysiology
Physician and Sportsmedicine
Psychological Medicine
Radiology
Scandinavian Journal of Rehabilitation Medicine
Science
Sports Medicine
Stroke

STANDARD ABBREVIATIONS

The following terms are abbreviated in this edition: acquired immunodeficiency syndrome (AIDS), cardiopulmonary resuscitation (CPR), central nervous system (CNS), cerebrospinal fluid (CSF), computed tomography (CT), deoxyribonucleic acid (DNA), electrocardiography (ECG), health maintenance organization (HMO), human immunodeficiency virus (HIV), intensive care unit (ICU), intramuscular (IM), intravenous (IV), magnetic resonance (MR) imaging (MRI), and ribonucleic acid (RNA).

NOTE

The YEAR BOOK OF SPORTS MEDICINE is a literature survey service providing abstracts of articles published in the professional literature. Every effort is made to assure the accuracy of the information presented in these pages. Neither the editors nor the publisher of the YEAR BOOK OF SPORTS MEDICINE can be responsible for errors in the original materials. The editors' comments are their own opinions. Mention of specific products within this publication does not constitute endorsement.

To facilitate the use of the YEAR BOOK OF SPORTS MEDICINE as a reference tool, all illustrations and tables included in this publication are now identified as they appear in the original article. This change is meant to help the reader recognize that any illustration or table appearing in the YEAR BOOK OF SPORTS MEDICINE may be only one of many in the original article. For this reason, figure and table numbers will often appear to be out of sequence within the YEAR BOOK OF SPORTS MEDICINE.

Introduction

The new millenium brings new challenges to the sports medicine practitioner, as the volume of published research continues to expand exponentially. The wonders of the electronic highway now bring 2000 journals into my home from the University of Toronto Library, some 3000 miles to the east. Downloading such articles is unbelievably easy—however, digesting and assimilating this vast array of literature is a task of an entirely different order. More than ever, there seems to be a need for the YEAR BOOK OF SPORTS MEDICINE, in which experts in various subdisciplines of the field perform a careful triage of the published reports, identify the key pieces of new information for presentation as succinct structured abstracts, and provide their personal editorial insights. I much appreciate the conscientious efforts of my several coeditors in this regard. I must also pay a warm tribute to Karen Moehlman and the entire Mosby team for the prompt and efficient manner in which they handle the complex task of distributing journal articles, collecting editorial comments, and preparing this volume.

What trends in sports medicine can we discern in the new millenium? In the surgical realm, as in other domains, experimental design and sample size are becoming critical issues in evaluating published research reports. Gene therapy and tissue engineering are particularly hot topics, with potential for future clinical application in the management of tissues with a poor healing capacity. Gene therapy offers a new way to deliver reparative proteins to injury sites, and tissue engineering allows the creation of scaffolds which may facilitate tissue regeneration in acute and chronic traumatic lesions. Chondrocyte transplants provide considerable promise in treating lesions of articular cartilage. However, hyperbaric oxygen is a less effective remedy for chronic injuries.

Looking at individual sport activities, mountain biking is becoming ever more popular (at least in this part of Canada) but a disturbing number of injuries to bikers' facial bones has prompted a call for the use of face guards. Full-face shields do not seem to increase neck injuries in hockey players. Snowboarding and telemark skiing still have high injury rates. Softer baseballs might increase rather than decrease the severity of eye injuries. Musicians (especially the inexperienced) are not immune to repetitive strain injuries.

Concussion remains a challenging problem in many sports, and there are disquieting suggestions of associations between repeated concussion and long-term mental impairment. Spinal injuries also continue to cause severe long-term morbidity in players of several major team sports. A randomized controlled trial has compared open diskectomy with video-assisted arthroscopic microdiskectomy. Complete acromioclavicular dislocation is now being treated with biodegradable cords. The timing of surgical intervention for suprascapular nerve entrapment is shown to be essential to successful treatment. Some authors now use laser treatment of inferior glenohumeral instability. An extensive literature review confirms the value of conservative treatment in mallett finger.

Lower abdominal and inguinal pain in high performance athletes has almost 40 possible causes. Diagnostic arthroscopy of the hip is both safe and worthwhile. Runners may develop sacral stress fractures, although healing is relatively rapid, leading to much underdiagnosis of this condition. Patellar dysfunction continues to attract much attention. Rainfall and evaporation influence the risk of anterior cruciate injuries; risks are also higher in women playing the same sports as men. Patient reports provide better assessments of anterior cruciate deficiencies than performance measures. Absorbable arrows are being used successfully in meniscal repair. Cryotherapy is shown to decrease pain and the need for analgesics following anterior cruciate ligament reconstruction. The long-term prognosis of knee surgery is substantially worsened if septic arthritis develops. Fasciotomy is not always indicated for lateral compartment syndrome. Likewise, chronic Achilles' tendinopathy sometimes responds well to percutaneous tenodesis or to non-surgical treatment. As runners become fatigued, a shift of loading from the heel to the tarsal region may predispose to injury. Taping may reduce ankle injuries by reducing inversion amplitudes and angular velocities of tilting. Weakness of the evertor muscles does not seem responsible for functional instability of the ankle. Fasciotomy for plantar fasciitis is not always an effective treatment.

The search for practical methods of promoting physical activity in primary practice continues. Measurement of physical activity continues to be a difficult technical problem, with evidence that both the Minnesota Leisure Time Physical Activity Survey and the Caltrac monitor underestimate total energy expenditures. Gastrointestinal disturbances are less prevalent during distance walking than during running. Many patients who are attempting to lose weight do not follow the recommended tactics of reduced energy intake and moderate physical activity. Search for the genetic determinants of athletic ability continues, although some of the research supposedly documenting major effects has significant flaws; in particular, the role of the gene controlling angiotensin-converting enzyme seems to have been overstated. Creatine supplements may enhance performance because such supplements permit more vigorous training. Attempts to detect erythropoietin administration in triathletes by hematocrit determinations have to date proven unsuccessful.

The World Wide Web now provides a very cost-effective tool in preparticipation examination. Debate continues on the extent of any cardiac dysfunction which may be induced by ultraendurance events. A study of orienteers cautions that in this sport, the incidence of osteoarthritis is twice that found in controls. The Framingham study also reports osteoarthritis can result from a lifetime of heavy physical activity. Sudden cardiac death in football players continues to attract attention. The possible impact of exercise on blood mononuclear cells and, thus, the development of ischemic heart disease is attracting increased interest. Exercise can precipitate epilepsy in some 10% of patients, but nevertheless most patients with this condition are overprotected. Contact dermatitis from sports equipment remains a toublesome problem.

At very high altitudes, the oxygen cost of breathing may be such that attempts to boost arterial oxygenation by hyperventilation are counterproductive. Plasma endothelin-1 levels may be useful in distinguishing those patients who are at particular risk of high-altitude pulmonary edema. The dangers of decompression sickness can be reduced if diving tables are adjusted for individual risk factors. Fluids significantly enhance performance in soccer, but the development of hyponatremia continues a problem in distance events. There is an uncomfortable suspicion that the problem often arises from an injudicious administration of fluids when treating heat casualties. The assumption that exercise will impair the shivering response in a cold environment is vigorously challenged. Exercise in bright light is shown to be an effective mood enhancing tactic. The idea that late-night exercise prevents sleep is exposed as an erroneous myth.

Somewhat in disagreement with earlier reports, carbohydrate supplements are found here to do little to boost immune function in soccer players, and the ingestion of triglycerides per-exercise fails to conserve glycogen. Nor does antibody production after influenza vaccination seem to be affected adversely by moderate exercise.

In women, menstrual disorders are associated with a low metabolic rate, presumably an attempt by the body to compensate for a negative energy balance. A reduction of body mass by a combination of dieting and increased exercise appears safe for lactating women. Articles continue to highlight the potential for large errors in both anthropometric and impedence estimates of body fat content. A detailed economic analysis shows the heavy costs associated with current national levels of obesity in the western world. An increase of fitness is beneficial not only to lean, but also to obese patients; likewise, smokers who are active enhance their active life expectancy. Smoking increases the risk of bone loss in premenopausal as well as in postmenopausal women. Greater symptom-reporting may contribute to the apparently higher injury rates of women who exercise. In the elderly, the emphasis continues on "aging successfully." At this stage in life, a walking program is quite effective in reducing coronary risk. Eccentric exercise also seems to be an effective method of increasing strength in the elderly, because aerobic demands in this activity are low. Regular activity also seems to prevent the age-related rise in systolic and pulse pressures. Creatine-based estimates of loss of lean tissue do not agree with estimates based on cross-sectional areas or fat free mass. Resistance exercise for the elderly neither impairs nor enhances immune function.

In terms of the secondary and tertiary prevention of disease, the long-term consequences of cardiac rehabilitation are now emerging from 20 to 30 year follow-up studies. More attention is being directed to dose-response relationships and resulting changes in quality-adjusted life expectancy. Discussion continues on the possibility of accumulating adequate physical activity through several brief sessions per day. Particularly in conditions with a metabolic basis, such as diabetes, even moderate intensities of physical activity appear to give a substantial decrease in risk.

Diabetes predisposes to osteoarthritis. Endurance exercise enhances the effect of fluvastatin in dyslipidemia. Regular physical activity appears to decrease the risk of gallstones. The impact of habitual physical activity on colon transit time continues to be controversial, with one report showing an acute decrease in colonic motility. For men with a family history of coronary heart disease, the weekly energy expenditure of 1.25 mJ is sufficient to induce an 8-fold reduction in the risk of a high serum Lp(a) level. The previously demonstrated favorable effect of exercise on depression in male cases of coronary heart disease has now been documented in women, who experience substantial improvements in the quality of life following rehabilitation. Smoking seems interlinked with inadequate physical activity in those who develop intermittent claudication. There is growing evidence that the risk of lung cancer may be reduced by a substantial volume of weekly exercise. Regarding chronic obstructive lung disease, an article challenges the conventional wisdom that the benefit of exercise comes from a strengthening of the limb muscles. In asthma, also, land exercises are shown to be as effective as pool exercises.

Documentation of infections associated with steroid injections is accumulating. Patients with HIV infection can enhance their exercise tolerance by a vigorous training program, without further compromising their immune status or increasing viral replication. Cognitive and physical impairments predict 5-year mortality in the elderly. Among centenarians, women are much more likely to be disabled than are men. Concerning stroke, the benefits of exercise in this condition appear to arise through an impact upon body mass, blood pressure, serum cholesterol and glucose tolerance. Leg rehabilitation is more beneficial than arm rehabilitation following stroke; the latter influences mainly dexterity. One-legged training may be helpful in developing muscle strength and, thus, overall fitness in patients with congestive heart failure. In patients with paraplegia, electrical stimulation of the paralyzed limbs can increase metabolic demand and, thus, enhance the response to training.

This is just a brief overview of the many exciting articles that are reviewed and discussed in the millennial edition of the YEAR BOOK OF SPORTS MEDICINE. I trust that you will find this entrée to current research as valuable as I do.

Roy J. Shephard, MD, PhD, DPE, FACSM

Can Insistence on Medical Clearance Inhibit the Adoption of an Active Lifestyle by Elderly Patients?

Roy J. Shephard, MD, PhD, DPE
Faculty of Physical Education and Health and Department of Public Health Sciences, University of Toronto, Ontario

This article's objectives are to explore when medical clearance is a necessary preliminary to an increase of physical activity in the older individual, and to consider whether insistence on universal medical clearance can be a significant barrier to the adoption of an active lifestyle by seniors. The editor-in-chief's position has been influenced strongly by recent discussions regarding the possible need to adapt the Physical Activity Readiness Questionnaire[1,2] to the needs of older individuals. The intent of this article is primarily to stimulate debate, because it is recognised that a consensus has yet to be reached on this important issue.[3,4]

Historical Background

The Canadian government began energetically to promote physical activity for Canadians some 35 years ago. It was quickly realized that the clearance procedures advocated by US physicians of that era, which included not only a complete clinical examination but also a stress electrocardiogram for every adult over the age of 35 years[5] were not only costly and inappropriate,[6] but could become an important barrier to the adoption of regular physical activity by senior citizens. If the US policy of that era were strictly adhered to, a person would need to schedule and keep an appointment with a physician before beginning even the mildest form of physical activity. Further, in part because of limitations in medical curricula, few physicians had any expertise in sports medicine. Ignorance was sometimes cloaked by an excessively conservative approach. Irrational fears were expressed about the possible consequences of any minor abnormalities that physicians thought they could detect on auscultation or by examination of a resting electrocardiogram, and the patient was more likely to receive a warning *against* exercise than any encouragement of their newfound desire to become more active. Cost was also a major consideration. Macauley[4] suggested that in Britain, the preseason examination of 10,000 adolescent athletes would at best detect some 47 minor abnormalities of questionable importance, at a cost of $1.5 billion. In the United States, many of the patients who wanted to exercise had to pay several hundred dollars for a specialized laboratory examination. In Canada, the prospect that our national system of Medicare might need to make similar payments for every Canadian adult who wished to adopt a more active lifestyle became a grave concern for our Ministers of Health and of Finance. So began the Canadian search for alternative methods of clearance prior to exercise testing and exercise prescription.

The Cardiovascular Risks Associated With Exercise

Some physicians were not very happy when it was suggested that patients might not need to visit them for medical clearance prior to beginning light physical activity. They argued that such a policy would expose individuals with undetected cardiac conditions to the risks of myocardial infarction and sudden exercise-induced death. Some maintained that it would be unethical not to insist on medical clearance.[7] Italian doctors went even further, making medical examination a binding legal requirement before a person began any type of sport.[8]

Stimulated by this controversy, our laboratory carried out various epidemiological studies of the risks associated with exercise in both ostensibly healthy patients and in individuals who had already sustained at least one myocardial infarction.[9,10] In both situations, we reached the conclusion that a myocardial infarction would be 5 to 6 times more likely to occur when an individual was exercising than when they were sedentary for an equivalent period of time. However, this could not be construed as an argument for continued sedentary behaviour, because between exercise bouts the physically active individual had a dramatic drop in risk relative to their sedentary counterparts. The net result was that relative to a sedentary person, the active individual had only about one third the overall risk of myocardial infarction and sudden death.[9,11] The difference in prognosis was such that it could be argued that an individual who intended to remain sedentary was in much greater need of preliminary medical clearance than the one who proposed to begin a mild exercise program!

Fallibility of the Stress Electrocardiogram

The next step in our analyses was to make a critical examination of the value of clinical examination and stress electrocardiography as a possible means of avoiding an exercise-induced catastrophe. Application of Bayes' theorem quickly demonstrated that for the average ostensibly healthy, middle-aged adult, the stress electrocardiogram was not only fallible, but was almost totally valueless.[12] The problem was inherent in the relatively low prevalence of ischemic heart disease in a random sample of the general population. Taking typical figures for the sensitivity and specificity of the exercise electrocardiogram relative to angiography, some two thirds of apparently positive tests were, in fact, false-positive results. Indeed, the proportion of false-positive diagnoses was so large that by insisting on preexercise stress testing, physicians were creating a great deal of unnecessary fear and iatrogenic disease in previously healthy individuals. To emphasize this conclusion, we suggested that physicians might make fewer diagnostic errors in medical clearance if they were to sell their treadmills and ECGs, and base their advice simply on the tossing of a coin!

Fallibility of Clinical Examination

We went on to expose the fallibility of the standard clinical examination in an ostensibly healthy population.[2,13] Trials were set up at the Pacific

National Exhibition in Vancouver[1] and at an office building in Toronto.[13] It immediately became apparent that there was no clinical consensus on findings that would require the exclusion of a patient from exercise testing or prescription. The proportion of ostensibly healthy individuals who were advised against undertaking a simple submaximal exercise test differed widely between physicians; the range of rejections was from 0.9% to 15% of the general population, depending on the conservatism of the examining physician. Moreover, there was almost no correlation between the proportion of individuals excluded by a given physician and the likelihood that these patients would develop electrocardiographic abnormalities in immediately subsequent performance of a simple submaximal exercise test. The original intent of our clinical examinations was to provide a gold standard against which we could validate other simpler procedures. However, the trials in Vancouver and Toronto demonstrated clearly that there was no commonly accepted and effective code of clincial practice that could be used to evaluate alternative methods of triage.[1,2,13]

The pièce de résistance of a family physician's clinical examination is often the determination of systemic blood pressure by means of a clinical sphygmomanometer. In about 20% of the population, a casual determination of blood pressure in the doctor's office yields values that appear to be above population norms. So, the patient is told "I think you ought to be careful about exercising—your blood pressure is a bit higher than it should be." The eager physician has perhaps forgotten the hypertensive effects of the hassle the patient encountered in driving to the office, waiting for an hour in a room filled with sick patients, finally to be examined by a person in a white coat.[13,14] In fact, the great majority of patients whom doctors have warned about hypertension have a perfectly normal blood pressure if the measurement is repeated in a relaxed setting.

Avoiding the Cardiac Catastrophe

Given the fallibility of current clinical and laboratory examinations, there is a need for a good method of detecting the vulnerable individual.[2,15] Although exercise-induced cardiac catastrophes are very rare, they receive wide publicity,[4,16]—like musculoskeletal injuries, they can have a strong negative impact on individuals' motivation to exercise.

Common features of exercise-induced myocardial infarction that our analysis of individual case histories have identified[9,15] include a bout of physical activity that is abnormally heavy or competitive for the individual, reluctance to admit tiredness in the face of a younger opponent, associated excitement or emotional distress, and a vague feeling of malaise experienced during the preceding 6 to 24 hours.

Considering again the implications of Bayes' theorem,[12] the number of false-positive diagnoses at stress electrocardiography (or indeed during any other laboratory test) diminishes with an increased prevalence of abnormalities in the population examined. Thus, one effective method both of reducing the costs of preliminary screening and of decreasing the proportion of the false-positive diagnoses is to undertake a preliminary triage of patients. Canadian investigators decided that most people were aware when something was wrong with their health, and could carry out the triage themselves with the use of a very simple self-administered questionnaire.[1,17] After trials of a number of potential questionnaires with 6 to 22 items, the 7-item Physical Activity Readiness Questionnaire (PAR-Q) was born.[1,17-19]

Given the fallibility of both clinical and laboratory examinations, it was decided that the most practical method of establishing the safety and efficacy of the PAR-Q approach was to apply it systematically to the clearance of potential exercisers across the entire Canadian population for a number of years, and to see if this caused the sudden epidemic of musculoskeletal injuries, myocardial infarctions and incidents of sudden death that some clinicians had predicted. The PAR-Q was thus used to clear more than 500,000 people for performance of a simple step test, carried to 70% to 80% of peak oxygen intake. We found no evidence that a preliminary screening by PAR-Q responses had allowed serious injury, myocardial infarction, or sudden death. The procedure thus became an accepted component of practice not only in Canada but also in the United States.[20]

ALTERNATIVE METHODS OF TRIAGE

After some 15 years of experience had been accumulated, the effectiveness of the PAR-Q instrument was reviewed.[18,19] Despite its safety, there were concerns that PAR-Q responses were still limiting exercise involvement in an excessive proportion of patients. In particular, about one in five individuals responded positively to the question "Has a doctor ever said your blood pressure was too high?" Small changes in the wording of the questionnaire were thus evaluated to determine if the safety of the PAR-Q-based triage could be conserved while enhancing its specificity as a means of detecting contraindications to exercise.[19] When the revised PAR-Q instrument was applied to the general adult population, it was successful in excluding a third less patients, and use of the new format over the past 5 years has raised no concerns regarding a deterioration in the safety of clearance procedures.

US epidemiologists have suggested an alternative method of triage.[20] In theory, this appears to have at least equal validity to the PAR-Q approach; it is based on the subject's age, the presence or absence of major cardiac risk factors (smoking, hypertension, a high serum cholesterol, and a lack of exercise) and the intensity of the proposed exercise program.[20] However, one immediate problem may be the patient's lack of appropriate knowledge about cardiac risk profile. Many people seem to be uninformed or misinformed about their personal cardiac risk factors and overall medical status. One recent study[21] noted that even children of cardiac patients often were unaware of their serum cholesterol, and frequently misdiagnosed the presence or absence of hypertension. The accuracy of simple cholesterol tests is now increasing rapidly, and in the future it seems likely that patients may indeed know if they have excessive levels of serum lipids.

EXTENDING THE AGE RANGE OF TRIAGE

The original PAR-Q test was devised for use on clients between the ages of 15 and 65 years, but, in response to public demand, the authorized range was subsequently extended to 69 years of age. However, the issue of exercise triage procedures for children and the elderly was still unresolved. During the past year, the Canadian Government developed and distributed widely a popular *Guide for Active Living*.[22] The official package incorporates the revised PAR-Q instrument. The guidance of the Canadian Society of Exercise Physiology (CSEP) was sought as the government contemplated developing appropriately modified guides for children and for seniors.[23] In particular, CSEP was asked whether there was a need to develop special versions of the Physical Activity Readiness Questionnaire for use in children and elderly adults.

After lengthy review, the committee appointed by the CSEP recommended that neither of these age groups required a specialized questionnaire. In the case of the children, the primary argument was based on Bayes' theorem. In ostensibly healthy youngsters, the incidence of dangerous abnormalities such as anomalous coronary artery or hypertrophic cardiomyopathy was so low that detection was virtually impossible, even with the most sophisticated techniques of diagnostic cardiology.[16] In one retrospective study of fatalities in young athletes, 115 of the 158 individuals who died had received a medical examination; only 4 of the 158 had been suspected of having cardiovascular disease, and in only one of these four patients was the diagnosis correct!

In the elderly, the problem with the use of such tools as the PAR-Q is the high proportion of positive responses to any potential form of triage. For example, if the original or the revised PAR-Q instrument were applied to a seniors'-aged group, 20% to 30% might yield a positive response because of angina of effort, 30% to 40% might report some degree of hypertension, and 40% to 50% would be likely to have some symptoms of arthritis. Others would report occasional giddiness, loss of consciousness, or occasional falls, which again might be interpreted as contraindications to physical activity. Thus, the triage could lead to an exclusion of almost all patients who had expressed an interest in adopting an active lifestyle.

The difficulty would not necessarily be resolved by referring the patient from a health professional to the family physician, because the latter would be unlikely to have expertise in exercise gerontology. The likely advice from the doctor would be "Well, at your age, you really should be very careful." Faced with obvious clinical and laboratory "abnormalities," few physicians would accept the perceived risk of litigation inherent in a whole-hearted endorsement of exercise.

Justification for NOT Requiring Exercise Clearance in Elderly Patients

Current Canadian medical protocol is to encourage physical activity in the elderly population without the constraint of a preliminary triage or clinical examination. There are at least three reasons behind this recommendation. First, it is recognized that senior citizens are by nature a cautious group, and when their behaviour is viewed in the broad perspective of public health, the main danger is a lack rather than an excess of physical activity. Among those who are persuaded to increase their habitual physical activity, the likely outcomes will include some walking at a moderate pace, gentle gardening, an occasional game of golf, and, in a few individuals, cycling, swimming, or pool exercise—hardly high-risk pursuits.[24,25]

Further, the risk that sudden death will occur during a bout of physical activity does not seem to increase greatly with age. In part because people pursue any form of physical activity with progressively greater caution as they become older, the number of deaths per million hours of activity does not increase appreciably from middle to old age,[26] and because the activity sessions of older people are usually shorter than those of younger individuals, the number of deaths per million sessions actually decreases with age. The overall risk of death increases exponentially as we get older, so that the ratio of deaths during physical activity to those occurring at rest shows a dramatic decline in the elderly. Data derived from exercise programmes for the frail elderly (those between the ages of 80 and 100 years) give no indication that such activity has provoked sudden death, myocardial infarction, or serious cardiovascular incident. Nor is there any evidence that existing hypertension or problems of metabolic control are exacerbated by physical activity.[27] Moreover, clinical trials have demonstrated that fears that regular physical activity might cause an epidemic of injurious falls and fractures are entirely unwarranted.

In fact, most of the conditions likely to be detected by any potential system of triage—arthritis, diabetes, coronary vascular disease, stable congestive heart failure, chronic obstructive lung disease, depression, disorders of gait and balance, susceptibility to falls and insomnia show a favourable response to a program of moderate progressive physical activity.[28] Indeed, the response of many of these conditions to regular physical activity of appropriate intensity and duration exceeds that realized by the use of medication.

Longevity, or Quality-adjusted Life Span?

The survival curves for active and inactive individuals appear to converge around the age of 80 years,[29] and there is at least one cross-sectional study which suggests that after the age of 80 years, life expectancy may be slightly shorter for those who are vigorously active than for sedentary individuals.[30] Even in this latter study, moderate physical activity was associated with a longer life expectancy than that for a sedentary lifestyle. But let us focus on the implications of the data for the senior who currently engages in vigorous exercise. What if we were to encourage an 80-year old to stop a pattern of regular vigorous physical activity and to sit around in an old folk's home? He or she might possibly sit there for a few months longer than if the exercise was continued, but the quality of life would deteriorate dramatically. The duty of the physician is to prevent premature death rather than to extend the life of the frail elderly needlessly. The focus should be on maximizing the quality-adjusted life expectancy rather than on mere extension of lifespan.

The quality of life of the senior is often threatened by depression, lack of sleep, and lack of social contacts. Regular physical activity can address each of these problems. Above all, the quality of life of a sedentary senior is likely to be compromised by a progressive decrease in aerobic power, muscular strength, flexibility, and balance.[28] The age-related decrease in aerobic power first causes severe dyspnoea when the individual is walking up hills. Walking on the level becomes progressively limited, until eventually the person finds it impossible to undertake the normal tasks of daily living.[28] Likewise, the age-related loss of muscular strength is such that it becomes impossible to carry groceries, to open a jar of conserves, or to lift oneself from a chair, a toilet seat, or a bed. The decrease in flexibility makes it difficult to climb steps, to sit in a car, or to dress without assistance. All of these changes contribute to a progressive decrease in the quality of life. Many seniors face increasing disability over a period of perhaps 10 years, and a final year of total dependency. The impact on quality of life varies with the personality of the individual and with his or her coping skills, but, on average, there may be a 3 to 4 year reduction in quality-adjusted lifespan.[31]

In the case of aerobic power, a sedentary person finds it difficult to perform the instrumental tasks of daily living[32] once values drop below 18 mL/[kg.min][33,34] and many seniors reach the threshold for loss of independence, a value of 12 to 14 mL/[kg.min], around the age of 80 years.[28] The typical rate of aging of aerobic power is some 5 mL/[kg.min] per decade, and if a progressive exercise program augments aerobic power by 10 mL/[kg.min], the threshold for loss of independence is not reached until 20 years later—in fact, many of the individuals concerned will die of some intercurrent condition before they reach the threshold.[28] And, if the factor limiting independence is aerobic power, their quality-adjusted life expectancy will be boosted by 3 to 4 years. This should be more than enough to offset any small decrease in gross life expectancy that may be associated with vigorous physical activity in the very old.

A similar argument can be made concerning the reversal of age-related losses in strength, flexibility and balance by appropriately designed exercise programs.

This is not to suggest that regular physical activity can reverse all of the problems that lead to a deterioration in the quality of life of the frail elderly. Nevertheless, exercise can make a difference to many of these factors, and this is what we must consider before advocating triage rules that might limit the exercise behaviour of the old and the very old. Is it not preferable for an 80-year-old to die suddenly on the golf course, perhaps caused by the excitement of having scored a birdie on a difficult hole, rather than to spend the final year in a nursing home watching the progression of a painful cancer, even if the age at death is a bit younger for the golfer than for the nursing home inmate?

Risks of Exercise

The significant risks of moderate physical activity are few, and in most risk-increasing conditions, there should be no question of triage, because the patient will already be in close contact with a physician, who should have given advice on an appropriate regimen of physical activity.

RELATIVE CONTRAINDICATIONS

Careful evaluation is warranted in patients with unstable chest pain, acute febrile illness, poorly controlled diabetes, severe hypertension, severe asthma, unstable congestive heart failure, acute musculoskeletal pain, and repeated falling episodes.[27] In such instances, it is unwise to engage in more than very light physical activity until the primary condition has resolved. But it is hard to believe that such individuals will not be in contact with their family physician, so that such cases do not constitute an effective argument for universal triage.

TEMPORARY CONTRAINDICATIONS

Hernias, cataracts, retinal bleeding and joint injuries are all potential reasons to avoid certain types of physical activity temporarily.[27] But again, patients with such conditions are likely to be receiving medical treatment during the period when activity is contraindicated.

PERMANENT CONTRAINDICATIONS

There are a few conditions that merit the more permanent avoidance of vigorous physical activity.[27] These conditions include an inoperable and enlarging aortic aneurysm, a malignant arrhythmia induced by exercise, severe aortic stenosis, end-stage congestive heart failure, and severe behavioural agitation induced by exercise.[27] The majority of these disorders cannot be reversed by treatment.

Although not very likely, it is conceivable that a patient who decides to begin exercising may be unaware of a ventricular arrhythmia or an aortic stenosis. In these few cases, progression to vigorous exercise could shorten life span, although even in such a situation it would probably add to the quality of the final months of life.

Conclusions

An elderly person who wishes to engage in light or moderate physical activity should be encouraged to do so without requiring any preliminary triage or special medical clearance. Probably the best, and certainly the simplest advice is to take a little more physical activity than during the previous week. Assuming that this can be accomplished with no more than pleasant tiredness a few hours later, then the initial intensity of physical activity is appropriate, and it may be reasonable to suggest progression to a slightly higher level of activity during the following week. Such progression can continue until the individual's fitness goals have been satisfied, or the US Surgeon General's recommendations are reached.

Very occasionally, there will be individuals who suddenly decide, at the age of 80 years, that they wish to prepare for a high performance event such as the Comrades' Marathon or the Vasa Loppet. Plainly, such people need a thorough medical examination. These are the rare exceptions, people who have selected themselves for special examination by virtue of a high level of motivation and a desire for unusual athletic achievement. There is little danger that such individuals will be dissuaded from training by the requirement of a preliminary medical examination. But, for the majority of older people who are thinking of beginning some gentle walking, medical examination is unnecessary, and, if it is made mandatory, is likely to have a negative influence on the adoption of an active lifestyle.

References

1. Chisholm DM, Collis ML, Kulak LL, et al: Physical activity readiness. *British Columbia Medical Journal* 17:375-378, 1975.
2. Shephard RJ: PAR-Q, Canadian Home Fitness Test and exercise screening alternatives. *Sports Med* 5:185-195, 1988.
3. Cantwell JD: Preparticipation physical evaluation: Getting to the heart of the matter. *Med Sci Sports Exerc* 30:S341-S344, 1998.
4. MacAuley D: Science or show business. *Br J Sports Med* 33:147-148, 1999.
5. Cooper KH: Guidelines in the management of the exercising patient. *JAMA* 211:1663-1667, 1970.
6. Wilson J, Jungner G: Principles and practice of screening for disease. Geneva: World Health Organisation, 1968.
7. Maron BJ: Considerations for preparticipation cardiovascular screening in young competitive athletes. In: Shephard RJ, Åstrand P-O (eds): *Endurance in Sport* (2nd ed.). Oxford, Blackwell Scientific Publications, 2000, pp 667-681.
8. Pelliccia A, Maron BJ: Preparticipation cardiovascular examination of the competitive athlete: Perspectives from the 30 year Italian experience. *Am J Cardiol* 75:827-831, 1995.
9. Shephard RJ: Sudden death: A significant hazard of exercise? *Br J Sports Med* 8:101-110, 1974.
10. Shephard RJ: Exercise and the recurrence of myocardial infarction. *Am Heart J* 100:404-405, 1980.
11. Siscovick DS: Risks of exercising: Sudden cardiac death and injuries. In: Bouchard C, Shephard RJ, Stephens T, Sutton J, McPherson BJ (eds): *Exercise, Fitness and Health*. Champaign, IL, Human Kinetics Publishers, 1900, pp 707-713.
12. Shephard RJ: Prognostic value of exercise testing for coronary heart disease. *Br J Sports Med* 16:220-229, 1982.
13. Shephard RJ, Cox MH, Simper K: An analysis of PAR-Q responses in an office population. *Can J Public Health* 72:37-40, 1981.
14. Young MA, Rowlands DB, Stallard TJ, et al: Effect of environment on blood pressure. *Br Med J* 286:1235-1236, 1983.
15. Shephard RJ, Kavanagh T: Predicting the cardiac catastrophe in the post-coronary patient. *Can Fam Phys* 24:614-618, 1978.
16. Maron BJ, Shirani J, Poliac LC, et al: Sudden death in young competitive athletes. Clinical, demographic and pathological profiles. *JAMA* 276:199-204, 1996.
17. Bailey DA, Shephard RJ, Mirwald RL, et al: A current view of Canadian cardiorespiratory fitness. *Can Med Assoc J* 111:25-30, 1974.
18. Shephard RJ, Thomas S, Weller I: The Canadian Home Fitness Test. 1991 Update. *Sports Med* 11:358-366, 1991.
19. Thomas S, Reading J, Shephard RJ: Revision of the Physical Activity Readiness Questionnaire (PAR-Q). *Can J Sport Sci* 17:338-345, 1992.

20. American College of Sports Medicine: *Guidelines for Graded Exercise Testing and Exercise Prescription.* (5th ed). Philadelphia, Lea & Febiger, 1995.
21. Shephard RJ, Kavanagh T, Kennedy J: Fitness and lifestyle: Offspring of MI patients. *Med Sci Sports Exerc* 30:S248 (abstr.), 1998.
22. Health Canada: *Handbook for Canada's Physical Activity Guide.* Ottawa, Ont, Health Canada/Canadian Society of Exercise Physiology, 1998.
23. Health Canada: *Canada's Physical Activity Guide to Healthy Active Living for Older Adults.* Ottawa, ON, Health Canada/Canadian Society for Exercise Physiology, 1999.
24. Skelton D, Young A, Walker A, et al: Physical activity in later life. London, Health Education Authority, 1999.
25. Stephens T, Craig CL: *The Well-being of Canadians: The 1988 Campbell's Survey.* Ottawa, Ont, Canadian Fitness & Lifestyle Research Institute, 1990.
26. Vuori I: Sudden death and exercise: Effects of age and type of activity. *Sports Sci Rev* 4(2):46-84, 1995.
27. American College of Sports Medicine: ACSM Position Stand: Exercise and physical activity for older adults. *Med Sci Sports Exerc* 30:992-1008, 1998.
28. Shephard RJ: *Aging, Physical Activity and Health.* Champaign, Ill, Human Kinetics Publishers, 1997.
29. Pekkanen J, Marti B, Nissinen A, et al: Reduction of premature mortality by high physical activity: A 20-year follow-up of middle-aged Finnish men. *Lancet* i:1473-1477, 1987.
30. Linsted KD, Tonstad K, Kuzma J: Self-report of physical activity and patterns of mortality in Seventh-Day Adventist men. *J Clin Epidemiol* 44:355-364, 1991.
31. Shephard RJ: Habitual physical activity and quality of life. *Quest* 48:354-365, 1996.
32. Heikkinen R-L: *The role of physical activity in healthy aging.* Geneva, World Health Organization, 1998.
33. Fletcher GF, Froelicher VF, Hartley H, et al: Exercise: A statement for health professionals from the American Heart Association. *Circ* 81:396-398, 1990.
34. Morey MC, Pieper CF, Coroni-Huntley J: Is there a threshold between peak oxygen uptake and self-reported physical functioning in older adults? *Med Sci Sports Exerc* 30:1223-1229, 1998.

1 Epidemiology, Prevention, and Treatment of Injuries, Lesions of the Head, the Neck, and the Spine

Sample Size and Statistical Power in Clinical Orthopaedic Research
Freedman KB, Bernstein J (Univ of Pennsylvania, Philadelphia)
J Bone Joint Surg Am 81-A:1454-1460, 1999   1-1

Objective.—Traditional orthopedic treatments have evolved from observation. Whether conclusions drawn from observations are valid is usually determined by statistical sampling and outcomes evaluations. The concepts of statistical sampling and hypothesis testing are reviewed, and statistical power and adequate sample size are discussed.

Methods.—Hypothesis testing involves determining whether different treatments actually produce different outcomes and whether those outcomes can be extrapolated to the general population being studied. Whether conclusions are correct is determined by controlling for type I (α) errors, when results indicate a difference between groups when there really is no difference, and for type II (β) errors, usually related to small sample size. Power calculation must be performed to be sure that statistical power is maximized (sample size is sufficient). Few studies perform such calculations. As the risk of type I error decreases, the risk of type II error increases. A statistically significant result is not always a clinically significant result. The clinically relevant effect size (the magnitude of the difference between groups), based on the best clinical judgment, must be determined to have a large enough sample size. Variance (how much a typical member of the group deviates from the mean) also influences sample size. Sample size also determines the power to detect a significant difference between groups with respect to results that have clinical significance. α, β, and effect size must be defined before sample size requirements can be estimated. Power calculations can be performed after the fact, a post hoc analysis, to determine the likelihood of a type II error.

Conclusion.—Proper study design necessitates appropriate statistical analyses that establish the validity of the study. Type I and type II errors can be avoided with a sample size large enough to yield statistically and clinically significant results. Type II errors are best prevented by performing a sample size calculation before starting the study.

▶ An understanding of sample size and statistical power has become a requirement for publication of study outcomes in creditable orthopaedic journals. The purpose of this article was to review the concepts of statistical sampling and hypothesis testing with particular emphasis on study results that are not statistically significant. The authors have accomplished this goal. The article is recommended reading for all those performing clinical research.

J. S. Torg, MD

Epidemiological Patterns of Musculoskeletal Injuries and Physical Training
Almeida SA, Williams KM, Shaffer RA, et al (Naval Health Research Ctr, San Diego)
Med Sci Sports Exerc 31:1176-1182, 1999   1–2

Objective.—Identification of specific injury risk factors for musculoskeletal injuries would provide a framework for the development of cost-effective and feasible preventive strategies. Diagnostically precise rates of training-related injuries were determined in a descriptive study, and hypotheses were generated regarding the potential role of physical training as an etiologic factor.

Methods.—Between January 12 and September 14, 1296 randomly selected male Marine recruits, aged 17 to 28 years, arriving at San Diego boot camp were followed prospectively through 12 weeks of training. Musculoskeletal injury data were collected for the 1143 boot camp graduates. The relationship between physical training volume and injury incidence was examined, and correlations between hours of vigorous physical training and cumulative incidence of injuries were calculated by training week and reported for acute and overuse injuries.

Results.—At least 1 musculoskeletal injury was documented in 453 (39.6%) recruits; the most common were lower extremity injuries (82%). Most injuries were ankle/foot (34.3%), knee (28.1%), leg (13.7%), and back/neck/trunk (9.9%). Overuse injuries accounted for 78% and acute injuries for 22% of reports. The most frequent overuse injury and the second most common overall injury was iliotibial band syndrome (5.3%), the second most common overuse injury was stress fracture (4.0%), and the most frequent acute injuries were ankle sprains (6.2%) and contusions (3.7%). Weekly hours of vigorous physical activity were significantly correlated with both acute ($r = 0.633$) and overuse ($r = 0.667$) injuries. Injuries were most frequently reported during weeks 3, 8, 10, and 11, during which there was a high volume of vigorous physical training, running, and marching.

Conclusion.—The volume of training appears to be related to the risk of musculoskeletal injury.

▶ The authors have done an excellent job of determining the overall injury rate in the US Marine Corp male recruits for musculoskeletal injuries, which they define as any problem involving bones, muscles, tendons, ligaments, and assorted connective tissues. They state that "the systematic identification of exercise injury risk factors through controlled, epidemiologic studies such as this will form the basis for development of injury prevention strategies that will benefit both the civilian and military communities." However, they fail to either identify or speculate as to what these injury prevention strategies might be.

J. S. Torg, MD

Differential Profile of Facial Injuries Among Mountainbikers Compared With Bicyclists
Gassner RJ, Hackl W, Tuli T, et al (Univ of Innsbruck, Austria; Univ of Pittsburgh, Pa)
J Trauma: Injury Infect Crit Care 47:50-54, 1999   1–3

Background.—Cross-country bicycling, or mountain biking, has grown steadily in popularity over the past 10 years. Mountain bikes differ from racing and street bikes in that they have broad, knobby tires under lower pressure, which creates more resistance to rolling. Mountain bikers also ride in a more-upright position because of differences in the handlebar and frame construction. Differences in patterns of oral and maxillofacial injuries in mountain biking accidents, as compared with accidents in racing or street riding, as a result of these differences in design and in the bikes' gear and braking systems are reported.

Methods.—From 1991 to 1996, 5466 oral and maxillofacial trauma patients were seen at a single institution in Austria. Sports-related trauma was the cause of injury in 1812 patients, and of this group, 502 (27.7%) suffered bicycling injuries (Fig 1) and 60 (3.31%) had mountain bike injuries. The records of these patients were reviewed and analyzed by age and sex distribution, accident cause, type of injury, frequency, and the location of injury. Injuries were classified as fractures, dentoalveolar trauma, and soft-tissue injuries. Data were then analyzed statistically for

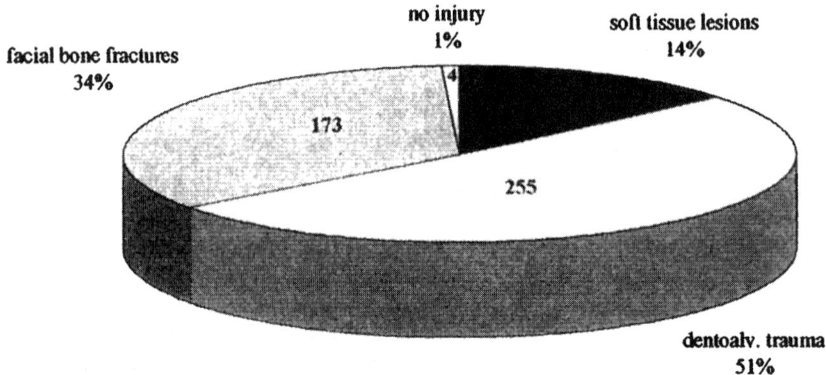

FIGURE 1.—Bicycle accidents 1991 to 1996, category of injury (*n* = 502). (Courtesy of Gassner RJ, Hackl W, Tuli T, et al: Differential profile of facial injuries among mountain bikers compared with bicyclists. *J Trauma: Injury Infect Crit Care* 47:50-54, 1999.)

proportional differences in injuries among bicyclists versus mountain bikers specifically.

Results.—The injuries among the 60 mountain bikers were more severe (Fig 2). Facial bone fractures accounted for 55% of mountain bike injuries, compared with 34.5% of bicyclist injuries. Soft-tissue injuries for the mountain bike group were 23% of injuries, compared with 14% for bicycle injuries. However, dentoalveolar injuries were higher in the bicycle group, accounting for 50.8% of injuries compared with 22% among the mountain bike group. The most frequent site of fracture for bicyclists was the zygoma (30%), while Le Fort I, II, and III fractures occurred at a high rate among mountain bikers (15%). Condyle fractures occurred more frequently among bicyclists (18.8%) than among mountain bikers (10.8%). The vast majority of both bicycle and mountain bike accidents resulted from falls (83.7% and 86.7%, respectively). Mountain bikers were older on average in this study, with a mean age of 30 versus a mean age of 18 among injured bicyclists. The male/female distributions were 1.35 to 1 for bicycle injuries and 3.6 to 1 for mountain bike injuries.

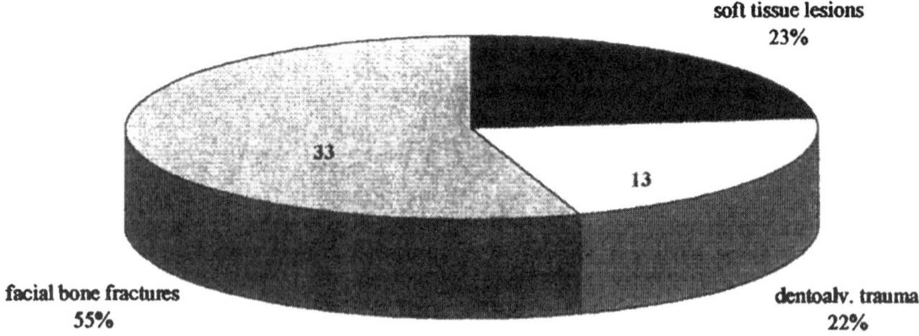

FIGURE 2.—Mountain bike accidents 1991 to 1996, category of injury (*n* = 60). (Courtesy of Gassner RJ, Hackl W, Tuli T, et al: Differential profile of facial injuries among mountain bikers compared with bicyclists. *J Trauma: Injury Infect Crit Care* 47:50-54, 1999.)

Conclusions.—Mountain biking accidents result in a higher rate of facial bone fractures and associated injuries, particularly among men over 30. Helmets should be designed appropriately and face guards should be used to reduce the incidence of facial injuries among cyclists, and use of helmets should be compulsory, particularly among mountain bikers.

▶ Among the 96 million cyclists in the United States, there are about 1000 deaths and 600,000 emergency room visits each year. Head injuries account for approximately two thirds of bicycling deaths and hospital admissions. The large increase in off-road or mountain bicycling has increased the need for safety measures, with injuries reported by 50% to 90% of participants each year.[1]

This study of cycling-related injuries revealed that mountain bike accidents resulted in a higher percentage of facial bone fractures, especially severe mid-face fractures, stressing the need for face guards in addition to helmets.

D. C. Nieman, DrPH

Reference

1. Kronisch RL, Pfeiffer RP, Chow TK: Acute injuries in cross-country and downhill off-road bicycle racing. *Med Sci Sports Exerc* 28:1351-1355, 1996.

The Circumstances and Scope for Prevention of Maxillofacial Injuries in Cyclists
Harrison MG, Shepherd JP (UMDS Guy's Dental Hosp, London; Univ of Wales College of Medicine, Cardiff)
J R Coll Surg Edinb 44:82-86, 1999   1–4

Background.—The researchers hypothesized that facial injuries caused by cycling accidents occur unevenly in the various facial zones. Variances are related to the age of the cyclist, the type of accident, and the presence of an accompanying head injury.

Methods.—The data accumulated on maxillofacial cycling injuries seen at 5 accident and emergency departments in South Wales during a 12-month period were reviewed prospectively. The type of injury (hematoma, abrasion, laceration, dental injury, or bone fracture) was determined, and the injury location was placed in 1 or more of 9 facial zones. Any alteration in consciousness was interpreted as a head injury. Finally, whether the cyclist was wearing a helmet and what specifically happened in the incident were noted.

Results.—The cyclists ranged in age from 2 to 41 years (mean, 14.2 years), and most of the cyclists were male. There were 201 recorded injuries of 104 cyclists. The central facial zone sustained the most injuries (almost 50%), and head injuries were noted more often in those who did not have bone fractures. Most accidents resulted after the cyclist lost control of the bicycle and involved no other vehicle.

Conclusions.—Only 14% of these cyclists wore helmets at the time of injury; this number was not enough to support inferences between helmet use and the other variables. Only 13% of those wearing helmets had head injuries, but 34% of those who did not wear helmets did. Facial injuries were seen significantly more in the central facial zone than in other areas.

▶ This is a prospective study in which injuries were accurately classified in terms of 9 facial zones as hematomas, abrasions, lacerations, dental injuries, or bone fractures. The authors also attempted to correlate maxillofacial injuries with head injuries. It should be noted that injuries were not categorized with regard to severity.

Only 15 of the injured cyclists were wearing a helmet at the time of injury; this precluded any statistical difference between helmet use and most of the other variables. Therefore the conclusion that "some of the injuries sustained in this investigation could have been prevented by the wearing of a cycle safety helmet . . ." is not supported by the data. Neither is the statement that " . . . this investigation demonstrates that significant reduction in morbidity could be achieved by . . . modifying cycle helmet design to incorporate a facebar and extending the facial aperture down over the frontal and temporal regions."

J. S. Torg, MD

Injury Patterns With Snowboarding
Ferrera PC, McKenna DP, Gilman EA (Albany Med Ctr, NY; Albany Med College, NY)
Am J Emerg Med 17:575-577, 1999   1–5

Objective.—The increased popularity of snowboarding has resulted in an increase in snowboarding injuries, with about 50% of all injuries occurring in less experienced snowboarders. Most of those injured are male and are younger than their skiing counterparts, and most injuries result from falling. Injury patterns associated with snowboarding seen in 1 ED are described, and recommendations for preventing injuries are made.

Methods.—During the 1994 through 1998 winter seasons, 71 snowboarders (13 females), aged 10 to 54 years (average age, 20 years), were injured, and 24 (79% male), average age, 22.0 years, required admission to the hospital.

Results.—The number of injuries has been increasing steadily from 1 in 1993 to 5 in 1994, 6 in 1995, 13 in 1996, and 46 in 1997. Contusions and fractures were the most common injuries. Simple sprains are the most commonly reported injuries, and upper extremity injuries occur more often than lower extremity injuries. Foot or ankle injuries and distal radius fractures are more common in snowboarders than in downhill skiers because of the soft boots that snowboarders wear. Deaths are rare. Injured snowboarders have a high rate (10%) of severe intracranial injuries.

Conclusion.—The overall incidence of snowboarding injuries is increasing. Because of the high incidence of head and spinal injuries, the possibility of such injuries must be considered in all injured snowboarders. Education, training, and wearing of stiffer boots, helmets, padding, and wrist guards can help prevent injuries.

▶ Most impressive is the number of severe injuries that occurred in this group of 71 snowboarders. Specifically, there were 6 closed head injuries, 5 intracerebral hemorrhages, 3 subdural hemorrhages, 1 fractured skull, 3 stomach lacerations, 3 liver lacerations, and 3 renal lacerations. Although it was not possible to present the data in terms of injury rates—and, granted, many minor injuries went either untreated or were managed closer to the ski resorts—the cases cited certainly declare the potential seriousness of snowboarding mishaps.

J. S. Torg, MD

Alpine Ski Bindings and Injuries: Current Findings
Natri A, Beynnon BD, Ettlinger CF, et al (Univ of Vermont, Burlington; Tampere Univ Hosp, Finland; Vermont Ski Safety Equipment Inc, Underhill; et al)
Sports Med 28:35-48, 1999

1–6

Objective.—Anterior cruciate ligament (ACL) skiing injuries are increasing while lower leg injuries are decreasing. The binding is one of the most important below-the-knee injury prevention devices. Current knowledge about alpine ski bindings and associated ski injuries was reviewed.

Epidemiology of Injuries.—Advances in the ski/binding/boot system dramatically lowered the injury rate from 5 to 8/1000 before 1970 to 2 to 3/1000 in the early 1990s. ACL injuries can be reduced in professional skiers with ACL awareness training. The incidence of severe knee injuries has increased with a female/male injury ratio of 2.3. Females are also 3.1 times more likely than males to have an ACL disruption.

Knee Injury Mechanisms.—The most common ACL injury mechanisms are valgus-external rotation, boot-induced anterior drawer mechanism, and flexion-induced rotation.

Lower Extremity Equipment-Related Injuries.—Most of these injuries are knee injuries and result from the ski acting as a lever to twist or bend the leg.

Development of Alpine Ski Bindings.—Release bindings, antifriction, and mechanical devices that have no boot-to-binding or boot-to-ski movement until the final point of release have contributed to the decrease the incidence of ankle injuries and tibia fractures.

Knee Injuries in Alpine Skiing and Their Possible Connection With Bindings.—The increase in knee sprains involving the ACL and binding release function are not related. The purpose of the release binding system is to prevent tibial shaft injuries. The load levels that cause serious knee injury are unknown, although optimal binding adjustments can substantially decrease the risk for lower leg injuries. Bindings with more than 2 release modes are associated with lower accident rates than bindings with 2 release modes. New upward release bindings should reduce the incidence of boot-top ACL injuries.

Problems With Bindings.—Bindings fail to protect the knee because the load needed to injure the hyperflexed knee is less than that required to execute skiing maneuvers, and bindings sense only forces translated to the boot and not forces that cause injury to the knee.

International Standards Organization (ISO) and American Society for Testing and Materials (ASTM) Standards.—These standards should be followed when release bindings are set.

Design-Related Studies of Ski/Binding/Boot Systems.—One new binding design has a heel release that is activated by the anterior/posterior bending moment at the boot sole. Another design has an electromechanical ski release with mechanical backup. None of the new designs address the injury mechanisms of the knee.

Conclusion.—The present binding designs do not address injury mechanisms of the knee, but, when adjusted according to ISO and ASTM standards, they do prevent many lower leg injuries.

▶ This is an excellent article dealing with the issue of the relationship of boot binding and skis to lower extremity injuries. It appears that the modern ski boot has protected the skier from tibia and ankle fractures at the expense of the ACL. As the authors point out, presently there is no binding design, setting, or function that can protect the knee from serious injury. They conclude "we are dealing with a system problem rather than just a single component of the system (ie, the binding). It is not until we address the entire scenario that we are going to make any headway on this problem from a hardware point of view."

J. S. Torg, MD

Injury Risk Factors Among Telemark Skiers
Tuggy ML, Ong R (Swedish Family Medicine, Seattle)
Am J Sports Med 28:83-89, 2000   1–7

Background.—Little research has been done on injury risk factors among telemark skiers. A population survey of telemark skiers conducted during 2 ski sessions was reported.

Methods and Findings.—Six hundred seventy-seven telemark skiing clubs contributed data on a total of 19,962 skier-days. One hundred seventy-eight injuries were self-reported. Thus, the overall self-reported injury rate was 8.9 per 1000 skier-days. Knee injuries were most common, occurring in 27%, followed by injuries to the thumb in 18% and the shoulder in 12%. Multivariate regression and survival analyses were performed. The skier's ski level and the use of plastic telemark boots had a significant injury-sparing effect. The boots' protective effect was probably attributable to their increased stability compared with traditional leather boots. The recently introduced releasable bindings for telemark skis reduced the number of knee injuries. Age and sex did not significantly affect injury rates. All reported deaths were attributed to environmental hazards.

Conclusions.—The use of the flexible plastic boots is the most significant factor affecting the telemark skier's risk of injury, followed by skill level and the use of releasable bindings. Telemark skiers must heed the environmental hazards in backcountry, as all reported deaths were attributable to such hazards.

▶ This is one of the few published articles dealing with injury risk and telemark skiing. A prior survey by Tuggy in 1994 to 1995 reported an injury rate of 10.6 per 1000 skier-days. However, because of the relatively small number of skier-days, lack of statistical power prevented definitive statements regarding injury rates. With regard to the current study, the response rate was 43% for the mailed survey and 94% for club meetings. Thus, the denominator for their injury rate calculations was 19,962 skier-days, which provided adequate statistical power to assess multiple risk factors for analysis. This, in itself, was a significant accomplishment for a retrospective survey of this nature.

J. S. Torg, MD

Baseball Hardness as a Risk Factor for Eye Injuries
Vinger PF, Duma SM, Crandall J (Tufts Univ, Medford, Mass; Univ of Virginia, Charlottesville)
Arch Ophthalmol 117:354-358, 1999   1–8

Objective.—Baseball is the leading cause of sports-related eye injury in children. Although softer baseballs decrease the risk for brain and cardiac injuries, they may increase the risk for eye injuries because they protrude into the orbit. Whether orbital intrusion and eye injury risk are increased with softer baseballs and whether players can feel the difference between hard and soft baseballs was investigated.

Methods.—Six different baseball hardnesses were tested. Eight balls of each hardness were pitched by an air cannon into an artificial orbit at velocities typical of young players. A soft baseball was pitched into 1 of a pair of matched unembalmed cadaver eyes at 120 km/h, and a hard baseball was pitched into the other eye at 88 km/h. Players aged 6 to 10 years (N = 4), 11 to 14 years (N = 4), adult men (N = 10), and adult women (N = 5) rated 3 samples of each test ball for relative hardness when pitching, batting, and catching.

Results.—The force increased with increasing ball hardness at all velocities except for the hardest balls. Peak orbital intrusion and velocity were weakly correlated for the soft balls but not for the hard balls. The eye hit by the soft ball remained intact. The eye hit by the hard ball was ruptured from the limbus to the optic nerve with almost total extrusion of the intraocular contents. Adults and children could tell that some balls were softer than others but could not detect hardness differences among the hardest balls. Young players could not detect differences in playability of balls.

Conclusion.—Although soft baseballs can cause significant eye injury, the injury is not greater than the injury produced by a hard ball. Players could not detect any playability differences between hard and soft baseballs. The wearing of eye protection is recommended for young ball players.

▶ As the authors have pointed out, eye and face protectors that meet the standard specifications of the American Society for Testing Materials have been available for more than a decade but are not commonly worn. Where are the rule makers? Also to be noted, it is speculated that softer baseballs would penetrate the orbit more deeply, increasing the severity and incidence of eye injuries.

J. S. Torg, MD

Risk Factors for Injuries and Other Health Problems Sustained in a Marathon
Satterthwaite P, Norton R, Larmer P, et al (Univ of Auckland, New Zealand)
Br J Sports Med 33:22-26, 1999   1–9

Objective.—Although injuries and other health problems are well documented in marathon runners, little information is available about modifiable risk and protective factors. The findings from a prospective cohort study of potential risk factors for injury while running the 1993 Auckland Citibank marathon are presented.

Methods.—Demographic, health history, and lifestyle data and information on injuries and other health problems during and after the marathon were collected from questionnaires completed by runners. Risk factors were identified with logistic regression analysis.

Results.—Men were at increased risk of calf and hamstring problems compared with women, and women were at increased risk of hip problems compared with men. First-time participation in the marathon, illness within 2 weeks before the marathon, current use of medication, and drinking alcohol more than once a month were associated with increased risk of problems. Although increased training increased the risk of thigh and hamstring problems, it probably decreased the risk of knee problems. Age and risk of injury or health problems were significantly associated in a complex way.

Conclusion.—Risk factors for injury and other health problems included illness before running the marathon and use of medication or alcohol.

▶ This study is one of the few controlled epidemiologic efforts undertaken to identify risk factors for injury and health problems sustained in a marathon. Of interest, the authors introduce the concept of a "survival phenomena" where, if an athlete is still running at an older age, it is because he or she has "survived" the injuries that cause many runners to leave the sport. This concept appears to apply also to "constitutional problems." Certainly, the conclusion is that those who have recently been ill or who are taking medications should carefully consider the pros and cons of participating in a marathon.

J. S. Torg, MD

Histopathology of Common Tendinopathies: Update and Implications for Clinical Management
Khan KM, Cook JL, Bonar F, et al (Univ of British Columbia, Vancouver, Canada; Victorian Inst of Sport, Melbourne, Australia; Douglass Hanly Moir Pathology, Sydney, Australia; et al)
Sports Med 27:393-408, 1999   1–10

Purpose.—Pathologic conditions involving the tendons are an important cause of pain and morbidity in athletes and nonathletes. The histopathologic findings in common tendon overuse syndromes involving the Achilles, patellar, extensor carpi radialis brevis, and rotator cuff tendons were reviewed.

Normal Tendon Anatomy.—Normal tendon anatomy consists of collagen arranged in increasingly complex tendons, beginning with the collagen fibril, through the primary, secondary, and tertiary fiber bundles, to the covering epitenon (Fig 1). To the naked eye, the tendon looks glistening white. Under the microscope, the parallel bundles of collagen fiber show a distinct pattern of reflectivity to polarized light. Few tenocytes and no fibroblasts or myofibroblasts are seen.

Tendonopathies.—Symptomatic tendons in athletes have a very different appearance. Macroscopically, they look gray and amorphous. Microscopy shows discontinuity and disorganization of collagen fibers, with loss of reflectivity under polarized light. The mucoid ground substance is increased, as shown by Alcian blue stain. Plump tenocytes with a chondroid appearance may be seen in areas of maximal mucoid change (exaggerated fibrocartilaginous metaplasia). Cells, mainly with a fibroblastic or myofibroblastic appearance, are seen within the tendon. Avidin biotin stain reveals the presence of smooth-muscle actin. At areas of maximal cellular proliferation, capillary proliferation is seen together with interrupted collagen fibers. Vascular and myofibroblastic proliferation may be abruptly interrupted immediately adjacent to the most abnormal-appearing area. Inflammatory cells are strikingly absent.

Discussion.—The histopathologic features of athletic overuse tendinopathies are very similar to those of the degenerative condition known as tendinosis. This pathologic picture has important implications for treat-

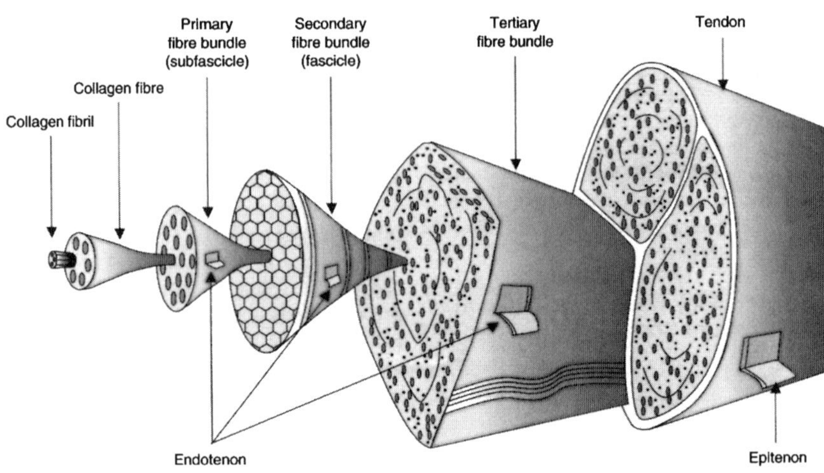

FIGURE 1.—The hierarchical organization of tendon structure from collagen fibrils to the entire tendon (reproduced from Józsa & Kannus,[5] with permission). (From Khan KM, Cook JL, Bonar F, et al: Histopathology of common tendinopathies: Update and implications for clinical management. *Sports Med* 27:393-408, 1999. Reprinted by permission from Józsa L, Kannus P: *Human* Tendons. *Anatomy, Physiology, and Pathology.* Champaign, Ill, *Human Kinetics*, 1997, p 50.)

ment and prognosis in athletes with tendon symptoms. The authors prefer the term tendinopathy to describe these overuse syndromes in athletes, as true tendinitis is rarely present. Tendinosis is a noninflammatory entity and should be treated as such. This concept warrants further consideration in clinical management and research.

▶ A comprehensive review article with 97 citations, the original article is recommended reading for the sports medicine practitioner. An interesting point brought out with regard to current treatment methods is that chronic overuse tendon conditions in athletes have been treated as inflammatory conditions when the histopathologic findings clearly reveal degenerative tendinosis. Hence, the observation that the efficacy of empirically based treatment protocols must necessarily be subjected to rigorous study.

J. S. Torg, MD

A Survey of Playing-related Musculoskeletal Problems Among Professional Orchestral Musicians in Hong Kong

Yeung E, Chan W, Pan F, et al (Hong Kong Polytechnic Univ, Kowloon, Hong Kong, China; Univ of Western Ontario, Canada)
Med Probl Perform Art 14:43-47, 1999
1–11

Background.—Previous research has attempted to define the intrinsic and extrinsic factors in the development of musculoskeletal disorders in musicians. The prevalence of and risk factors for playing-related musculoskeletal complaints (PRMCs) in symphony orchestra musicians in Hong Kong were reported.

Methods.—A validated questionnaire was distributed to all 170 professional orchestral musicians in Hong Kong. Thirty-nine returned the questionnaire, for a response rate of 23%.

Findings.—The 1-year prevalence of PRMCs was 64%, consistent with previously reported findings. The musicians reporting PRMCs in the preceding 12 months were relatively young (mean, 26 years) with less playing experience (mean, 8.9 years). In a stepwise logistic regression analysis, less playing experience and lack of regular exercise predicted PRMCs.

Conclusion.—These data suggest that young professional musicians are likely to have PRMCs. Regular exercise may prevent such symptoms. However, the sample size in the study was small, indicating the need for hypothesis testing on a larger sample.

▶ Interestingly, the younger musicians with lesser experience were more likely to have playing-related musculoskeletal complaints. With regard to this study, however, the small sample size appears to have had insufficient power to detect other important determinants in the development of these conditions.

J. S. Torg, MD

Cytokines and the Role They Play in the Healing of Ligaments and Tendons
Evans CH (Univ of Pittsburgh, Pa)
Sports Med 28:71-76, 1999   1–12

Background.—Cytokines behave like locally acting hormones, and play a key role in connective tissue healing. These small proteins trigger a cellular response when they engage with their specific receptors, also proteins, on target cells. There are many different types of cytokines with complex patterns of interaction, making it difficult to make simple statements about their properties. The author reviews the role of cytokines in ligament and tendon healing.

Cytokines in Ligament and Tendon Healing.—Although tendon and ligament healing has traditionally been considered from a biomechanical point of view, these structures must be understood as biological entities. Tendons and ligaments that heal follow the same healing pattern as other connective tissues, including the release of key cytokines—such as platelet-derived growth factor and transforming growth factor β—by platelets. Other cytokines probably play important roles in the inflammatory and reparative phases. However, very few studies have scientifically demonstrated the role of cytokines in healing. Most studies have examined responses to cytokines in culture. Despite the limitations of such in vitro studies, platelet-derived growth factor appears to be a potent stimulator of cell division and migration, whereas basic fibroblast growth factor and insulin-like growth factor (IGF) inhibit these activities. Both transforming growth factor β and IGF-I and IGF-II appear to stimulate matrix synthesis.

There is some evidence that topical application of cytokines may stimulate healing in vivo.

Other cytokines with specific effects on tendons and ligaments have recently been described. These include various growth and differentiation factors, which appear to be involved in embryonic organ development. They may become important in the search for biologically based methods of ligament and tendon healing, repair, and regeneration. Various anti-inflammatory cytokines, such as interleukin-10 and interleukin-1 receptor antagonist may help to promote healing when persistent inflammation is present. Local delivery of cytokines will pose major challenges, however. Gene-based approaches may be useful in addressing this problem.

Discussion.—Mounting evidence suggests that cytokines are very important for ligament and tendon healing. Delivery of various cytokines in the proper sequence may be necessary to optimize the progressive, multifunctional healing process. Gene delivery systems may play an important role in the clinical application of cytokines to ligament and tendon healing.

Gene Therapy and Tissue Engineering in Sports Medicine
Martinek V, Fu FH, Huard J (Univ of Pittsburgh, Pa)
Physician Sportsmed 28:34-51, 2000   1–13

Introduction.—Despite advances in many areas, treatment of sports injuries is limited by the poor healing capacity of certain tissues, such as ligaments, tendons, and articular cartilage. Growth factors can promote musculoskeletal healing and, directly applied, can be beneficial to healing in some situations. However, there is a need for some mode of delivery to maintain adequate levels of these proteins at the injured site. Gene transfer techniques are the most promising delivery system. The potential uses of gene therapy and tissue engineering in sports medicine were described.

Gene Therapy.—The goal of gene therapy in sports medicine is to promote therapeutic levels of beneficial proteins by transformed cells at the site of the injury. Gene therapy requires insertion of the DNA into some type of viral or nonviral vector delivery system. Viral gene vectors provide a more efficient method for gene transfer, although nonviral vectors are simpler and safer. Local delivery of gene vectors into the musculoskeletal system can be achieved by direct injection, or indirectly through removal, genetic manipulation, and replacement of cells from the injured tissue. Safety is the main concern in using gene therapy for sports medicine; the risk of side effects may simply be too high. These techniques may come into clinical use as new therapeutic vectors are developed.

Tissue Engineering.—Tissue engineering seeks to develop biological substitutes for repair, reconstruction, or replacement of tissues. Shaped polymers that serve as the scaffold or matrix for new tissue growth are combined with selected growth factors and responsive cells. So far, tissue engineering has been applied mainly to bone, in situations involving large defects or impaired vascularization. Cartilage has poor intrinsic repair capacity. Biological scaffolds have also been developed for meniscus regeneration and anterior cruciate ligament replacement.

Discussion.—Gene therapy and tissue regeneration have many potential uses in sports medicine. Injuries to skeletal muscle may be treated with growth factor gene therapy techniques. Gene therapy and tissue engineering approaches may one day be used to treat cartilage defects. Growth factor–based methods may also prove useful in the restoration of anterior cruciate ligament, meniscus, and bone deficits.

▶ These 2 articles (Abstracts 1–12 and 1–13) are essentially primers explaining the basic concepts of gene therapy, tissue engineering, and molecular biology in the facilitation of tissue healing. Although these modalities are clearly in the formative stages, it is hoped that they represent, so to speak, the wave of the future with regard to management of sports medicine problems that affect the musculoskeletal system.

J. S. Torg, MD

Transfer of LacZ Marker Gene to the Meniscus
Goto H, Shuler FD, Lamsam C, et al (Univ of Pittsburgh, Pa)
J Bone Joint Surg Am 81-A:918-925, 1999   1–14

Objective.—Lesions in the relatively avascular inner two thirds of the meniscus are associated with poor healing. Healing may be enhanced by the use of growth factors that promote meniscus cell proliferation and matrix synthesis, but problems with delivery have limited the clinical use of such growth factors. One way to achieve sufficient growth factor concentrations at the site of the lesion may be the transfer of genes encoding the growth factor. Vectors for gene delivery to the meniscus were evaluated.

Methods.—The researchers used the bacterial marker gene *lacZ*, which expresses β-galactosidase. Transfer was attempted with the use of vectors developed from an adenovirus and a retrovirus. Gene transfer was evaluated in an in vitro model with the use of rabbit, dog, and human meniscal cells, as well as intact rabbit and human menisci. In vivo studies were performed in rabbits and dogs. The gene was delivered by an adenovirus in a blood clot or by a retrovirally transduced allogeneic meniscal cells embedded in collagen gels, respectively.

Results.—Monolayer cultures showed successful *lacZ* gene transduction by both the adenovirus and retrovirus. Successful gene transfer was also noted in intact menisci, delivered directly by adenovirus and indirectly by retrovirus. In vitro gene expression persisted for at least 20 weeks. In the in vivo rabbit study, *lacZ* gene expression persisted within the blood clot and in some adjacent meniscal cells for at least 3 weeks. In the dog model, gene expression by the transduced, transplanted meniscal cells persisted for at least 6 weeks.

Conclusions.—These experiments showed the successful transfer of genes to the site of meniscal injuries, followed by local gene expression for several weeks. These methods may be useful to promote the healing of lesions in the avascular portion of the meniscus. In vivo studies are needed to assess the effect of growth factor gene transfer techniques on meniscal healing.

▶ As concluded by the authors, this study "permits cautious optimism regarding the possibility that these techniques could form the basis of gene-transfer approach to the repair of meniscal lesions." Presumably, the future could hold a dramatic transformation in the manner in which surgical problems of the knee joint are managed.

J. S. Torg, MD

Insulin-like Growth Factor I Accelerates Functional Recovery from Achilles Tendon Injury in a Rat Model
Kurtz CA, Loebig TG, Anderson DD, et al (Allegheny Univ, Pittsburgh, Pa; Minneapolis Sports Medicine Ctr, Minn)
Am J Sports Med 27:363-369, 1999   1–15

Introduction.—Insulin-like growth factor I (IGF-I) is an important mediator in all stages of wound healing, including inflammation. Its absence dramatically affects wound healing across several parameters. It directly influences all cells involved in repair of musculoskeletal soft tissue. The effects of IGF-I on Achilles tendon healing were examined in a rat model of Achilles tendon injury.

Methods.—Forty-eight male Sprague-Dawley rats were used; 18 underwent functional and biochemical evaluation, 20 were used to evaluate inflammation, and 10 underwent histologic examination. Rats were randomized into groups of 6 animals each for sham surgery (Achilles and plantaris tendons dissected free), transection alone (the plantaris was excised in its entirety and the Achilles tendon was transected transversely 0.5 cm proximal to its insertion), and transection plus IGF-I. Rats underwent functional evaluation. The Achilles functional index was determined. Baseline measurements were compared with those of postoperative days 1, 2, 3, and subsequent odd-numbered days until postoperative day 15. Tissues underwent biomechanical, inflammation, and histologic evaluations.

Results.—Rats treated with IGF-I had a significantly smaller maximum functional deficit and a shorter time to functional recovery compared with untreated animals. Biomechanical testing showed no significant between-group differences in the measured parameters after transection. To determine the mechanism of action, 6 additional rats received an Achilles tendon injection of carrageenan alone and 6 others received carrageenan plus IGF-I. Animals treated with IGF-I did not experience the inflammation-induced functional deficit experienced by control animals. Spectrometric myeloperoxidase assays on the remaining 8 animals after Achilles tendon transection showed no significant difference between treated and untreated growth factor groups, suggesting a mechanism other than neutrophil recruitment by which the growth factor limits inflammatory response. Histologic evaluations were performed on carregeenan-injected animals on postinjection day 2 and on surgically treated animals on postoperative day 15. No gross histologic differences were observed between treated and untreated growth factor groups.

Conclusion.—IGF-I diminishes maximum functional deficit and accelerates recovery after Achilles tendon injury, possibly by an anti-inflammatory mechanism.

Enhanced Repair of Extensive Articular Defects by Insulin-like Growth Factor-I-Laden Fibrin Composites

Nixon AJ, Fortier LA, Williams J, et al (Cornell Univ, Ithaca, NY)
J Orthop Res 17:475-487, 1999   1–16

Introduction.—Insulin-like growth factor I (IGF-I) has frequently been shown by in vitro cartilage explant and isolated cell cultures to be important in the cartilage anabolic process. Investigations on the repeated intra-articular administration of IGF-I to treat cartilage disease are rare. It is possible that IGF-I may facilitate chondrogenesis of bone marrow stem cells in long-term cultures and may thus enhance chondrogenesis in healing cartilage lesions in vivo. The impact of IGF-I, gradually released from fibrin clots polymerized in situ in large cartilage lesions, on the recruitable stem cell pool was examined in an equine full-thickness cartilage defect.

Findings.—Twelve full-thickness articular defects were created in the femoropatellar joints of 6 normal horses aged 2 to 6 years. The defects were repaired by an injection of autogenous fibrin containing 25 µg of human recombinant IGF-I or fibrin without IGF-I (controls). Animals were killed at 6 months. Cartilage repair tissue and surrounding cartilage were examined by histochemistry, types I and II collagen immunohistochemistry, types I and II collagen in situ hybridization, and matrix biochemical determinations.

Results.—Morphologic analysis revealed that white tissue filled treated and control lesions. The IGF-I–treated defects were more completely filled and securely attached to subchondral bone. A moderately improved chondrocyte population, more columnar cellular organization, and better attachment to the underlying bone were obvious on histologic examination of IGF-I–treated defects. Type II procollagen messenger RNA was plentiful in the deeper half of the treated sections, compared with the moderate messenger expression observed in control tissues. Immunolocalization of type II collagen revealed a preponderance of the collagen in IGF-I–treated defects, confirming translation of type II messenger to protein. Composite histologic healing scores for treated defects were significantly better than those of controls. The DNA content was similar for both groups. Matrix proteoglycan content was similar in the defects for both groups and lower in the defects, than in the intact surrounding and remote cartilage of the treated and control joints.

Conclusion.—Fibrin polymers laden with IGF-I augmented the hyaline repair of critical sized defects in a horse model of cartilage resurfacing. The overall quality of repair was superior to that of fibrin-grafted control defects, yet was not typical of normal hyaline articular cartilage.

▶ These 2 articles (Abstracts 1–15 and 1–16) are of no clinical relevance other than to indicate the potential of molecular biology in the facilitation of tissue healing.

J. S. Torg, MD

PT-12, a Putative Ras-activated Proliferation-dependent Gene, Is Expressed in Patellar Tendon and Not in Anterior Cruciate Ligament
Gommer RS, Maris T, Ostrander R, et al (Univ of California, San Diego, La Jolla)
J Orthop Res 17:745-747, 1999   1–17

Introduction.—The patellar tendon is commonly used to reconstruct the anterior cruciate ligament (ACL). Tendons and ligaments have different biochemical environments. The primary cells from the ACL proliferate and migrate at a slower rate, compared with the patellar tendon and medial collateral ligament. A subtractive hybridization technique was used to identify genes that are differently expressed in the patellar tendon and ACL.

Methods.—Patellar tendon and ACL tissues were dissected from mature New Zealand White rabbits. Messenger RNA was extracted from snap-frozen tissues. Representational difference analysis, a newly developed polymerase chain reaction (PCR)-based subtractive complementary DNA, was used to identify genes expressed in the patellar tendon and not the ACL. The RNA free of total DNA and purified from the ACL ligament and ACL was reverse-transcribed and amplified by PCR with the use of deferentially expressed gene-specific oligonucleotide primers to examine patellar tendon–specific expression of deferentially expressed genes. Genes expressed in proliferating cells and nonproliferating cells were examined by sequence analysis.

Results.—Six clones isolated after 2 rounds of hybridization during representational difference analysis showed an insert. Only the twelfth clone had sequence similarity to a proliferation-dependent gene. This clone was named PT-12. A comparison of the 221 bp of the PT-12 sequence with that of the Gen EMBL databank showed that the PT-12 was highly homologous (>87%) to the human *S2* or mouse LLPep3 ribosomal gene. The homology region included the S2-LLRep3 coding region (190 bp) and approximately 30 pb of the 3'-untranslated region. The PT-12–specific oligonucleotides amplified a specific product in the patellar tendon, yet did not yield a specific product when first-strand synthesis products from the ACL were amplified. β-Actin gene was amplified to act as a positive control from the same RNA samples. It yielded a specific product that did not vary from either sample.

Conclusion.—The PT-12 is a homologue of human *S2* or mouse LLPep3 ribosomal gene that is overexpressed in the patellar tendon and not the ACL. These data may provide further explanation of why the patellar tendon heals and the ACL does not heal.

Expression of the Gene Encoding the Matrix Gla Protein by Mature Osteoblasts in Human Fracture Non-unions
Lawton DM, Andrew JG, Marsh DR, et al (Univ of Manchester, England)
J Clin Pathol Mol Pathol 52:92-96, 1999   1–18

Introduction.—Osteoblast phenotype abnormality, primarily the expression of collagen type III, has been reported earlier in fracture nonunion woven bone. The matrix gla protein (MGP) is a consistent component of bone matrix, yet no reports have indicated that there are osteoblasts in the skeleton expressing the gene for MGP. The site of skeletal MGP synthesis remains unknown. Osteoblasts from fracture nonunion were evaluated for evidence of gene expression of noncollagenous bone matrix proteins involved in mineralization: MGP, osteonectin, osteopontin, and osteocalcin.

Methods.—Biopsy specimens from normally healing human fractures and nonunions were assessed by in situ hybridization by S labeled probes and autoradiology to determine levels of gene expression.

Results.—In normally healing fractures, mature osteoblasts on woven bone did not express MGP messenger RNA and did express osteonectin, osteopontin, and osteocalcin messenger RNA molecules. In nonunion fractures, osteoblasts showed a novel phenotype. They expressed MGP messenger RNA and osteonectin, osteopontin, and osteocalcin messenger RNA molecules.

Conclusion.—An unusual phenotype is observed in mature osteoblasts of slowly healing fractures. They express the gene encoding MGP, which suggests that control of osteoblast gene expression in nonunions is abnormal. This may be a significant factor in the pathogenesis of nonuniting human fractures.

▶ Although these 2 articles (Abstracts 1–17 and 1–18) have no current clinical applications of significance, they certainly suggest the potential for genetic engineering in the management of soft tissue and bone injury. Importantly, the clinical application of gene therapy is a matter of when and not if.

J. S. Torg, MD

Use of Recombinant Human Bone Morphogenetic Protein-2 to Enhance Tendon Healing in a Bone Tunnel

Rodeo SA, Suzuki K, Deng X-h, et al (Cornell Univ, New York; Genetics Inst Inc, Andover, Mass)
Am J Sports Med 27:476-488, 1999   1–19

Background.—The firm healing of tendon or ligament to bone is crucial to the success of a number of reconstructive surgical procedures. The hypothesis that bone ingrowth into a tendon graft placed in a bone tunnel can be enhanced by human bone morphogenetic protein-2 was investigated.

Methods.—Researchers used 65 male adult mongrel dogs for this study. They detached the long digital extensor tendon of the knee joint from its femoral insertion in both hindlimbs. A drill hole was made in the proximal tibia, and the tendon was transplanted through the bone tunnel into the proximal tibial metaphysis. Two different doses of morphogenetic protein-2 were applied to the tendon-bone interface in hindlimb with an absorbable type I collagen sponge. One subgroup received a lower dose and 1 a higher dose. In the contralateral limb, only the sponge was applied. The animals were then evaluated at serial times between 3 days and 8 weeks, using radiography, histologic examination, and biomechanical testing to evaluate the healed tendon-bone attachment.

Results.—Histologic examination and radiography showed more extensive formation of bone around the tendon and close apposition of new bone to the tendon in the limbs treated with morphogenetic protein-2 compared with the contralateral control limb. Results of the biomechanical testing also demonstrated improvements in the treated limbs, with higher tendon pull-out strength in the protein-treated limbs at all time points. There was a statistically significant difference in the protein-treated limbs versus the control limbs in the low-dose–treated subgroup at 2 weeks of follow-up. Data from the histologic and biomechanical examinations indicated that the lower protein dose provided superior healing results compared with the higher dose.

Conclusion.—The healing process after a tendon graft is transplanted into a bone tunnel can be accelerated by use of bone morphogenetic protein-2.

The Effect of Cytokines on the Proliferation and Migration of Bovine Meniscal Cells

Bhargava MM, Attia ET, Murrell GAC, et al (Cornell Univ, New York)
Am J Sports Med 27:636-643, 1999   1–20

Background.—A number of studies have reported on the potential value of cytokines in the healing process after meniscal injury. In this study, researchers investigated the effects of cytokines on the proliferation and migration of bovine meniscal cells, to characterize the nature of cytokine's effects on meniscal tissue. The cells under investigation were isolated from the inner (peripheral), middle, and avascular thirds of the meniscus.

Methods.—Bovine stifle joints from skeletally mature animals were used. After harvesting and sharp dissection, the meniscal specimens were immersed in medium M199, then sectioned into outer, middle, and inner thirds. The sections were diced, placed in M199 solution containing 10% antibiotic-antimycotic solution, and incubated at 37°C in a humidified atmosphere. Migration and confluence of the cells occurred within 2 to 3 weeks. The cells were then tested for DNA synthesis and chemotactic response to various cytokines.

Results.—The outer, or peripheral, cells showed a significantly higher rate of DNA synthesis in response to 10% serum than was seen in cells from the middle or inner (avascular) regions. DNA synthesis was stimulated in a dose-dependent manner in response to recombinant human platelet–derived growth factor-AB, hepatocyte growth factor/scatter factor, and bone morphogenic protein-2. Cytokines also stimulated cell migration. Migration of cells increased in cells from all 3 zones in response to platelet-derived growth factor and hepatocyte growth factor, but interleukin-1 only stimulated migration of cells derived from the outer third of the meniscus. Cell migration was stimulated only by 40% to 50% in the inner and outer zones by epidermal growth factor. Bone morphogenic protein-2 and insulin-like growth factor-1 produced a 40% to 50% stimulation of cell migration in cells derived from the middle third of the meniscus.

Conclusion.—Improvement in the ability to modulate meniscal healing is aided by identification of cytokines that stimulate growth and migration of meniscal cells.

▶ Like recent studies dealing with gene therapy in the management of soft-tissue and bone injury, these 2 articles (Abstracts 1–19 and 1–20) have no current clinical application. However, they do represent the prelude or potential of molecular biology in management of soft-tissue and bone injury. Again, we note that clinical application of this approach is a matter of *when* and not *if*.

J. S. Torg, MD

Evidence of Inappropriate Application of Autologous Cartilage Transplantation Therapy in an Uncontrolled Environment

Mont MA, Jones LC, Vogelstein BN, et al (Good Samaritan Hosp, Baltimore, Md)
Am J Sports Med 27:617-620, 1999   1–21

Purpose.—Initial studies have shown promising results with autologous chondrocyte transplantation for the management of patients with focal articular cartilage defects in the knee. However, in the absence of prospective randomized trials, the appropriate indications for and limitations of this procedure remain to be defined. Cases rejected for insurance reimbursement for autologous cartilage transplantation were analyzed to determine whether the referred patients met appropriate criteria for this procedure.

Methods.—The analysis included 24 consecutive cases in which reimbursement for autologous cartilage transplantation was refused by an insurance company. In each case, the decision of the medical reviewer was appealed by the recommending orthopedic surgeon. The investigators reviewed each case to determine whether it met appropriate criteria for this procedure. The evaluation included the number and size of cartilage defects, the presence of tricompartmental arthritis, the recommendation of transplantation for patellar lesions, the age of the patient, and the presence of sagittal plane deformity.

Results.—All but 1 of the cases reviewed either failed to meet the criteria for autologous cartilage transplantation or had specific contraindications. In 15 cases, multiple contraindications were present. The most common reasons for not meeting the criteria were lesions larger than 10 cm², more than 2 areas of involvement, tricompartmental arthritis, and recommendation of transplantation for patellar lesions. Of the recommending surgeons, 44% would be performing autologous cartilage transplantation for the first time.

Conclusion.—The results suggest that many patients are being referred for autologous cartilage transplantation without meeting the general indications for this procedure. Such uncontrolled use of a new procedure may give an inaccurately negative impression of the results possible in properly selected cases. Controlled application-limited experience is needed before new procedures such as this are allowed to come into widespread clinical use.

▶ Although the seemingly good results attributed to this procedure did not involve a randomized, prospective study, the indications included small-to-medium sized hyaline cartilage lesions ranging from 1 to 10 cm² in patients between the ages of 15 and 55 years. Clearly, these indications are empirical and without scientific foundation. The statement that "uncontrolled use of this procedure may negatively skew the overall results for this technique, prejudicing a procedure that may be successful for the correct indications" is valid. However, who is to say what the correct indications are?

J. S. Torg, MD

Effects of Hyperbaric Oxygen on a Human Model of Injury
Staples JR, Clement DB, Taunton JE, et al (Univ of British Columbia, Vancouver, Canada)
Am J Sports Med 27:600-605, 1999
1–22

Purpose.—Studies have suggested that adjunctive hyperbaric oxygen (HBO) therapy can promote soft-tissue healing in severely injured patients.

However, few studies have addressed the use of HBO therapy for athletic injuries, and those studies have lacked randomization and double-blinding. A randomized controlled study of HBO therapy for induced delayed-onset quadriceps muscle soreness was reported.

Methods.—The study included 66 untrained young men. Quadriceps muscle soreness was induced by having the subjects exercise on a KIN-COM Dynamometer (Chattax, Chattanooga, Tenn). The volunteers then underwent treatment in an HBO chamber over a 5-day period. During the first phase, 1 group received immediate HBO, consisting of 100% oxygen for 1 h/d at 2.0 standard atmosphere 1 received delayed HBO; and 1 received sham treatment, consisting of 21% oxygen for 1 h/d at 1.2 standard atmosphere. A fourth group served as a control. During the second phase, subjects received 3 or 5 days of HBO treatment or sham treatment. Recovery was assessed by testing eccentric torque of the non-dominant quadriceps before and immediately after exercise, as well as 48 and 96 hours post exercise. Daily visual analogue pain scores were recorded.

Results.—The phase 1 data showed significantly faster recovery of eccentric torque in the immediate HBO group compared with the sham, control, and delayed HBO groups. The difference was significant from immediately to 96 hours post exercise. During phase 2, recovery of eccentric torque was significantly greater in the 5-day treatment group than in the sham treatment group or in the 3-day treatment group. Pain scores did not differ significantly at any time during either phase of the study.

Conclusion.—In this human study, HBO therapy appears to promote recovery of eccentric quadriceps muscle torque in subjects with delayed-onset muscle soreness. This benefit is achieved with 1 hour of HBO therapy started within 20 minutes after exercise and continued for 3 to 5 days. However, HBO treatment does not appear to alter pain scores associated with this injury.

▶ It is my observation that, other than its use in the management of acute decompression syndrome, hyperbaric oxygen therapy is a treatment looking for a disease, particularly with regard to the management of musculoskeletal injuries.

J. S. Torg, MD

Concussion in Sports
Wojtys EM, Hovda D, Landry G, et al (AOSSM Concussion Workshop Group, Rosemont, Ill)
Am J Sports Med 27:676-687, 1999   1–23

Objective.—The recognition and management of concussion is a medical challenge. Accurate diagnosis, time to recover, second-impact syndrome, occurrence, frequency, cumulative effects of repeated injury, individual recovery, persistence of symptoms, and pathobiology of cerebral

1. Orientation		
Month: ___________________	0	1
Date: ___________________	0	1
Day of week: ___________	0	1
Year: ___________________	0	1
Time (within 1 hr): _________	0	1

Orientation Total Score _____ / 5

2. Immediate Memory (all 3 trials are completed regardless of score on trial 1 & 2; total score equals sum across all 3 trials)

List	Trial 1		Trial 2		Trial 3	
Word 1	0	1	0	1	0	1
Word 2	0	1	0	1	0	1
Word 3	0	1	0	1	0	1
Word 4	0	1	0	1	0	1
Word 5	0	1	0	1	0	1
Total						

Immediate Memory Total Score __ / 15

(Note: Subject is not informed of Delayed Recall testing of memory)

NEUROLOGICAL SCREENING:

Recollection if injury (pre- or post-traumatic amnesia)

Strength:

Sensation:

Coordination:

Loss of Consciousness:

3. Concentration

Digits Backward (If correct, go to next string length. If incorrect, read trial 2. Stop after incorrect on both trials.)

4-9-3	6-2-9 _________	0	1
3-8-1-4	3-2-7-9 _________	0	1
6-2-9-7-1	1-5-2-8-6 ___	0	1
7-1-8-4-6-2	5-3-9-1-4-8 ___	0	1

Months in reverse order (entire sequence correct for 1 point)
Dec-Nov-Oct-Sep-Aug-Jul
Jun-May-Apr-Mar-Feb-Jan ___ 0 1

Concentration Total Score __ / 5

EXERTIONAL MANEUVERS:
(when appropriate):

5 jumping jacks	5 push-ups
5 sit-ups	5 knee bends

4. Delayed Recall

Word 1	0	1
Word 2	0	1
Word 3	0	1
Word 4	0	1
Word 5	0	1

Delayed Recall Total Score __ / 5

Summary of Total Scores:

Orientation __________	/	5
Immediate Memory _____	/	15
Concentration _______	/	5
Delayed Recall _______	/	5
Overall Total Score _______	/	30

APPENDIX 1.—The SAC form for evaluating concussion. (Courtesy of Wojtys EM, Hovda D, Landry G, et al: Concussion in sports. *Am J Sports Med* 27:676-687, 1999.)

concussion have not been well studied. In December 1997, the Concussion Workshop, sponsored by the American Orthopaedic Society for Sports Medicine, examined areas of agreement and disagreement in the detection and management of concussion in sports.

Methods.—The workshop on the neurobiology of cerebral concussion examined why the brain is so vulnerable after a concussion, and identified metabolic dysfunction as the primary physiologic event that produces and maintains the brain in a vulnerable state for minutes or days after injury. The workshop section on initial evaluation—anticipation, awareness, preparation—called for measures to be performed on the playing field and on the sidelines. Assessment of spontaneous breathing, pulse, and a Glasgow Coma Scale rating should be performed. On the bench, symptoms should be reviewed, and a neurologic examination and neuropsychological testing should be performed. The Standardized Assessment of Concussion (SAC), a valid, standardized, systematic sideline evaluation, should be performed on the sidelined athlete (App 1). Recommendations for concussion evaluation and return to play call for observation and evaluation for at least 15 minutes and disqualification for a day for those players whose symptoms do not resolve. The recommendations contain return-to-play classifications.

Results.—The workshop generated 9 recommendations.

Conclusion.—Concussion in sports is a challenging medical problem that needs a systematic acute and long-term management approach.

▶ This article is a comprehensive review of the current concepts relating to concussion in sports. It is a well written and evenly balanced presentation of the subject matter. Worth noting is the section on sideline evaluation of the athlete using the standardized assessment of concussions. "The SAC takes approximately 5 minutes to administer and is designed for use by the nonneuropsychologist with no prior expertise in psychometric testing. . . . Orientation is assessed by asking the subject to provide the day of the week, month, year, and time of day to within 1 hour. A 5-word list is used to measure immediate memory; the list is read to the subject for immediate recall and the procedure is repeated for 3 trials. Concentration is tested by having the subject repeat, in reverse order, strings of digits that increase in length from 3 to 6 numbers. Reciting the months of the year in reverse order is also used to assess concentration. Delayed recall of the original 5-word list is also assessed. A composite total test score is computed to derive the index of the subject's overall level of impairment after concussion."

J. S. Torg, MD

Relationship Between Concussion and Neuropsychological Performance in College Football Players
Collins MW, Grindel SH, Lovell MR, et al (Henry Ford Health System, Detroit, Univ of Pittsburgh, Pa; Univ of Florida, Gainesville; et al)
JAMA 282:964-970, 1999   1–24

Objective.—Research on the consequences of mild traumatic brain injury (MTBI) in athletics is lacking. Although few data on any association between long-term cognitive morbidity and concussion are available, it is known that a prior history of head injury increases the risk for future MTBI. The relationship between prior discussion and diagnosed learning disability in college football players and the influence of these variables alone and in combination on baseline neuropsychologic performance were investigated. The use of a neuropsychologic test battery for diagnosing concussion and delineating recovery of cognitive function following MTBI was evaluated in athletes. The relationship between learning disability (LD) and concussion was investigated.

Methods.—Preseason neurologic evaluations were performed between May 1997 and February 1999 in 393 male college football players, average age, 20.4 years, from 4 Division IA football programs. Those players who sustained concussion playing football were reevaluated.

Results.—At baseline, 179 (46%) players had no history of concussion, 129 (34%) had 1 concussion, and 79 (29%) had 2 or more concussions. Years playing football and number of concussions were significantly correlated ($r = 0.15$). Quarterbacks and tight ends had the highest concussion rates (68% and 65%, respectively). There was no significant relationship between LD and concussion history. Athletes with multiple concussion and LD demonstrated significantly poorer performance on neuropsychologic tests than athletes with multiple concussion and no LD. A history of concussion and LD independently contribute to poorer cognitive performance in football players. There was a significant association between players with 2 or more concussions and long-term deficits in executive functioning, speed of information processing, and self-reported symptoms.

Conclusion.—Multiple concussions can lead to neurologic and cognitive deficits. Neuropsychologic tests are useful for assessing cognitive functioning.

▶ According to the Centers for Disease Control and Prevention (CDC), an estimated 300,000 sports-related MTBIs of mild to moderate severity, most of which can be classified as concussions (ie, conditions of temporarily altered mental status as a result of head trauma), occur in the United States each year.[1] The proportion of these concussions that are repeat injuries is unknown; however, there is an increased risk for subsequent MTBI among persons who have had at least 1 previous MTBI (case in point, NFL quarterback Steve Young). As emphasized in this article, repeated MTBIs occurring over an extended period (ie, months or years) can result in cumulative neurologic and cognitive deficits. The CDC warns, however, that repeated MTBIs occurring within a short period (ie, hours, days, weeks) can be catastrophic or fatal.[1]

D. C. Nieman, DrPH

Reference

1. Sports-related recurrent brain injuries—United States. *Morbid Mortal Weekly Rep* 46:224-227, 1997.

Neuropsychological Impairment in Amateur Soccer Players
Matser EJT, Kessels AG, Lezak MD, et al (St Anna Hosp, Geldrop, The Netherlands; Erasmus Univ, Rotterdam, The Netherlands; Univ Hosp of Maastricht, The Netherlands; et al)
JAMA 282:971-973, 1999
                                                                1–25

Background.—Chronic traumatic brain injury (CTBI) is generally associated with boxing, but may also occur in soccer players. Factors related to CTBI include concussions that occur during practice and during matches and frequent subconcussive blows to the head from the soccer ball that occur when the player does headers. Evidence of CTBI among amateur players was sought.

Methods.—Interviews and neuropsychological testing of 33 amateur soccer players and 27 amateur athletes (control subjects) who were involved in swimming and track in the Netherlands were conducted. The performances of these 2 groups on the neurological tests were compared, and impaired performance was attributed to possible CTBI.

Results.—The soccer players had significant impairment on planning and memory tests compared with controls. The results for concussions unrelated to soccer, alcohol intake, level of education, and number of general anesthesias were adjusted for, and significantly poorer performances were seen among soccer players for the Complex Figure Test, the Digit Span Test, and 3 subtests of the Wechsler Memory Scale (Logical Memory, Visual Reproduction, and Associate Learning). There was an inverse correlation between the number of concussions incurred in soccer and several test performances.

Conclusions.—The concussions amateur soccer players repeatedly have may lead to the development of cognitive impairment. Mild CTBI was seen as impaired performance on tests of memory and planning ability.

▶ My interpretation of the results of this study is that at one point in time a group of 27 swimmers and track runners were better at performing psychometric tests than were 33 amateur soccer players. The mild cognitive changes demonstrated, if they were in fact real, were not absolutely correlated with head trauma. The differences were described by the authors as "mild" and the designation of "neuropsychological impairment" appears to be a stretch.

J. S. Torg, MD

Traumatic Brain Injury in High School Athletes
Powell JW, Barber-Foss KD (Med Sports Systems, Iowa City, Iowa)
JAMA 282:958-963, 1999
                                                                1–26

Background.—Mild traumatic brain injury (MTBI) can be serious. Little is known about the frequency of such injuries among high school athletes.

The type, frequency, and severity of MTBI in selected high school sports activities were reported.

Methods and Findings.—Between 1995 and 1997, 246 certified athletic trainers at 235 US high schools recorded injury and exposure data for high school varsity athletes in boys' football, wrestling, baseball, and field hockey; girls' volleyball and softball; boys' and girls' basketball; and boys' and girls' soccer. During the 3-year period, a total of 23,566 injuries occurred in the 10 sports. Of these, 1219 (5.5%) were MTBIs. Football accounted for 63.4% of the MTBIs; wrestling, 10.5%; girls' soccer, 6.2%; boys' soccer, 5.7%; girls' basketball, 5.2%; boys' basketball, 4.2%; softball, 2.1%; baseball, 1.2%; field hockey, 1.1%; and volleyball, 0.5%. Injury rates per 100 player-seasons were 3.66 for football; 1.58 for wrestling; 1.14 for girls' soccer; 1.04 for girls' basketball; 0.92 for boys' soccer; 0.75 for boys' basketball; 0.46 for softball; 0.46 for field hockey; 0.23 for baseball; and 0.14 for volleyball. A median of 3 days were lost from sports participation because of MTBIs. Six cases of subdural hematoma and intracranial injury occurred, all among football players.

Conclusions.—An estimated 62,816 MTBIs occur annually among high school varsity athletes participating in the 10 sports studied. About 63% of these injuries occur in football players.

▶ This article presents a huge problem with regard to terminology. As stated, concussion is defined as a trauma-induced alteration in mental status that may or may not involve a loss of consciousness. *Mild head injury, traumatic brain injury,* and *mild traumatic brain injury* have been used to describe brain injuries. Powell et al characterized players removed from participation and evaluated for traumatic brain or head injury by an athletic trainer, physician, or both before returning to participation as having MTBI. Clearly, we are equating apples with pineapples. Therefore, the data presented only identify individuals removed from a contest and do not correlate with the existence of a defined injury pattern.

J. S. Torg, MD

Head and Neck Injuries Among Ice Hockey Players Wearing Full Face Shields vs Half Face Shields

Benson BW, Mohtadi NGH, Rose MS, et al (Univ of Calgary, Alta, Canada)
JAMA 282:2328-2332, 1999   1–27

Purpose.—Full face shields have been introduced for use by ice hockey players across many different levels of play, and have helped to reduce the rate of facial and eye injuries. However, some reports have suggested that the use of full face shields may somehow have contributed to an increase in the rate of neck injuries. This prospective cohort study compared rates of head or neck injuries among college ice hockey players wearing full-face shields versus half-face shields.

Methods.—The study sample comprised 642 men playing during 1 Canadian intercollegiate hockey season. Of the 22 teams participating, 11 wore full-face shields throughout the season, whereas 11 wore half-face shields. The 2 groups were compared for their rates of reportable injuries, (ie, any event requiring attention by the team therapist or physician). Also assessed were incidents of mild traumatic brain injury or brachial plexus stretch.

Results.—During the season, at least 1 injury occurred in 61.6% of athletes wearing full-face shields versus 63.2% of those wearing half-face shields. The rate of facial laceration or dental injury was more than twice as high for players wearing half-face shields, with relative risks of 2.31 and 9.90, respectively. However, there were no differences in the rates of other injuries, including neck injuries or concussions. Players wearing half-face shields lost more time because of concussions than those wearing full-face shields.

Conclusion.—This prospective study finds no evidence that full-face shields increase the risk of head and neck injuries in college ice hockey players. The results also confirm reduced rates of dental and facial injuries with full-face shields. The findings support the use of full-face shields for intercollegiate ice hockey players.

▶ The National Collegiate Athletic Association requires that a full-face shield and mouth piece be worn by hockey players. Frequently, proposals are made to change this legislation so that athletes would be required to wear only a half-face shield. The reasoning of the proponents for this change is that the full-face shield changes the nature of the game and encourages the athletes to use the helmet as a weapon. Therefore, rather than preventing injuries, they state, it causes serious injuries. This study indicates that full-face shields definitely reduce the number of facial and dental injuries and do not increase head or neck injuries. Hopefully, studies such as this will put the matter to rest, and the full-face shield will be worn at all levels of ice hockey.

F. J. George ATC, PT

Cervical Spine Injuries in Football Players
Thomas BE, McCullen GM, Yuan HA (Naval Med Ctr, San Diego, Calif; Univ of California, San Diego; Univ of New York, Syracuse)
J Am Acad Orthop Surg 7:338-347, 1999   1–28

Objective.—Ten percent to 15% of football players, mostly linemen, defensive ends, and linebackers, incur cervical spine injuries. Although most of these injuries are self-limiting and heal completely, some players with "neck injuries" show radiographic evidence of compression fractures, neural arch fractures, and abnormal motion segments. Clinical syndromes, field evaluation, and management of cervical spine injuries are discussed.

Clinical Syndromes.—Neuropraxia of the nerve roots or brachial plexus is the most common injury, affecting about half of the injured players. Any persistent burning or stinging sensation must be carefully examined to rule out compressive or traction injuries to multiple roots or to the brachial plexus. A thermoplastic total-contact neck-shoulder-chest orthosis beneath well-fitting shoulder pads can decrease the severity and recurrence of these injuries. Acute cervical sprain is a ligamentous injury, resulting from nonradiating pain in the neck. Intervertebral disk lesions can lead to temporary or complete paralysis and may require anterior diskectomy with interbody fusion. Cervical spondylolytc changes without herniation can be treated nonsurgically with activity modification. Symptoms of transient quadriplegia, after axial load with hyperextension or hyperflexion, include bilateral burning or tingling and can result from congenital stenosis, Klippel-Feil syndrome, or intervertebral disk disease or acquired stenosis. Congenital abnormalities, such as failure of segmentation and failure of formation, increase the risk of injury. Deaths from unstable cervical fractures and dislocations have dropped dramatically with better-designed helmets and rules against head butting. Axial loading accounts for most of these injuries.

Field Evaluation and Early Treatment.—Immobilize the injured play, remove the face mask with tools, if necessary, perform CPR, and transport the player to a medical facility.

Rehabilitation.—The program consists of isometric contractions, followed by concentric resistance exercises, and later, gentle passive stretching. Eccentric muscle strengthening begins when painless full range of motion is attained.

Return to Play.—Players can return to play when paresthesias, and any radicular pain or neurologic deficits resolve and individuals demonstrate full strength and painless neck mobility. Individuals with congenital anomalies or type I injuries must not play contact sports.

Conclusion.—Avoiding head-down tackling techniques and wearing proper equipment can reduce the risk of injury. After injury, return to play must be evaluated on a case-by-case basis. Individuals with type I injuries or congenital anomalies should not play contact sports.

▶ This article is a comprehensive review of the current literature dealing with cervical spine injuries in football. I certainly agree that "severe cervical injuries share a common mechanism of application of an axial load to the straightened spine." Also, avoiding techniques that use head-down "spear" tackling . . . markedly reduces the risk of serious injury.

J. S. Torg, MD

Spinal Cord Injuries in Ice Hockey in Finland and Sweden From 1980 to 1996

Mölsä JJ, Tegner Y, Alaranta H, et al (LIKES Research Ctr for Sports and Health Sciences, Jyväskylä, Finland; Ermine Clinic, Luleå, Sweden; Käpylä Rehabilitation Centre, Helsinki; et al)

Int J Sports Med 20:64-67, 1999   1–29

Objective.—Sports-related spinal cord injuries (SCIs) in hockey are caused by collisions with the boards or other players. The frequency and mechanisms of SCIs in ice hockey were retrospectively investigated.

Methods.—A medical records review found 8 ice hockey SCIs in Sweden and 8 in Finland between 1980 and 1996. Injured players were interviewed to gather additional details.

Results.—Injured players were aged 14 to 33 years, and all were male. All but 1 injury occurred during supervised games, and all players were wearing helmets. Body checking from behind followed by a blow to the head on the boards was the cause of 50% of SCIs. Vertebral fractures or luxation occurred between C5 and C7 in 11 players, in C3 in 1, C4 in 1, T5 in 1, T7 in 1, and there was 1 herniated disk between C3 and C4. Ten patients were operated on. Ten had tetraplegia/paresis and 6 had paraplegia/paresis.

Conclusion.—Most SCI injuries in ice hockey result from body checking followed by head contact with the boards (Fig 1). The results were cata-

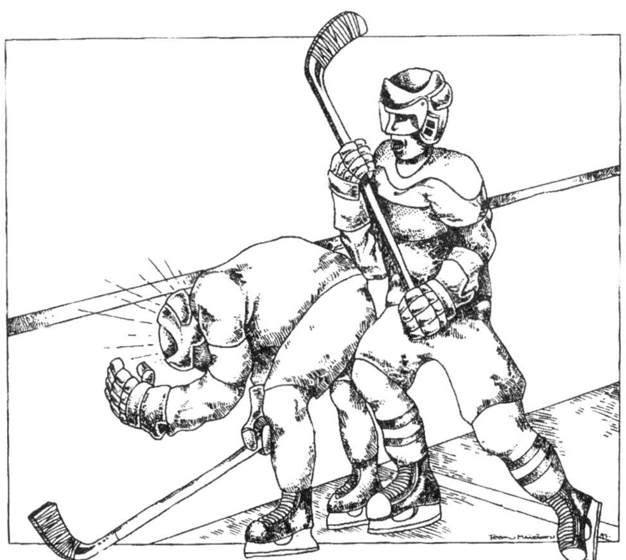

FIGURE 1.—Body checking from behind is usually the precipitating event in the mechanism of spinal cord injury in ice hockey. (Courtesy of Mölsä JJ, Tegner Y, Alaranta H, et al: Spinal cord injuries in ice hockey in Finland and Sweden from 1980 to 1996. *Int J Sports Med* 20:64-67, 1999. Copyright 1999, Georg Thieme Verlag.)

strophic in all cases. Strict refereeing accompanied by rule changes may prevent many of these serious injuries.

▶ Contrary to the practice of some investigators who mix oranges with apples, Mölsä et al limit their report to severe spinal cord injuries, excluding those involving transient neurologic deficits. They also clearly understand the mechanism of cervical spine and cord injury, and their position that "these serious injuries may be prevented by changing rules with strict refereeing and education of trainers and players" is well founded. However, it is my impression that attempts to prevent spinal cord injuries in ice hockey by such measures have not followed the course demonstrated by rule changes in American football.

J. S. Torg, MD

Disabling Injuries of the Cervical Spine in Argentine Rugby Over the Last 20 Years
Secin FP, Poggi EJT, Luzuriaga F, et al (Clínicas Norberto Quirno, Buenos Aires, Argentina; Medical Committee of the Argentine Rugby Union; Norwalk Hosp, Conn)
Br J Sports Med 33:33-36, 1999   1–30

Background.—Cervical spine injuries occur in rugby more commonly than in other sports, perhaps because of the extensive use of the head in this sport. The number of Argentinian players with this injury, the circumstances under which the injuries occurred (including age, field position, and phase of play), and possible rule changes were studied.

Methods.—The researchers obtained data by reviewing cases reported to the Argentine Rugby Union and the Rugby Amistad Foundation and described the circumstances for all rugby players who had had a disabling cervical spine injury, whether permanent or transient.

Results.—The age range of the injured players (with a total of 18 injuries) in this study was 15 to 27 years, and fractures or dislocations between the fourth and sixth cervical vertebrae were seen most often. The incidence among forwards (14 cases) exceeded that among backs (4 cases); hookers had the highest risk of injury. The plays that were most likely to produce injury were scrummaging (11 cases) and tackling (5 cases). All but one of the injuries occurred during match play, and neurological damage resulted from all of the injuries. One patient died and 2 recovered completely. The rest of the players had some degree of impairment. Rule changes during the period when these injuries occurred appeared to have no effect on reducing the risk of cervical spine injuries in Argentina.

Conclusions.—The forwards are particularly susceptible to cervical spine injuries, and the risk hookers have is higher than for any other players. Scrummaging is the most common time when injury occurs. Currently, no rule changes have protected rugby players from these injuries.

▶ This article verifies that rugby injuries to the cervical spine that result in paralysis are not limited to the English-speaking nations. Unfortunately, the data are not presented in terms of injury rates. Also, it appears that the authors do not understand the axial load mechanism. This obviously presents a problem in the implementation of prophylactic measures.

J. S. Torg, MD

A Prospective, Randomized Study Comparing the Results of Open Discectomy With Those of Video-assisted Arthroscopic Microdiscectomy

Hermantin FU, Peters T, Quartararo L, et al (Med College of Pennsylvania and Hahnemann Univ Hosps, Philadelphia)
J Bone Joint Surg Am 81:958-965, 1999   1–31

Objective.—Video-assisted arthroscopic microdiskectomy was compared with conventional open laminotomy and diskectomy for treatment of a herniated lumbar disk in a prospective, randomized study.

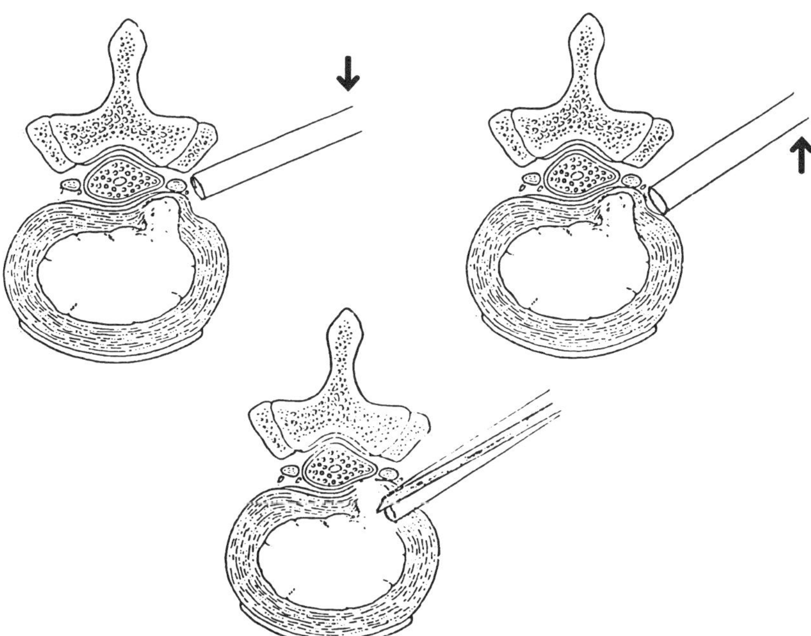

FIGURE 2.—Schematic drawings showing the operative technique. *Top left*: The external end of the cannula is tilted anteriorly, thus rotating the tip posteriorly for inspection and localization of the contents of the spinal canal. *Top right*: The external end of the cannula then is tilted posteriorly, thus rotating the tip anteriorly, and the cannula is held firmly against the annulus in preparation for an annulotomy adjacent to the spinal canal. *Bottom*: A 30- or 70-degree arthroscope is used for final inspection of the operative site, the anterior surface of the dural sac, and the fibers of the posterior longitudinal ligament in a contained subligamentous herniation. (Courtesy of Hermantin FU, Peters T, Quartararo L, et al: A prospective, randomized study comparing the results of open discectomy with those of video-assisted arthroscopic microdiscectomy. *J Bone Joint Surg Am* 81:958-965, 1999.)

Methods.—Sixty patients, aged 15 to 67 years, with a single intracanalicular disk herniation were randomly allocated to treatment with laminotomy and diskectomy (group 1) (n = 30, 13 females) or arthroscopic microdiskectomy (group 2) (n = 30, 8 females) (Fig 2). No patient had central or lateral stenosis or previous back surgery. Conservative treatment had failed in all patients. Patients were followed up at 2 weeks, 3 months, 6 months, 1 year, and 2 years.

Results.—The average postoperative disability period was 49 days for group 1 and 27 days for group 2. One patient in group 1 had spinal fluid leakage necessitating reoperation, and the procedure failed in 1 group 1 patient. One group 2 patient required a 2-level laminotomy and partial facetectomy. There were no postoperative infections or neurovascular injuries. Six group 1 patients and 7 group 2 patients had reflex abnormalities, 18 and 16 patients had sensory deficits, and 10 and 5 had motor weakness. The outcome was satisfactory in 28 (93%) group 1 patients and in 29 (97%) group 2 patients. Patient evaluation questionnaires revealed that 20 (67%) group 1 patients and 22 (73%) group 2 patients were very satisfied. When patients rated their pain scores on a scale from 0 to 10, the mean pain score was 1.9 for group 1 and 1.2 for group 2.

Conclusion.—Video-assisted arthroscopic microdiskectomy is a satisfactory alternative for operative treatment of lumbar disk herniation in selected patients. The technique is technically demanding and should be attempted only after specific instruction and training.

▶ Having been professionally associated with the authors, I can attest to both their credibility and the authenticity of their work. To be emphasized is their caution that arthroscopic microdiskectomy is a demanding technique and should not be attempted without specific instruction and training.

J. S. Torg, MD

Age-related Changes in the Cervical Spines of Front-line Rugby Players
Berge J, Marque B, Vital J-M, et al (Hôpital Pellegrin, Bordeaux, France)
Am J Sports Med 27:422-429, 1999   1–32

Objective.—Cervical spine injuries are relatively common in rugby players. Changes in the cervical spines of high-level rugby players at different points in their careers were analyzed to determine the cumulative effects of repeated microtrauma.

Methods.—Cervical spine MRIs were performed on 47 forwards and hookers (21 senior, 14 veteran or retired, 7 cadet, and 5 junior players) free of cervical spine symptoms and on 40 age-matched controls. Results were compared between groups using the Mann-Whitney U test.

Results.—Fourteen (66%) senior players showed advanced osteosclerosis, and a large number of young players showed complete disappearance of their hemopoietic bone marrow. Only 1 (3%) control subject showed a similar disappearance. Degeneration of the vertebral endplate was found in 27 (77%) of 35 rugby players older than 21 and in 4 (13%) control subjects in the same age group, and cortical hypertrophy of the posterior processes in 26 (74%) senior and veteran players and in 5 (17%) controls. One (20%) junior rugby player had anterior corporeal osteophytes. Posterior and anterior osteophytes were seen in 29 (83%) senior and veteran players and 10 (33%) age-matched controls. Disk degeneration was found in 109 (56%) of 193 disks in rugby players and in 27 (15%) of 180 disks in controls. Compared with controls, older rugby players had significantly decreased constitutional sagittal diameters of the cervical canal. Young rugby layers had larger vertebral bodies than age-matched controls. Height of vertebral bodies and width of cervical canal decreased with age in rugby players but remained stable in controls. Cervical canal width (Torg index) was decreased in older rugby players compared with younger players. Compared with younger players and controls, the cord/canal ratio was increased in older players, indicating potential repercussion of the narrowed canal on the cervical cord. For detection of a narrowed cervical canal, the Torg index has a sensitivity, specificity, and positive and negative predictive values of 100%, 86%, 69%, and 100%, respectively.

Conclusion.—Chronic cervical spine injuries in rugby players decrease the width of the cervical canal.

▶ This interesting article compares the dimensions of various components of the cervical spine—the sagittal diameter of the vertebral body, the vertebral cervical canal, and spinal cord. Basically, the authors demonstrate that the effect of chronic degenerative changes is to decrease the caliber of the cervical canal. However, there is no correlation of the data with such clinical findings as pain, decreased spinal motion, occurrence of cord neurapraxia, or permanent neurologic sequelae. It is gratifying to observe that the authors conclude that "the Torg index is, therefore, an excellent screening test for detecting a narrow cervical canal."

J. S. Torg, MD

2 Injuries of Shoulder Girdle and Upper Limbs

Injuries of the Pectoralis Major Muscle: Evaluation With MR Imaging
Connell DA, Potter HG, Sherman MF, et al (Hosp for Special Surgery, New York)
Radiology 210:785-791, 1999   2–1

Background.—As participation in sports becomes more common, rupture of the pectoralis major muscle will become more prevalent (Fig 1).

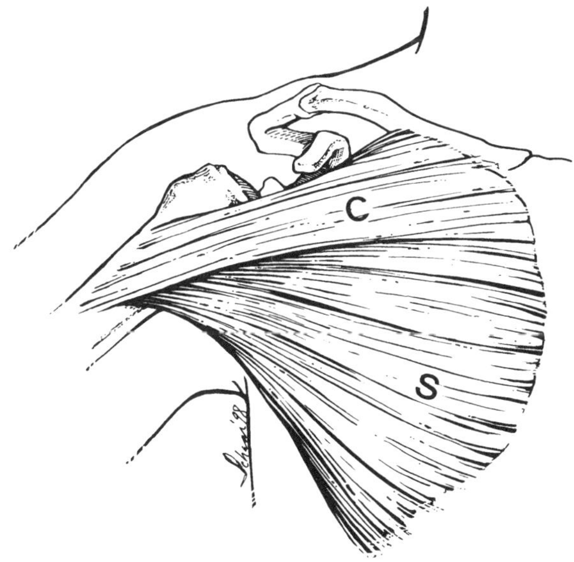

FIGURE 1.—Normal anatomy of the pectoralis major muscle. Frontal diagram of the chest wall shows the distinct orientation of the clavicular head (C) a the superior margin of the chest, as well as the sternal head (S) more inferiorly. The insertional fibers from the sternal head pass deep to those arising from the clavicular head. (Courtesy of Connell DA, Potter HG, Sherman MF, et al: Injuries of the pectoralis major muscle: Evaluation with MR imaging. *Radiology* 210:785-791, 1999. Radiological Society of North America.)

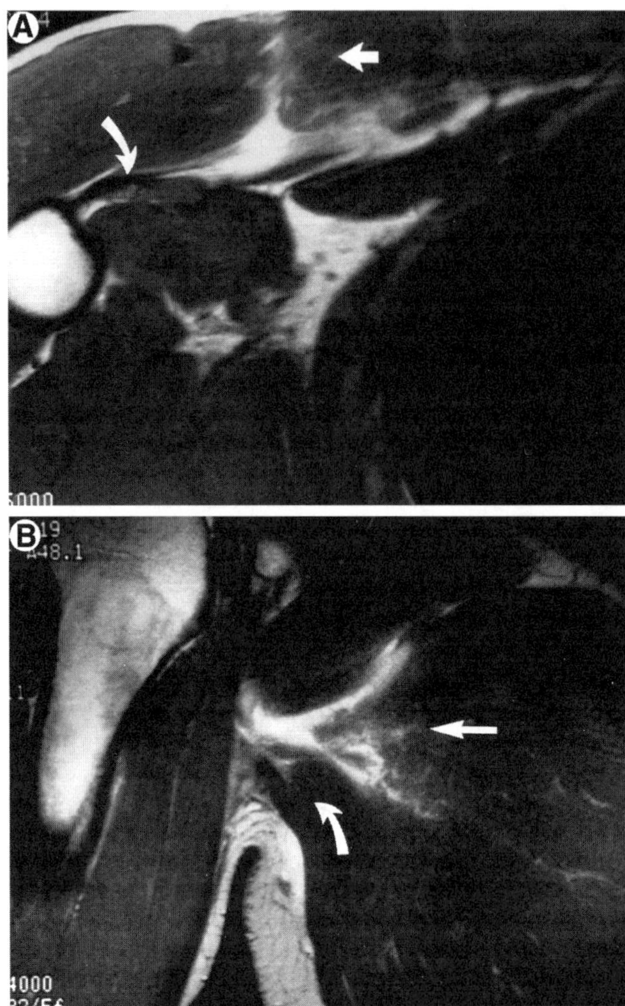

FIGURE 3.—Musculotendinous junction injury in a 27-year-old professional quarterback who was tackled while attempting to throw. A, Axial fast spin-echo MRI (4000/45) of the right pectoralis major muscle show a tear at the musculotendinous junction (*straight arrow*). Note the intact tendon insertion (*curved arrow*). B, Oblique coronal fast spin-echo MRI (4000/45) shows a high-grade tear of the clavicular head (*straight arrow*) with relative preservation of the sternal head (*curved arrow*).

(*Continued*)

The use of MRI in the assessment of injuries to the pectoralis major muscle was described.

Methods.—Fifteen men with injuries to the pectoralis major muscle underwent MRI. Nine were injured while weight lifting, specifically benchpressing. Abnormal morphology, signal intensity, injury site, degree of tearing, and amount of tendon retraction were recorded.

FIGURE 3 (cont.)

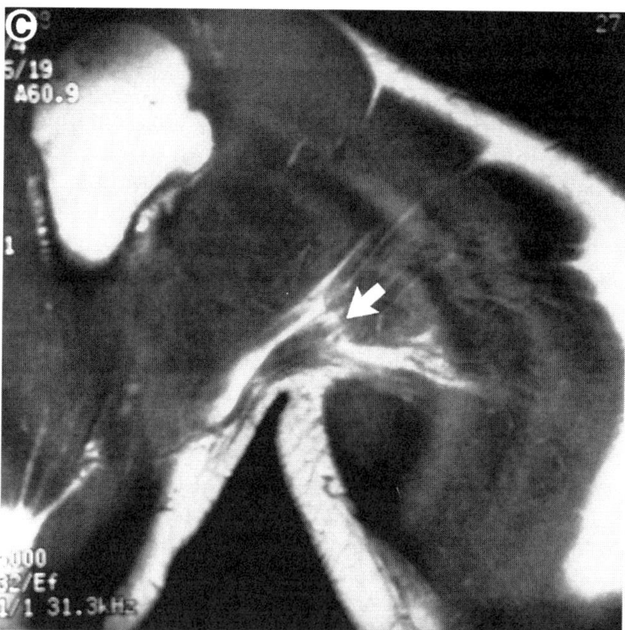

C, Far anterior oblique coronal fast spin-echo MRI (4000/45) shows some intact muscle fibers arising from the clavicular head (*arrow*). This finding confirms that the injury is a high-grade partial tear, not a complete tear. (Courtesy of Connell DA, Potter HG, Sherman MF, et al: Injuries of the pectoralis major muscle: Evaluation with MR imaging. *Radiology* 210:785-791, 1999. Radiological Society of North America.)

Findings.—Six injuries were found at the musculotendinous junction (Fig 3). Five patients were treated conservatively. Eight of 9 patients with distal tendon avulsion underwent primary surgical repair. Tearing was complete in 3 patients and partial in 12. In 10 patients, both the sternal and clavicular heads were torn. Two had only clavicular head tearing, and 3 had only sternal head tearing. Acute tears, occurring in 10 patients, showed hemorrhage and edema, whereas chronic tears, occurring in 5, showed fibrosis and scarring. The amount of tendon retraction was variable.

Conclusions.—MRI is an accurate modality for assessment of injuries of the pectoralis major muscle. This examination enables the clinician to identify patients who would benefit from surgical repair.

▶ The observations and conclusions of this study are in keeping with my own clinical experience.

J. S. Torg, MD

Rupture of the Pectoralis Major Muscle: Outcome After Repair of Acute and Chronic Injuries

Schepsis AA, Grafe MW, Jones HP, et al (Boston Med Ctr)
Am J Sports Med 28:9-15, 2000   2–2

Objective.—There has been a significant increase in ruptures of the pectoralis major muscle in the past 2 decades. All pectoralis major muscle ruptures repaired by 1 surgeon were retrospectively reviewed for operative versus nonoperative repair and outcomes after operative repair of chronic and acute injuries.

Methods.—Between 1983 and 1996, 17 patients (all male), aged 19 to 37 years, were treated for complete or nearly complete distal pectoralis major muscle rupture. All were injured in athletic events, and 10 were injured as a result of weight lifting. Eight patients had acute injuries. Patient follow-up ranged from 18 months to 6 years; patients were evaluated by subjective questionnaire, examination, and strength testing.

Technique.—An anterior axillary approach was used. The deltoid muscle was retracted laterally, and a 5-cm trough was cut into the humerus at the insertion of the pectoralis major muscle. The muscle was repaired (Fig 2). Drill holes were made for passage and typing of sutures (Figs 3 and 4).

Results.—Subjective results showed that strength had returned to 85% to 100% of preinjury levels in the group with acute injuries, to 80% to 100% in the chronic injury group, and to 55% to 85% in the nonoperated group. Subjective pain relief ranged from 85% to 100% in the acute group, 75% to 100% in the chronic group, and 50% to 80% in the nonoperated group. Subjective cosmesis assessments ranged from 75% to 95% in the acute injury group, 70% to 95% in the chronic injury group,

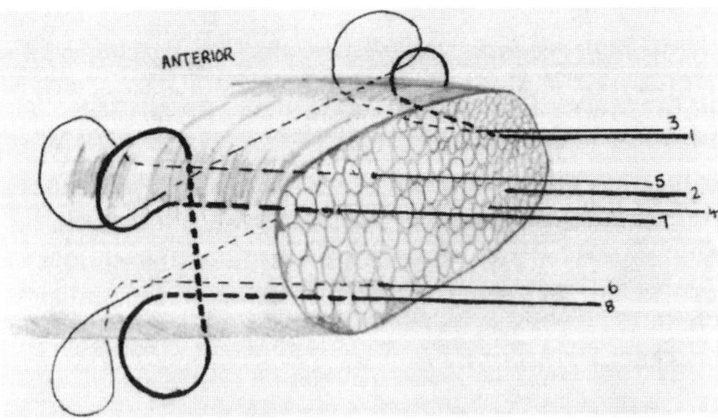

FIGURE 2.—Configuration of the two sets of horizontal and vertical modified Kessler sutures used to capture the whole muscle and its surrounding fascia. (Courtesy of Schepsis AA, Grafe MW, Jones HP, et al: Rupture of the pectoralis major muscle: Outcome after repair of acute and chronic injuries. *Am J Sports Med* 28:9-15, 2000.)

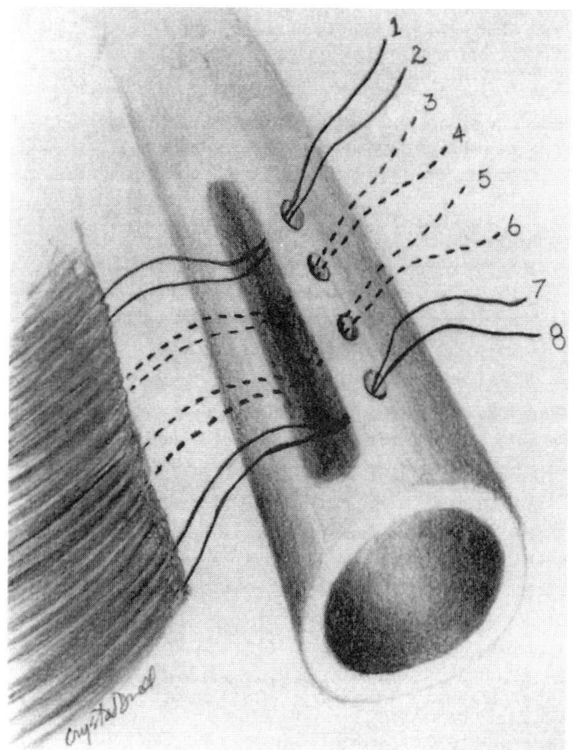

FIGURE 3.—The sequence of suture passage through the 4 drill holes. (Courtesy of Schepsis AA, Grafe MW, Jones HP, et al: Rupture of the pectoralis major muscle: Outcome after repair of acute and chronic injuries. *Am J Sports Med* 28:9-15, 2000.)

and 40% to 70% in the nonoperated group. Overall satisfaction with outcome was rated as 90% to 100% in the acute injury group, 85% to 100% in the chronic injury group, and 40% to 70% in the nonoperated group. Objective results showed that all operated patients had 5/5 strength on adduction and internal rotation. Three of 4 nonoperated patients scored 4/5 on horizontal adduction, 1 scored 5/5 for horizontal adduction, 2 scored 4/5, and 2 scored 5/5 for internal rotation. One patient in the chronic injury group had some muscle deformity. All nonoperated patients had obvious deformities. Peak torque levels were between 74% and 110% for acute and chronic injury patients and between 63% and 75% for nonoperated patients. Work per repetition ranged from 82% to 108% for the acute injury and chronic injury groups but dropped to 58% to 82% for the nonoperated group. Respective fatigue levels were 86% to 121% and 52% to 78%.

Conclusion.—Both the acute and chronic injury groups scored significantly higher in all parameters than the nonoperated groups. There were no differences between the acute and chronic injury groups with respect to torque, work per repetition, and fatigue index.

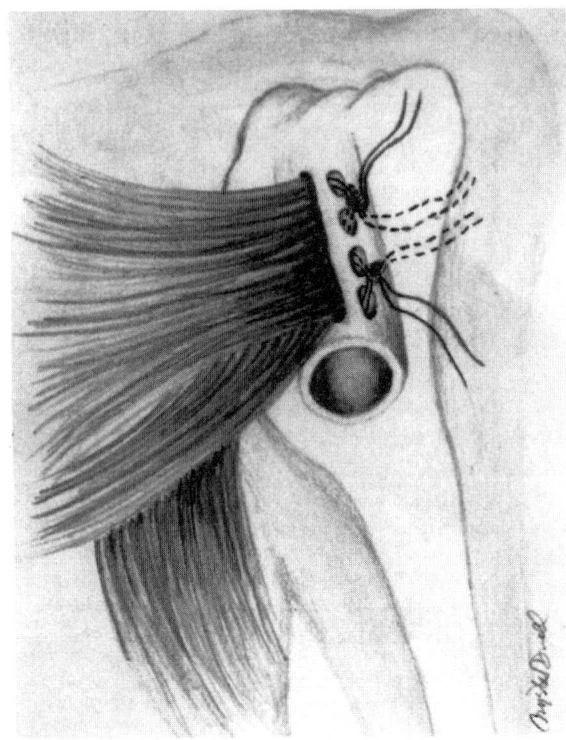

FIGURE 4.—The final repair. (Courtesy of Schepsis AA, Grafe MW, Jones HP, et al: Rupture of the pectoralis major muscle: Outcome after repair of acute and chronic injuries. *Am J Sports Med* 28:9-15, 2000.)

▶ An interesting and well-documented study. However, several questions remain unanswered. How should partial ruptures of the muscle be handled? Is there an explanation for the gender specificity of the injury? What is the relation of anabolic steroid use to the apparent increased incidence?

J. S. Torg, MD

Multiplanar Analysis of Acromion Morphology

MacGillivray JD, Fealy S, Potter HG, et al (Cornell Univ Med Ctr, New York)
Am J Sports Med 26:836-840, 1998
2–3

Background.—The analysis of acromion morphology in several planes should reveal how it relates to impingement syndrome. In addition, the presence of acromioclavicular joint osteophytes inferiorly may play a role in impingement syndrome.

Methods.—Forty women and 92 men (a total of 132 shoulders) underwent MRI or CT). Twenty-five asymptomatic shoulders were also studied. Each decade of life from the second to the eighth was represented in the patient sample. Images were evaluated for the anterior slope of the acro-

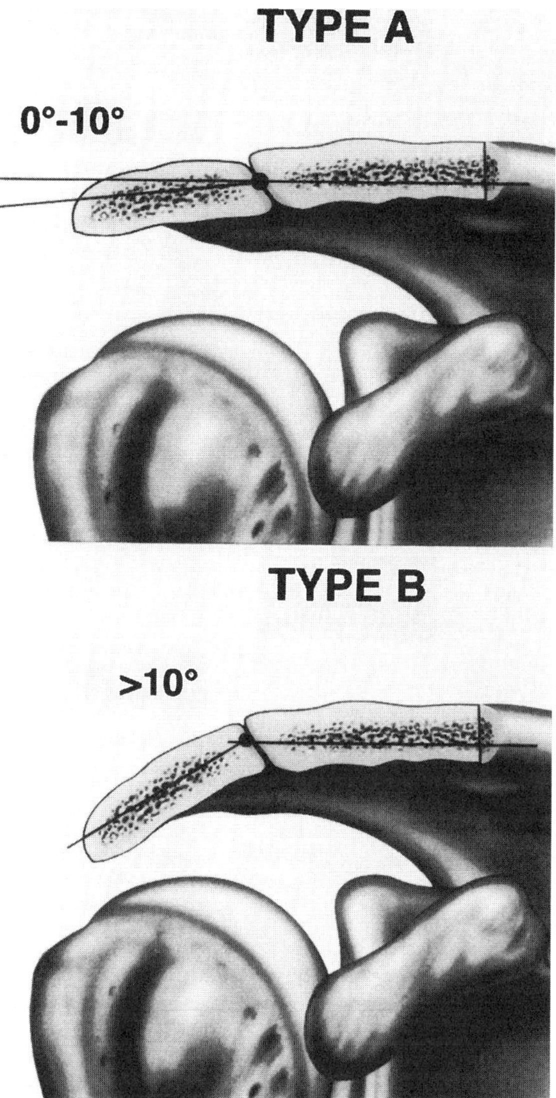

FIGURE 2.—Method of determining lateral acromion angulation in the coronal plane. (Courtesy of MacGillivray JD, Fealy S, Potter HG, et al: Multiplanar analysis of acromion morphology. *Am J Sports Med* 26:836-840, 1998.)

mion in the midsagittal and lateral-sagittal planes, lateral acromial angulation in the coronal plane, and the presence or absence of medial encroachment. The Neer classification was used to assign stages of impingement.

Results.—Imaging results showed no significant differences, so the results were combined. The mean acromion angle was 19.4 degrees midsagittally and 20 degrees in the lateral-sagittal plane. Ninety-seven neutral coronal acromions were noted, and 35 coronal acromions had downward slopes (most often in the shoulders of older patients). Encroachment was noted in 31 shoulders. Younger patients had flat acromions, whereas older patients had progressively more hooked acromions in the midsagittal and lateral-sagittal planes. Coronal lateral acromion angulation was defined as either type A or type B (Fig 2). Impingement was noted to be stage II or III in 98 patients; of those 98 patients, 39 had type I acromions, 51 had type II acromions, and 8 had type III acromions. Impingement was seen in 28 of the 33 acromions with coronal lateral downward slope and in all of those with medial encroachment.

Conclusions.—During a period of years (the second through eighth decades) a gradual transition from a flat to a hooked acromion seems to occur. A downward angled acromion also seems to develop with increasing age. These changes can be seen with MRI, and acromion findings can be classified in a way that correlates with clinical findings.

▶ The purpose of this study was "to more completely describe acromion morphology in several planes and to document the relationship of acromion morphology to impingement syndrome." The authors have accomplished that. Of note, there was no attempt to correlate the MRI or CT reconstructions with routine radiography. Thus whether lateral acromion angulation and acromioclavicular joint osteophytes can be visualized on routine roentgenograms should be questioned. Certainly, this would be the more cost-effective approach for those patients with signs and symptoms of impingement with clinically intact rotator cuffs.

J. S. Torg, MD

The Value of Weighted Views of the Acromioclavicular Joint: Results of a Survey
Yap JJL, Curl LA, Kvitne RS, et al (Johns Hopkins Hosp, Baltimore, Md; Univ of Maryland, Baltimore; Kerlan-Jobe Clinic, Santa Monica, Calif)
Am J Sports Med 27:806-809, 1999   2–4

Background.—A great deal of controversy continues to surround the acute treatment of grade III acromioclavicular (AC) injuries. Most recent studies have reported good to excellent results with nonoperative treatments for grade I, II, or III injuries, but other studies have reported poor long-term results with nonoperative treatment of chronic grade III AC separations. Weighted AC views have been used to diagnose occult grade III injuries and continue to be recommended in many standard orthopedic textbooks. In this study, a select group of shoulder surgeons was surveyed regarding the necessity and usefulness of weighted AC views in their practices and in the emergency department.

Methods.—Questionnaires were sent to 112 practicing members of the American Shoulder and Elbow Surgeons in the United States and Canada, who were asked about their preferences for surgical treatment of grades II and III AC separations in the dominant and nondominant arms of laborers and nonlaborers, throwers and nonthrowers. The questionnaires also asked about the number of times in the past year and in the past 5 years the surgeons had changed their treatment of AC separations on the basis of weighted views.

Results.—Completion and return rate for the surveys was 94%, with 105 of 112 questionnaires returned. The average years of practice of the respondents was 18, and the average number of AC separations seen yearly was 29, with a range of 7 to 90. Average percentage of each type of AC separations seen in 1 year were grade I, 29%; grade II, 26.4%; grade III, 34%; grade IV, 3.8%; grade V, 6.2%; and grade VI, 0.28%. Most respondents said that weighted views were unnecessary and of no value in deciding treatment options. Weighted views were used by 45 of the 105 respondents (43%). Eighty-five of the respondents (81%) indicated that they would not recommend weighted views for an acutely injured patient in the emergency department. Only 9 of the respondents had, in the past year, changed their nonoperative treatment of a grade II AC separation when stress radiographs indicated a grade III separation. These 9 surgeons estimated that in a 5-year period they had changed their treatment on the basis of weighted views in 86 patients. Respondents said overwhelmingly that they would not change their initial treatment choice if weighted views showed a grade III AC separation when the shoulder was initially thought to have a grade II separation or less. Regarding certain patients, 99 of 105 surgeons (94%) said that they would not change their initial choice of nonsurgical treatment of grade III AC separations, no matter what the arm dominance in a nonathletic, nonlaboring patient.

Conclusions.—Appropriate treatment of grade III AC separations remains controversial. Surgeons who had been in practice longer were more inclined toward operative intervention and thus recommended the use of weighted views more often than surgeons with fewer years of practice. However, only 9% of the surgeons in this survey consistently use weighted views when selecting surgical treatment. It was also discovered that weighted views for AC sprains are also not widely used by the surgeons surveyed. Disadvantages of this study were that it was subjective and required respondents to rely on recall without the benefit of chart review. However, the opinion of the surgeons in this survey is that weighted views of the AC joint are of limited clinical value. They should probably not be used in the emergency department for purely diagnostic purposes because of the radiation exposure, increased pain to the patient, and additional cost. Weighted views should not be done routinely but should be left to the discretion of the treating surgeon.

▶ I would agree with the opinion that "weighted views of the AC joint have limited clinical value in evaluation of AC separations." However, it should be kept in mind that the views expressed were those of the most experienced shoulder and elbow surgeons and not that of the orthopedic generalist, who may find them valuable in his decision-making process. What's good for the goose may not necessarily be good for the gander. Although the authors state that they found "provocative results," they recognize that the study is limited by the very nature of a retrospective survey. Also, the article does not deal with criteria to be used in determining when surgery is indicated.

J. S. Torg, MD

Treatment of Complete Acromioclavicular Dislocation: Present Indications and Surgical Technique With Biodegradable Cords

Mönig SP, Burger C, Helling HJ, et al (Cologne Univ, Germany)
Int J Sports Med 20:560-562, 1999   2–5

Objective.—Of the 3 types of acromioclavicular (AC) dislocations, Tossy I and II can be treated conservatively. Whether surgical treatment of Tossy III complete dislocations is appropriate is controversial. Long-term results of surgical treatment with polydioxanone augmentation of Tossy III injuries were retrospectively reviewed.

Methods.—Between 1989 and 1997, 54 patients underwent surgery with PDS-augmentation, and 48 (10 female), aged 20 to 63 years, were followed up for an average of 39.5 months. Injuries resulted from contact sports in 51% of patients, traffic accidents in 31%, and other means in 18%. All patients had a 1.5-mm PDS augmentation with the AC joint fixed temporarily by a Kirschner wire. Reconstructed ligaments were augmented

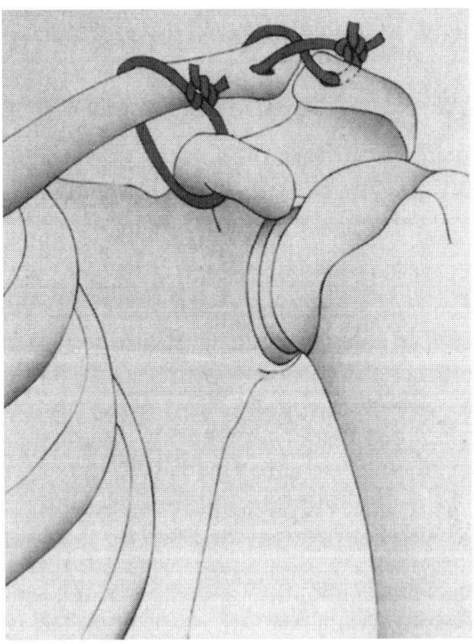

FIGURE 1.—PDS augmentation technique. (Courtesy of Mönig SP, Burger C, Helling HJ, et al: Treatment of complete acromioclavicular dislocation: Present indications and surgical technique with biodegradable cords. *Int J Sports Med* 20:560-562, 1999. Georg Thieme Verlag.)

by two 1.5-mm PDS cords (Fig 1). Early movement was begun on postoperative day 1, and full range of motion was permitted at week 6. Patients were allowed to return to sports activities at 3 months. Patients were rated on the Taft scale.

Results.—There were no perioperative complications. There were 2 wound healing complications that resolved uneventfully. On the Taft scale, 69% of patients scored 10 to 12 points. 23% scored 7 to 9 points, and 6% scored less than 7 points. Patients rated their outcomes as excellent (54%), good (33%), or fair (13%). Radiologically, 25% of patients had subluxation of the clavicula, and 17% had arthrosis.

Conclusion.—PDS-augmentation for Tossy III shoulder dislocations is safe and produces good to excellent long-term results.

▶ It is pointed out that there is a lack of consensus both with regard to indication for surgery in complete AC dislocations as well as the preferred surgical technique. In my view, it is the rare AC joint dislocation that requires surgical reduction and stabilization. However, the use of biodegradable cords to maintain reduction is most intriguing in view of the problems associated with pins, wires, and screws. The latter devices can migrate, cut through the clavicle, and require removal. It appears that these problems would be obviated by the technique described by Mönig et al.

J. S. Torg, MD

MR Observations of Posttraumatic Osteolysis of the Distal Clavicle After Traumatic Separation of the Acromioclavicular Joint
Yu JS, Dardani M, Fischer RA (Ohio State Univ, Columbus)
J Comput Assist Tomogr 24:159-164, 2000   2–6

Background.—Acromioclavicular (AC) joint injuries are common, and the prevalence of posttraumatic disorders in this articulation is increasing. The MRI features of posttraumatic osteolysis of the distal clavicle in patients with previous separation of the ipsilateral AC joint were reported.

Methods.—Eight men (mean age, 25 years) with intractable pain in the AC joint after traumatic joint separation underwent MRI. The Rockwood classification system was used, and the separations were categorized as type 1 in 1 patient, type 2 in 2, and type 3 in 5. Osteolysis of the distal clavicle was verified pathologically in 7 patients and during surgery in 1.

Findings.—The incidence of osteolysis was about 6%. Findings on MRI were soft-tissue swelling, bone marrow edema in the distal clavicle, and cortical irregularity associated with periarticular cystlike erosions in 8 patients, joint space widening in 6, clavicular periostitis in 3, and marrow edema in the cromion in 5. Osteophyte formation was present in 1 patient. Prospective radiographic diagnosis was possible in only 4 patients. Radiographic findings were periarticular soft-tissue swelling, osteopenia of the distal clavicle, articular erosions, and joint space widening.

Conclusions.—MRI findings are characteristic of posttraumatic osteolysis. Patients with chronic AC joint pain who have had a previous AC joint dislocation should undergo MRI, especially if follow-up radiographs are non-specific, equivocal, or show no secondary osteoarthritis.

▶ Although I am not certain that changes associated with osteolysis of the distal clavicle cannot be adequately demonstrated on routine roentgenograms, the subtle MRI changes are certainly interesting. Unfortunately, there is no correlation between these changes and response to management. Also, it should be pointed out that posttraumatic osteolysis of the clavicle is usually not associated with a previous AC joint separation but, rather, is associated with the rigors of weight lifting and similar mechanical stresses on the joint.

J. S. Torg, MD

Noncontrast Magnetic Resonance Imaging of Superior Labral Lesions: 102 Cases Confirmed at Arthroscopic Surgery
Connell DA, Potter HG, Wickiewicz TL, et al (Hosp for Special Surgery, New York)
Am J Sports Med 27:208-213, 1999   2–7

Background.—Superior labrum anterior and posterior (SLAP) lesions reportedly result from an injury to the superior labrum that begins posteriorly and extends anteriorly, stopping before or at the midglenoid notch and including the anchor of the biceps tendon to the labrum. The Snyder classification system includes 4 types, although other classification systems have been proposed to accommodate the SLAP lesions that do not fit into Snyder's system. That noncontrast MRI reliably diagnoses SLAP lesions with the use of sequences routinely obtained for shoulder assessment was shown.

Methods.—One hundred four patients with SLAP lesions who were undergoing MRI and subsequently having arthroscopic surgery were included in the analysis. Lesions were classified according to Snyder's system, and MRI findings were correlated with surgical findings (Figs 1, 2A, 3, 4, and 5).

Findings.—One hundred tears were confirmed surgically. Four findings were false positive, and 2 were false negative. The former occurred in 1 patient with a normal labrum, 2 with meniscoid-type labra, and 1 with a

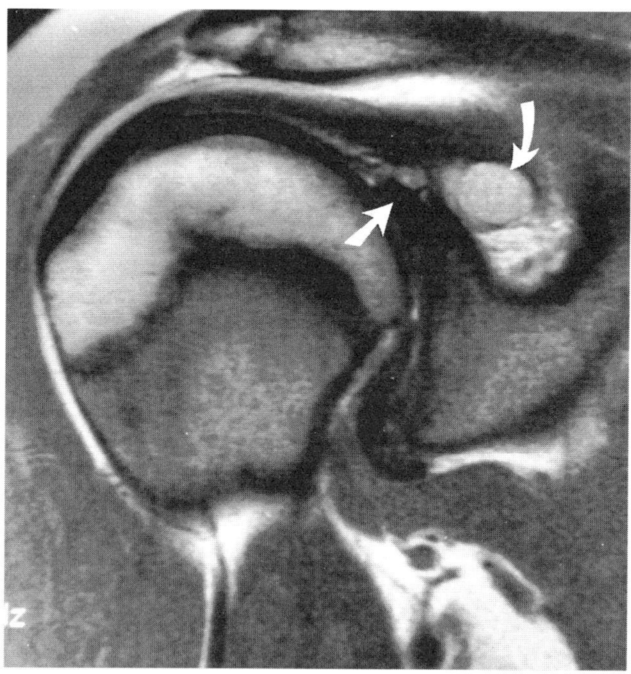

FIGURE 1.—A type I SLAP lesion in an 18-year-old tennis player who had sudden onset of pain and clicking after an audible pop during a match. He had since complained of intermittent recurrent pain, particularly in the overhead position. Coronal images demonstrate a frayed, hyperintense superior labrum (*short arrow*) with decompression into a large paralabral cyst (*curved arrow*). (Courtesy of Connell DA, Potter HG, Wickiewicz TL, et al: Noncontrast magnetic resonance imaging of superior labral lesions: 102 cases confirmed at arthroscopic surgery. *Am J Sports Med* 27:208-213, 1999.)

sublabral foramen. Using arthroscopic surgery as the standard, MRI was 98% sensitive, 89.5% specific, and 95.7% accurate in detecting superior labral lesions.

Conclusions.—Advances in surface coil and software design have improved soft-tissue contrast in high-resolution imaging, which aids in labral visualization. High-resolution noncontrast MRI accurately diagnoses SLAP lesions and aids in surgical management.

▶ An excellent article correlating MRI with arthroscopic findings in patients with superior labral lesions.

J. S. Torg, MD

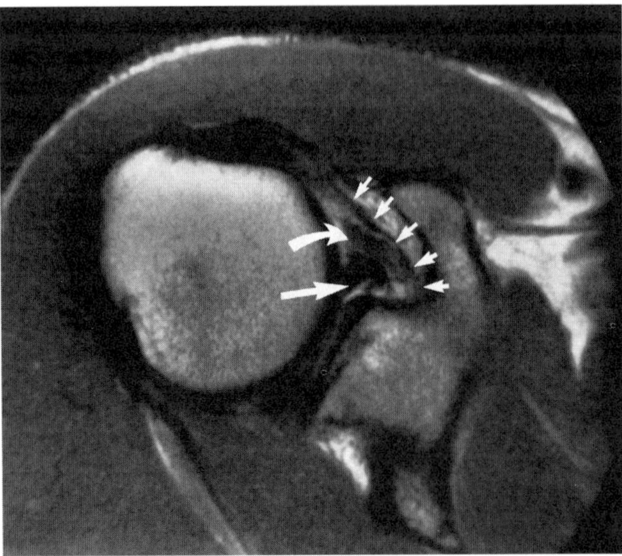

FIGURE 2A.—A type II SLAP lesion in a 33-year-old man who had a long history of right shoulder pain that was exacerbated by a recent skiing injury. The MR images demonstrate a tear of the anterosuperior labrum (*straight arrow*) at the insertion of the middle glenohumeral ligament (*curved arrow*). Note the frayed superior capsule (*small arrows*). (Courtesy of Connell DA, Potter HG, Wickiewicz TL, et al: Noncontrast magnetic resonance imaging of superior labral lesions: 102 cases confirmed at arthroscopic surgery. *Am J Sports Med* 27:208-213, 1999.)

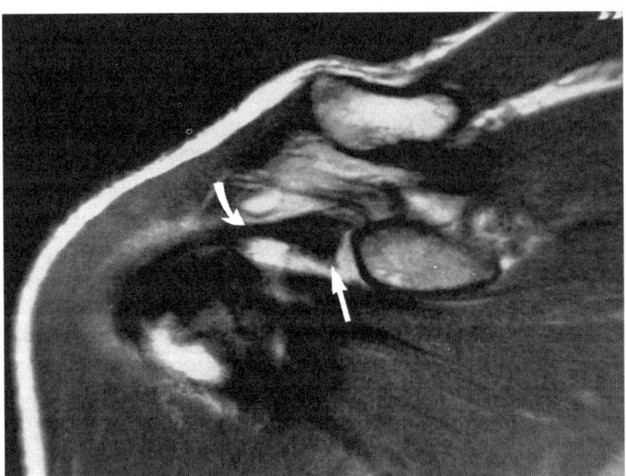

FIGURE 3.—A type II SLAP lesion in a 46-year-old man, a high-level recreational tennis player, who had shoulder pain. The coronal image demonstrates avulsion of the superior labrum from the glenoid (*straight arrow*). Note the retracted biceps tendon (*curved arrow*) attached to the avulsed labrum. (Courtesy of Connell DA, Potter HG, Wickiewicz TL, et al: Noncontrast magnetic resonance imaging of superior labral lesions: 102 cases confirmed at arthroscopic surgery. *Am J Sports Med* 27:208-213, 1999.)

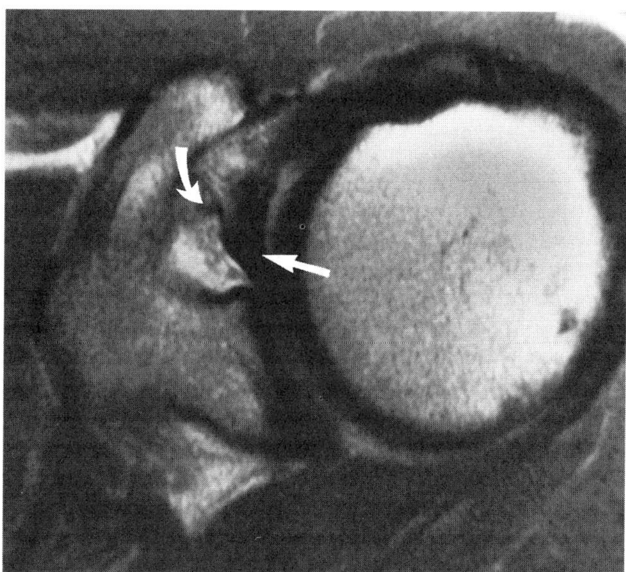

FIGURE 4.—A type III SLAP lesion in a 24-year-old male patient who sustained a fall while skiing. He had since experienced pain during overhead activities. An axial image through the labrum demonstrates a detached labral fragment (*straight arrow*), as well as a frayed superior glenohumeral ligament (*curved arrow*). (Courtesy of Connell DA, Potter HG, Wickiewcz TL, et al: Noncontrast magnetic resonance imaging of superior labral lesions: 102 cases confirmed at arthroscopic surgery. *Am J Sports Med* 27:208-213, 1999.)

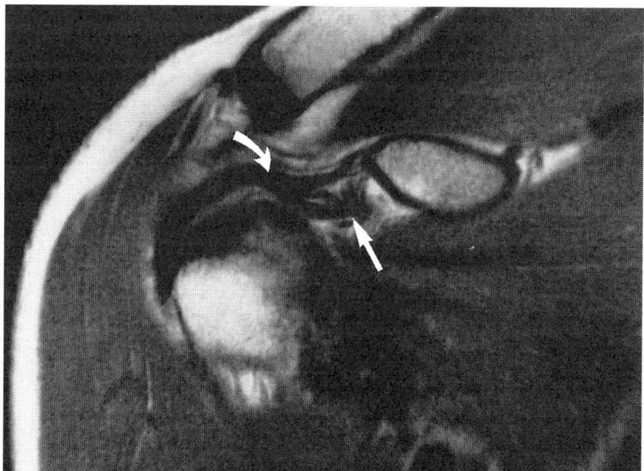

FIGURE 5.—A type IV SLAP lesion in a 20-year-old baseball pitcher who had pain and discomfort related to throwing in the early acceleration phase. Far anterior coronal image demonstrates the displaced superior labral flap (*straight arrow*) with tearing and fraying of the biceps tendon (*curved arrow*). (Courtesy of Connell DA, Potter HG, Wickiewicz TL, et al: Noncontrast magnetic resonance imaging of superior labral lesions: 102 cases confirmed at arthroscopic surgery. *Am J Sports Med* 27:208-213, 1999.)

Arthroscopic Findings in the Overhand Throwing Athlete: Evidence for Posterior Internal Impingement of the Rotator Cuff

Paley KJ, Jobe FW, Pink MM, et al (Centinela Hosp Med Ctr, Inglewood, Calif)
Arthroscopy 16:35-40, 2000

2–8

Introduction.—Surgical decompression of the subacromial space is the procedure of choice for classic refractory impingement symptoms. The exception is the young overhand-throwing athlete for whom the outcome of surgical decompression has been disappointing. The surgical procedure that allows these athletes to return to their former competitive level of activity is anterior capsular labral reconstruction (ACLR). A separate site of impingement has been suggested for overhand-throwing athletes. The biomechanics of the overhand throw make the athlete susceptible to varying degrees of anterior shoulder instability and excessive humeral external rotation that can lead to impingement or compression of the undersurface of the supraspinatus and infraspinatus tendons against the posterosuperior glenoid rim—thus, the term *posterior internal impingement of the rotator cuff.* The outcome of an arthroscopic examination and the pathologic findings in symptomatic shoulders of 41 professional overhand-throwing athletes are described.

Methods.—Forty baseball players and 1 football quarterback with an average age of 25 years (range, 18-36 years) were seen for complaints of shoulder pain during the late cocking, acceleration, or both phases of the throwing motion that limited their throwing ability. All athletes had not responded to an extensive physical therapy program focusing on rotator cuff and scapular stability strengthening of at least 3 months' duration. All participants underwent a diagnostic arthroscopic evaluation before ACLR.

Results.—All arthroscopic examinations revealed either contact between the rotator cuff undersurface and the posterosuperior glenoid rim or osteochondral lesions. Additional important findings were 93% undersurface cuff fraying, 88% posterosuperior labral fraying, and 36% anterior labral fraying.

Conclusion.—These findings confirm that internal impingement of the humeral head and rotator cuff undersurface occur along the posterosuperior glenoid rim in the overhand-throwing athlete. The primary pathologic findings include undersurface rotator cuff fraying and posterosuperior labral fraying.

▶ This is an interesting article, the purpose of which was to "describe the arthroscopic findings of the shoulder. . . and to determine if posterior internal impingement of the rotator cuff" exists in a group of overhand-throwing athletes. Importantly, it is pointed out that conventional surgery for "outlet impingement" is not rewarding. It is inferred that ACLR corrects capsular laxity, inferring that "shoulder instability may play a role in rotator cuff injury [in this group of patients]." However, this is not supported by the data.

J. S. Torg, MD

Symptomatic Thrower's Exostosis: Arthroscopic Evaluation and Treatment
Meister K, Andrews JR, Batts J, et al (Univ of Florida, Gainesville; Alabama Sports Medicine Inst, Birmingham)
Am J Sports Med 27:133-136, 1999
2–9

Objective.—Whether posterior glenoid exostosis is the primary cause of posterior and lateral shoulder pain in throwers is controversial. The significance of thrower's exostosis was reviewed in a large series of throwing athletes, and a technique for the arthroscopic débridement of those lesions is described.

Methods.—Preoperative radiographs of anteroposterior views in internal and external rotation, a West Point axillary view, and a Stryker notch view revealed exostosis in 22 male throwing athletes who had shoulder pain during throwing. Average age at onset of pain was 16 to 44 years, and the average duration of symptoms before surgery was 2.3 years. Eleven patients underwent arthroscopic removal of the posterior glenoid osteophyte, with débridement of the extra bone back to normal contour. Patients underwent physical therapy. The status of 18 patients was followed up for an average of 6.3 years.

Results.—In addition to the presence of an osteophyte, 21 patients had partial-thickness undersurface tears of the rotator cuff; 15 had fraying in the posterior labrum, 4 in the anterior labrum and 1 in the superior labrum. Ten athletes returned to the preinjury level of performance after a year. At latest follow-up, 5 players were still playing and 5 had retired. One retired player had recurrent pain that required repeat arthroscopic débridement of a torn rotator cuff and posterior labrum and excision of a recurring exostosis. Patients with an exostosis greater than 100 mm^2 tended to have a poorer outcome. Three of 7 patients with a successful outcome and 3 of 4 patients with a poor outcome had asymmetric shoulder laxity.

Conclusion.—Shoulder exostosis in throwers should be treated with arthroscopic débridement of the rotator cuff and labral lesions if the shoulder is stable and with arthroscopic excision of the exostosis if the shoulder is painful or tender. Patients with exostosis greater than 100 mm^2 tended to have a poor outcome.

▶ The fact that there was concomitant undersurface tearing of the rotator cuff in 21 of the patients and tear of the posterior labrum in 15 raises the question as to what exactly was responsible for the symptoms. Also, the authors point out that the finding of a posterior glenoid exostosis is a definite marker of internal impingement. Thus, what came first, the chicken or the egg? Did the exostosis cause the impingement or vice versa? The authors have described a plethora of pathologies in the glenohumeral joint of the symptomatic throwing athlete; however, although they are attributed to the exostosis, there is clearly no definite correlation.

J. S. Torg, MD

Entrapment of the Suprascapular Nerve
Fabre Th, Piton C, Leclouerec G, et al (Groupe Hospitalier Pellegrin, Bordeaux, France)
J Bone Joint Surg Br 81-B:414-419, 1999   2–10

Background.—The shoulder pain experienced by a patient with entrapment of the suprascapular nerve can be incorrectly attributed to cervical disk disease, rotator cuff tear, or tendinitis. This often delays treatment until atrophy of the supraspinatus, infraspinatus, or both has occurred. This delay and subsequent muscular atrophy then impede postsurgical functional recovery. Causes of suprascapular nerve entrapment include sports activities—especially those that involve repetitive arm motion—and enlargement of the suprascapular nerve, which may be associated with rotator cuff tear. Cases of suprascapular nerve compression by a ganglion have also been described in the literature. This article reported on a series of 35 patients who underwent surgical release for entrapment of the suprascapular nerve.

Methods.—The patient group consisted of 26 men and 9 women with an average age of 40 years (range, 17-67 years). The cause of entrapment was direct injury in 10 patients. Eighteen patients reported that their work placed significant demands on their shoulders. In 3 patients, no cause for the entrapment could be identified. The average time from onset of symptoms to surgery was 10 months. Patients were evaluated by means of the Constant score both before surgery and at an average of 30 months after surgery. Before surgery, the average Constant score, unadjusted for age or gender, was 47%. Atrophy of the infraspinatus and supraspinatus muscles was evident in 25 patients, and 7 had isolated atrophy of the infraspinatus muscle. The average conduction time from Erb's point to the supraspinatus muscle was 5.7 msec, the average time from Erb's point to the infraspinatus muscle was 7.4 msec. MRI indicated a ganglion in the infraspinatus fossa in 2 patients and complete rupture of the rotator cuff in 1 patient. Surgery was performed using a posterior approach.

Results.—This average Constant score improved to 77% after operative release of the suprascapular nerve. Outcomes were graded as excellent in 10 patients, good in 14 patients, fair in 2 patients, and poor in 2 patients. After surgery, 22 of 34 patients reported no pain at final follow-up. One patient had slight pain, and 8 reported moderate pain; however, all 8 indicated that the pain was significantly less than before surgery. There were similar improvements in the majority of patients in resumption of everyday activities, range of motion, strength, and muscle atrophy.

Conclusion.—The efficacy and safety of operative release for entrapment of the suprascapular nerve is confirmed by the results achieved in this series of patients.

► The indications and timing of operative management of suprascapular nerve entrapment are important. Patients with symptoms but without muscle atrophy should be placed on a nonoperative regimen consisting of rest and physical therapy. Fabre et al advocate operative decompression if symptoms persist 3 to 4 months. In affected patients with evidence of muscle atrophy, surgery is indicated. It should be noted that patients who were operated on within 6 months of the onset of symptoms show better recovery than those who had surgery after a longer interval.

J. S. Torg, MD

Biceps Load Test: A Clinical Test for Superior Labrum Anterior and Posterior Lesions in Shoulders With Recurrent Anterior Dislocations
Kim S-H, Ha K-I, Han K-Y (Sungkyunkwan Univ, Seoul, Korea)
Am J Sports Med 27:300-303, 1999   2–11

Background.—Few physical tests are available for diagnosing isolated superior labral anterior and posterior (SLAP) lesions. A new clinical test for SLAP lesions in shoulders with recurrent anterior dislocations was reported.

Methods.—Seventy-five patients with proven unilateral anterior shoulder dislocations were studied prospectively. In a double-blind fashion, the patients underwent arthroscopic examination and the biceps load test. To

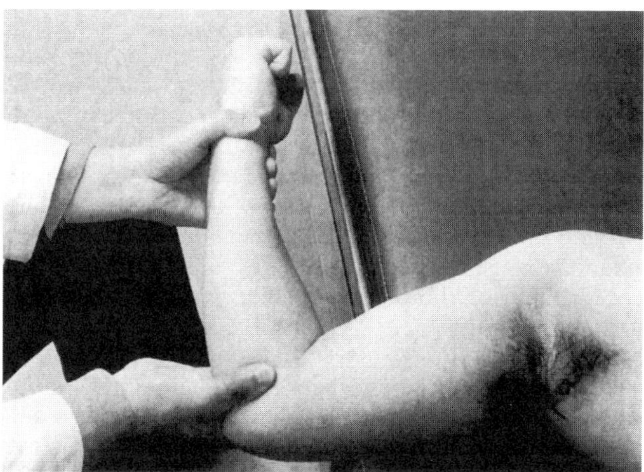

FIGURE 1.—In the biceps load test, the forearm is supinated during the biceps muscle contraction with the shoulder in abduction and external rotation. (Courtesy of Kim S-H, Ha K-I, Han K-Y: Biceps load test: A clinical test for superior labrum anterior and posterior lesions in shoulders with recurrent anterior dislocations. *Am J Sports Med* 27:300-303, 1999.)

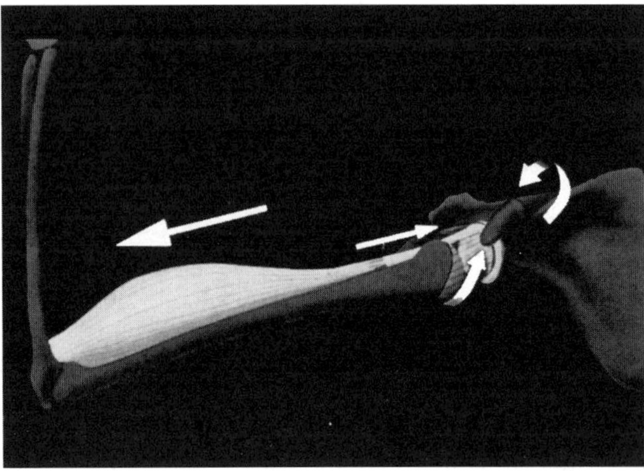

FIGURE 2.—Contraction of the biceps muscle causes tension on the biceps tendon–superior labrum complex and increases glenohumeral stability with the arm in the abducted and externally rotated position. (Courtesy of Kim S-H, Ha K-I, Han K-Y: Biceps load test: A clinical test for superior labrum anterior and posterior lesions in shoulders with recurrent anterior dislocations. *Am J Sports Med* 27:300-303, 1999.)

perform the biceps load test, the examiner sits adjacent to the patient, resisting the active elbow flexion of the patient only in the direction opposite the vector of the biceps tendon force, in line with the arm. Throughout the test, the forearm is maintained in a supinated position. The patient is told not to simply pull the whole upper extremity, but to bend the forearm (Figs 1 and 2).

Findings.—Sixty-three patients had negative test results; 62 of them had an intact biceps tendon–superior labrum complex. The last patient had a type II SLAP lesion. Of the 12 patients with positive test results, 10 had superior labral lesions, and 2 had intact superior labra. The biceps load test had a 90.9% sensitivity, a 96.9% specificity, and positive and negative predictive values of 83% and 98%, respectively. The κ coefficient was 0.846.

Conclusions.—The biceps load test is a reliable tool for diagnosing SLAP lesions in shoulders with recurrent anterior dislocations. To perform this test, the clinician has the patient hold the shoulder in an abducted, externally rotated position with the forearem supinated. Active flexion of the elbow against resistance relieves the discomfort of a standard apprehension test for anterior shoulder instability.

▶ As pointed out by the authors, physical findings and MR examinations are not specific for the SLAP lesion. Certainly, knowledge of a coexisting SLAP lesion when one is planning surgery for anterior instability is a definite plus. It should be pointed out, however, that a determination of the result of the test is subjective in nature; that is, the patient is asked to report "if the apprehension is lessened" or if he or she "feels more comfortable than before the test".

J. S. Torg, MD

Intra- and Interobserver Reproducibility of the Shoulder Laxity Examination
Levy AS, Lintner S, Kenter K, et al (Ctr for Advanced Sports Medicine, Knee and Shoulder, Newark, NJ; Univ of Indiana, Indianapolis; Univ of Missouri, Columbia; et al)
Am J Sports Med 27:460-463, 1999   2–12

Background.—Assessment of the degree of shoulder laxity can be a useful diagnostic tool in the examination of a patient with suspected instability of the shoulder. Several techniques for assessing shoulder laxity have been described, but no data have been presented regarding the intraobserver or interobserver reproducibility of these techniques. The interobserver and intraobserver reproducibility of the clinical examination of shoulder laxity was studied.

Methods.—The study group comprised 43 Division I college athletes at 4 institutions. Both shoulders of each athlete were examined in the anterior, posterior, and inferior directions. For the anterior and posterior examinations, the subjects were supine and the shoulder held in 20 degrees of flexion in the scapular plane, at 90 degrees of abduction, and at neutral rotation. The sulcus test was used to examine the shoulder in the inferior position, with the patient supine. Glenohumeral laxity in each patient was scored from 0 to 3+. The subjects were reexamined in 3 months, with investigators blinded to their own previous grading and the grading of other examiners.

Results.—Intraobserver reproducibility was 46% overall. After grades 0 and 1 were equalized, the overall score for intraobserver reproducibility improved to 74%. However, κ values for intraobserver correlation for both equalized and nonequalized reproducibility values were less than 0.5. This suggests that the correlations observed were only marginally better than may have been obtained by chance. Interobserver reproducibility overall was 47%, and improved to 78% after grades 0 and 1 were equalized. In interobserver reproducibility, κ values greater than 0.5 were only found in equalized posterior and inferior laxity.

Conclusion.—These results indicate that the reproducibility of the laxity examination in an unanesthetized shoulder is not easy to accomplish in terms of either intraobserver or interobserver comparison. Reproducibility can be improved by equalization of grades 0 and 1; however, the authors of this study advise caution when using this examination as a basis for diagnosis and treatment of shoulder instability.

▶ The conclusion that "caution is recommended when using results of laxity examination of unanesthetized shoulders to determine the diagnosis and treatment for shoulder disorders" is unquestioned. However, I would add that laxity examinations performed when the patient is under anesthesia can also be misleading or inconclusive. Perhaps that is what the arthroscope is for.

J. S. Torg, MD

Anesthetic Methods for Reduction of Acute Shoulder Dislocations: A Prospective Randomized Study Comparing Intraarticular Lidocaine With Intravenous Analgesia and Sedation
Kosnik J, Shamsa F, Raphael E, et al (Wayne State Univ, Detroit)
Am J Emerg Med 17:566-570, 1999   2–13

Objective.—Whether intraarticular lidocaine (IAL) is as effective as IV analgesia/sedation (IVAS) for facilitating shoulder reduction in acute anterior shoulder dislocation (AASD) was investigated in a prospective, randomized, nonblinded clinical trial.

Methods.—Ease of reduction and pain of reduction were evaluated in 49 patients treated at a large urban Level I trauma center for reduction of AASD facilitated by IVAS (n = 20, 16 males) or IAL (n = 29, 20 males).

Results.—There was no significant difference between groups with respect to pain of reduction or ease of reduction. The reduction rate of 5.5 hours delayed time for the IAL group was significantly shorter than for the IVAS group (78.24 vs 100%). Four of 5 patients in whom IAL failed had successful reduction with IVAS. Half of the IAL patients who had experience with IVAS preferred IVAS.

Conclusion.—Although there were no significant differences between results for IAL and IVAS, patients who were familiar with both preferred IVAS for reduction of AASD. IAL is an alternative for patients who do not want systemic analgesia.

▶ Lippitt et al[1] were the first to describe the use of intraarticular lidocaine to facilitate reduction of acute glenohumeral joint dislocation. Importantly, it should be noted that 15 minutes should be allowed between injection and attempt at reduction. It is interesting to note that the small sample size was the result of patient refusal to be enrolled in the study. In addition to sample size, other limitations of the study were related to physician experience and verification of injection.

J. S. Torg, MD

Reference

1. Lippitt et al: Orthopaedic Transactions 15:804, 1991.

Arthroscopic Bankart Repair of Anterior Detachments of the Glenoid Labrum: A Prospective Study
O'Neill, DB (St John Sports Medicine Ctr, Nassau Bay, Tex)
J Bone Joint Surg Am 81-A:1357-1366, 1999   2–14

Objective.—The outcomes of a standardized arthroscopic transglenoid suture-stabilization technique for the treatment of recurrent unidirectional anterior dislocations of the shoulder and an isolated anterior detachment of the glenoid labrum in athletically active patients were prospectively assessed.

Methods.—Forty-four of 50 patients with at least 2 documented episodes of anterior unilateral dislocation and failure of physical therapy had arthroscopic repair of the anterior aspect of the glenoid labrum. Forty-one were followed annually with examinations, radiographs, isokinetic strength-testing, and shoulder rating (Rowe and Zarins scale and the American Shoulder and Elbow Surgeons) for an average of 52 months.

Technique.—The anterior aspect of the scapular neck was abraded, and the anteriorly detached labrum and inferior glenohumeral ligament are advanced to the prepared bone surface. A Beath pin is drilled through the cannulated grasper instrument, and a transcapular suture is passed through the pin, knotted posteriorly, and pulled to the posterior aspect of the scapular neck. A second suture is placed above the first and knotted posteriorly. Extraarticular knots are made to secure the capsulolabral complex to the anterior aspect of the scapular neck. Intraarticular knots are secured. Pais of sutures are placed above the first knot. Four to 6 sutures were used in patients.

Results.—Forty (98%) patients returned to their athletic activities. Two (5%) football players each had 1 postoperative subluxation but were able to return to their sport. There were 32 (78%) patients who finished the complete rehabilitation program. Compliance with the rehabilitation program, presence of preoperative, and posterior labral tears without detachment did not affect outcome. Complex labral tears, subluxation, and loose bodies were each associated with poorer outcomes. There were 2 complications, including a posterior suture abscess requiring reoperation for removal of a foreign body and sterile posterior foreign-body granulomas, which were excised. There were 37 (90%) patients with a score of more than or equal to 80 points on the Rowe and Zarins' scale and 34 (83%) with a score of more than or equal to 90. There were 39 (95%) patients with a score of more than or equal to 80 points on the American Shoulder and Elbow Surgeons' scale and 25 (61%) with a score of more than or equal to 90. Full range of motion and full strength were achieved by 22 (54%) and 18 (44%) patients, respectively. There was a significant association between the presence of a Hill-Sachs or Bankart lesion and scores on both function scales. The presence of loose bodies was significantly associated with decreased strength and range of motion. Strength was also related to arm dominance and number of dislocations.

Conclusion.—Most athletic patients with shoulder instability were able to return to their sport after arthroscopic transglenoid repair of isolated anterior labral detachments.

▶ The author presents a well-documented series of patients who were treated for recurrent unilateral unidirectional anterior dislocation of the shoulder with an associated anterior detachment of the glenoid labrum treated by arthroscopic transglenoid suture stabilization. One complication associated with transglenoid suture fixation is that of injury to the suprascapular nerve. Although O'Neill does not report this complication in this series, I can attest to my own experience that this can happen. Of course, this is not a problem if one uses the variety of absorbable and nonabsorbable suture anchors now available.

J. S. Torg, MD

The Effects of Laser-induced Collagen Shortening on the Biomechanical Properties of the Inferior Glenohumeral Ligament Complex
Selecky MT, Vangsness CT Jr, Liao W-L, et al (Univ of Southern California, Los Angeles)
Am J Sports Med 27:168-172, 1999   2–15

Objective.—Laser shrinkage of shoulder ligaments/capsule has recently been used to treat shoulder laxity. No studies have investigated the effects of lasing on the structural properties of the inferior glenohumeral ligament complex. The effects of laser-induced collagen shortening on the tensile and cyclic properties of the inferior glenohumeral ligament complex were investigated.

Methods.—The shoulder capsule was isolated in 20 fresh-frozen human cadaveric shoulders, aged 74 to 91 years, and the inferior glenohumeral ligament complex was exposed and kept moistened. A total of 57 bone blocks containing the insertion sites of the anterior superior band, the anterior axillary pouch, and the posterior axillary pouch were harvested. The bone blocks were embedded in resin. All specimens were attached to a hydraulic testing machine and subjected to uniaxial tensioning to 10% strain. The specimens were randomly allocated to a lased or nonlased group. The lased group was treated with a holmium:yttrium-aluminum-garnet laser at energy levels sufficient to cause a 10% decrease in ligament length. Tensioning tests were repeated, and then each specimen was loaded to failure. Strain, stress, and elastic modulus values were compared for the 2 groups.

Results.—Mean ultimate stress, mean ultimate strain, and mean modulus of elasticity were nonsignificantly greater for the lased specimens than for the unlased specimens. Student's *t*-test showed that ultimate strain and yield strain were significantly higher in lased specimens than in nonlased specimens. Failure of the nonlased specimens occurred 41.7% of the time at the humeral attachment, 33.3% of the time in ligament tissue, and 25% of the time at the glenoid attachment. Failure of the lased specimens occurred at the humeral attachment 36.4% of the time, in ligament tissue 33.3% of the time, and at the glenoid attachment 30.3% of the time.

Conclusion.—In this cadaver load-to-failure study of shoulders treated by laser-induced collagen shortening, failure did not occur at the lased sites, and strength of the ligament complex was not significantly affected by the lasing procedure.

Histologic Evaluation of the Glenohumeral Joint Capsule After the Laser-assisted Capsular Shift Procedure for Glenohumeral Instability
Hayashi K, Massa KL, Thabit G III, et al (Univ of Wisconsin-Madison; Sports, Orthopedic and Rehabilitation Medicine Associates, Menlo Park, Calif)
Am J Sports Med 27:162-167, 1999   2–16

Objective.—Use of the holmium:yttrium-aluminum-garnet (Ho:YAG) laser to shrink the redundant joint capsule in patients with glenohumeral instability is controversial. Higher temperatures have been shown to decrease tissue stiffness in animal studies. The short- and long-term histologic properties of the glenohumeral joint capsule in patients treated with the laser-assisted capsular shift procedure were evaluated.

Methods.—Between 1993 and 1996, 53 joint capsule specimens collected before and at various times after surgery from 42 patients (19 men; age, 18-44 years) with glenohumeral instability and from 3 patients without joint capsule pathologic abnormalities underwent histologic evaluation. Quality of collagen, quality and quantity of synovial cells and fibroblasts, and vascularity in the subsynovial region and ligament tissue were scored. Groups were compared by means of the Kruskal-Wallis test.

Results.—Before laser treatment, joint capsule specimens showed no significant histologic lesions and no inflammation. After laser treatment, collagen had lost its fibrous structure and bundles were fused. Synovial cells, fibroblasts, and smooth muscle and endothelial cells were necrotic and fragmented. Lumina of blood vessels were constricted. At 3 months, significant repair had occurred. By 7 to 38 months, the joint capsule was almost normal, although the fibroblast level remained high. In 6 patients with stiff shoulder (postoperative arthrofibrosis), there were dramatic reactive responses at 3 months. Reactive responses were still apparent at 1 year.

Conclusion.—After Ho:YAG laser surgery to repair glenohumeral instability, there is significant tissue repair and remodeling, although reactive responses continue after 1 year in a subset of patients with postoperative stiff shoulder. Additional longer-term studies are needed to evaluate the advantages and disadvantages of this procedure.

▶ Selecky et al point out that there is minimal published information regarding laser-induced ligament/capsular shrinkage and none regarding the effects of structural and material properties of the inferior glenohumeral ligament complex and joint capsule caused by lasing. Thus, they have attempted to determine the effects of laser-induced collagen shortening on the cyclical and tensile properties of the IGF ligament complex. Hayashi et al attempted to evaluate short- and long-term histologic properties of the glenohumeral joint capsule after the laser-assisted capsular shift procedure. Although both studies report positive conclusions (ie, Selecky et al state that they "interpret results to suggest that the viscoelastic properties and strength of the inferior glenohumeral ligament complex were not significantly compromised by lasing"), Selecky et al acknowledged that the mechanical and biochemical properties were not evaluated and that clinical follow-up was also necessary.

J. S. Torg, MD

Position of Immobilization After Dislocation of the Shoulder

Itol E, Hatakeyama Y, Urayama M, et al (Akita Univ, Japan)
J Bone Joint Surg Am 81-A:385-390, 1999   2–17

Objective.—There is no evidence to support the tradition position of immobilization after treatment for acute dislocation of the shoulder. How the coaptation of the edges of a Bankart lesion changes with alterations in the position of the arm were investigated in cadaveric shoulders.

Methods.—A simulated Bankart lesion was created in the exposed joint capsule of 10 fresh-frozen cadaveric shoulders. The humerus was elevated to 0, 30, 45, and 60 degrees relative to the scapula and manually rotated from neutral to full internal rotation, back to neutral, and then to full external rotation at each angle. Opening and closing of the lesion was measured using linear transducers attached to the anteroinferior and inferior portions of the lesion (Fig 1).

Results.—Rotation at elevations of 60 degrees created an opening greater than the 6-mm measurement capacity of the transducers. Displacement of the edges of the lesion at 30 degrees of external rotation was significantly larger than at 0, 10, and 20 degrees of internal rotation. Displacement at 45 degrees of abduction was significantly larger than at 0 degrees of internal rotation and 30 degrees of external rotation. With the arm in 30 degrees of external rotation, displacement at 30 degrees of abduction was significantly larger than at 0 degrees of abduction. Results were similar for the inferior part of the lesion.

Displacement at the anteroinferior part of the lesion increased significantly with increased rotation when the shoulder was in 30 degrees of flexion, and displacement was significantly larger than that at 0 degrees of flexion. Displacement at 45 degrees was larger than at 0 degrees through-

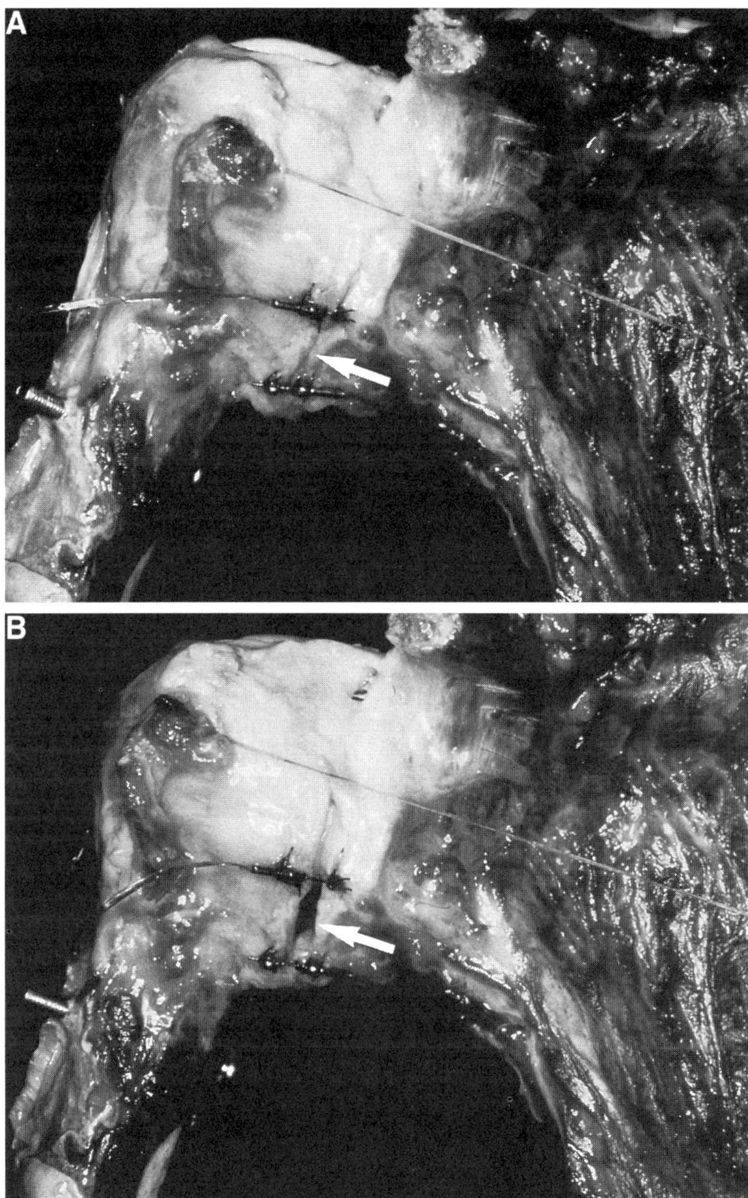

FIGURE 1.—Photographs showing the positions of the differential variable reluctance transducers with the arm in 30 degrees of abduction. One transducer is at the anteroinferior portion (the 4:30 position) of the simulated Bankart lesion, and the other is at the inferior portion (the 6:00 position). Fig. 1-A: The edges of the lesion (*arrow*) were approximated with the arm in neutral rotation. Fig. 1-B: The edges of the lesion (*arrow*) were separately with the arm in external rotation. (Courtesy of Itol E, Hatakeyama Y, Urayama M, et al: Position of immobilization after dislocation of the shoulder. *J Bone Joint Surg Am* 81-A:385-390, 1999.)

out the entire range of rotation. Results tended to be similar for the inferior portion of the lesion during flexion.

Conclusion.—An immobilization position that increases tension in anterior soft tissue may be better than the traditional immobilization position.

▶ This interesting article is somewhat confusing in that the authors do not define the "conventional position of immobilization." They do describe the traditional position of immobilization as one of adduction and internal rotation to be within the so-called coaptation zone. However, the point is made that there are "no experimental data to support immobilization of the arm to the trunk" and to this observer, it appears that the "traditional" position should coaptate a simulated Bankart lesion. Of course, the question as to whether the position alone will effect successful healing of the Bankart lesion is both doubtful and not dealt with here.

J. S. Torg, MD

Operative Treatment of Ulnar Collateral Ligament Injuries of the Elbow in Athletes
Azar FM, Andrews JR, Wilk KE, et al (American Sports Medicine Inst, Birmingham, Ala)
Am J Sports Med 28:16-23, 2000   2–18

Introduction.—Baseball pitchers are prone to injury to the ulnar collateral ligament. These injuries likely result from the tremendous static forces placed on the ligament during overhead throwing. An experience with ulnar collateral ligament reconstruction in athletes was reported.

Technique.—The repairs were performed by a technique similar to that of Jobe et al, except that the medial condyle and flexor-pronator mass were not detached, and ulnar nerve transposition was performed subcutaneously. The definition of ulnar collateral ligament tear was arthroscopically documented laxity of 2 mm or greater. The nerve was exposed through a medial approach, with protection of the medial antebrachial cutaneous nerve. The tear was identified and the ligament remnants preserved. An autogenous graft using palmaris longus, plantaris, or toe extensor tendon was obtained, and posterior olecranon osteophytes were removed if necessary. Tunnels were made in the medial epicondyle for graft placement (Figs 4 and 5). The subcutaneous ulnar nerve was transposed and secured with the use of fascial slings elevated from the flexor pronator mass (Fig 6).

Experience.—A total of 78 ulnar collateral ligament reconstructions and 13 repairs were performed over a 9-year period. All patients were male; 86% were collegiate or professional baseball players. Preoperative ulnar

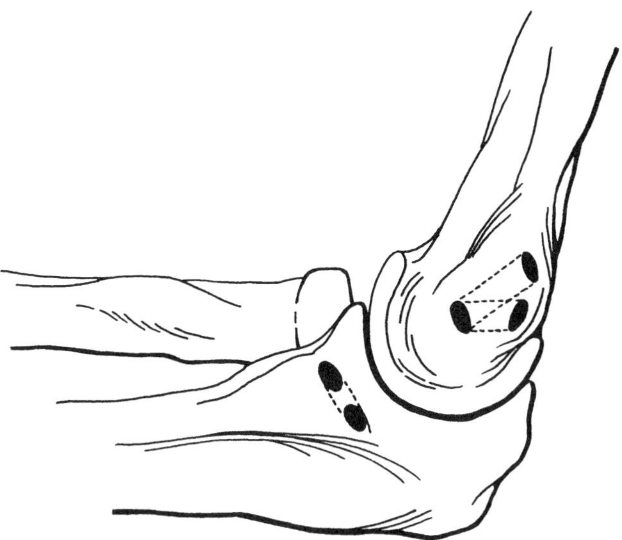

FIGURE 4.—Placement of bone tunnels for ulnar collateral ligament reconstruction. (Courtesy of Azar FM, Andrews JR, Wilk KE, et al: Operative treatment of ulnar collateral ligament injuries of the elbow in athletes. *Am J Sports Med* 28:16-23, 2000.)

nerve symptoms were completely eliminated after surgery in 9 of 10 patients. The complication rate was 9%, including problems at the graft harvest site in the wrist in 4 patients. The patients started an interval throwing program at an average of 3.4 months, and returned to competition at average of 9.8 months. Sixty-seven patients were followed up for an average of 35 months. Seventy-nine percent resumed at least their former level of competition.

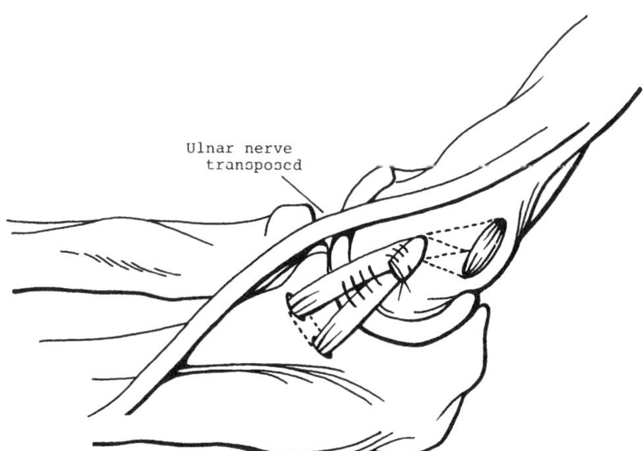

FIGURE 5.—Graft placement for ulnar collateral ligament reconstruction. (Courtesy of Azar FM, Andrews JR, Wilk KE, et al: Operative treatment of ulnar collateral ligament injuries of the elbow in athletes. *Am J Sports Med* 28:16-23, 2000.)

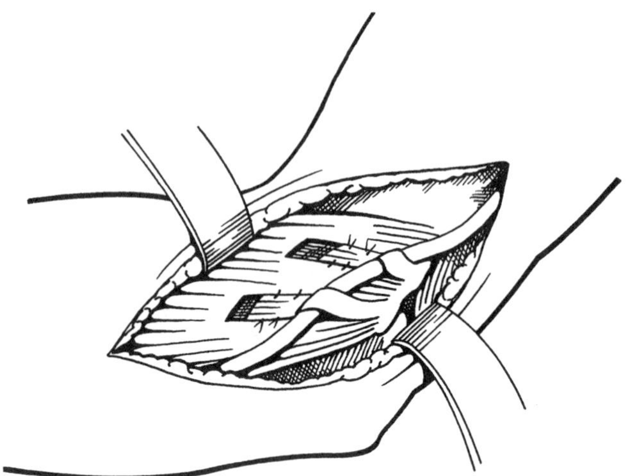

FIGURE 6.—Fascial slings for ulnar nerve transposition. (Courtesy of Azar FM, Andrews JR, Wilk KE, et al: Operative treatment of ulnar collateral ligament injuries of the elbow in athletes. *Am J Sports Med* 28:16-23, 2000.)

Conclusion.—The authors' technique yields good results in reconstruction of the ulnar collateral ligament in throwing athletes. Most patients are able to return to their previous level of play within less than a year. The authors recommend autograft augmentation even if ligament repair is possible. The use of subcutaneous rather than submuscular transposition of the ulnar nerve appears to reduce the complication rate.

▶ The authors state that indications for surgery "included a complete tear of the anterior bundle of the ulnar collateral ligament as documented by positive findings on the history, physical examination, and imaging studies." However, 44% of the group had a positive ulnar nerve Tinel's sign, whereas only 26% demonstrated preoperative laxity with valgus stress. In that the operation really consisted of a number of procedures in addition to the ulnar collateral ligament reconstruction (ie, ulnar nerve transposition, posterior medial olecranon osteophyte excision, etc.), the procedure appears to be somewhat of a shotgun approach to pitchers with medial elbow problems.

J. S. Torg, MD

Snowboarder's Wrist: Its Severity Compared With Alpine Skiing
Sasaki K, Takagi M, Kiyoshige Y, et al (Saiseikai Yamagate Hosp, Oki-machi, Japan; Yamagata Univ, Iida-Nishi, Japan)
J Trauma Injury Infect Crit Care 46:1059-1061, 1999   2–19

Objective.—Although wrist injuries are the most common snowboard injuries reported, the severity of these injuries is not known. The severity of snowboarding wrist injuries was compared with those of alpine skiing during the past 7 years.

Methods.—Between 1990 and 1997, 1446 injured snowboarders (456 female), aged 9 to 62 years, and 10,152 injured skiers (4253 female), aged 3 to 89 years, were treated at 1 clinic in Japan. There were 271 snowboarders and 257 skiers with wrist pain and 184 and 176, respectively, with radiographic evidence of wrist injury. Severity of fractures was compared.

Results.—The incidence of injuries was significantly higher for snowboarders than for skiers (0.35 vs 0.11). Wrist joint injuries accounted for 18.7% of snowboarding injuries and 2.5% of skiing injuries. The rate of wrist joint fractures was 0.28/1000 for snowboarders and 0.008/1000 for skiers. Comminuted fractures accounted for 49.4% of snowboarding wrist fractures and 23.8% of skiing wrist fractures.

Conclusion.—Snowboarders are significantly more likely to have fractures of the distal radius than skiers and significantly more likely to have comminuted fractures.

▶ The authors have clearly demonstrated, as would be expected, that in addition to snowboarder's foot, spear tackler's spine, and tennis elbow, we now have snowboarder's wrist.

J. S. Torg, MD

Conservative Versus Surgical Treatment of Mallet Finger: A Pooled Quantitative Literature Evaluation
Geyman JP, Fink K, Sullivan SD (Univ of Washington, Seattle)
J Am Board Fam Pract 11:382-390, 1998   2–20

Objective.—Optimal treatment for mallet finger is controversial. A pooled quantitative literature evaluation of published studies was performed to investigate the outcomes of treatment according to patients and physicians, outcomes of surgical versus conservative treatment, and outcomes after treatment for chronic or recurrent mallet finger.

Methods.—A search of MEDLINE and EMBASE databases uncovered 41 observational and randomized trials published in English between January 1966 and February 1998. Outcome criteria included extensor lag, flexion arc, pain or stiffness, functional impairment, and overall patient evaluation.

Results.—There were 26 studies that met the inclusion criteria for initial acute treatment (n = 21, 1146 digits) and chronic or recurrent treatment (n = 5, 148 digits). In the acute treatment group, 20 studies encompassed conservative splinting treatment and 3 encompassed surgical treatment. Outcomes were successful in more than 77% of patients. Of 315 patients polled, satisfaction level averaged 83.4%. In the surgery treatment group, outcomes were successful in 85% of patients in 3 studies (60 digits).

Patient satisfaction was 73% in 5 studies that investigated chronic or recurrent injuries.

Conclusion.—Conservative splinting treatment is effective for the vast majority of closed mallet finger injuries, and most patients have a high level of satisfaction with their outcomes. Patient education is extremely important. Surgical treatment is effective for the small number of complex acute injuries or chronic or recurrent injuries that require operative management.

▶ This study strongly indicates that acute mallet finger injuries should be treated conservatively. The authors state some basics of treatment that must be adhered to closely. The involved finger should be splinted in slight hyperextension of the distal interphalangeal joint and moderate flexion of the proximal interphalangeal joint for at least 6 to 8 weeks. Careful changing of the splint to avoid distal interphalangeal joint flexion is a must. This can be accomplished by placing the extended finger on a firm surface and then sliding the splint on and off carefully, always avoiding distal interphalangeal joint flexion.

F. J. George ATC, PT

3 Injuries of Hips, Pelvis, and Lower Limbs

Management of Severe Lower Abdominal or Inguinal Pain in High-Performance Athletes
Meyers WC, and the PAIN Study Group (Performing Athletes with Abdominal or Inguinal Neuromuscular Pain Study Group) (Univ of Massachusetts, Worcester)
Am J Sports Med 28:2-8, 2000   3–1

Background.—Lower abdominal pain can end athletic careers. The management of severe lower abdominal or inguinal pain in high-performance athletes was investigated.

Methods and Findings.—Two hundred seventy-six high-performance athletes with severe lower abdominal or inguinal pain were included in the study. One hundred seventy-five had pelvic floor repairs. Seventy-nine percent of the 157 athletes who had not had previous surgery were professional or highly competitive athletes. Eighty-eight percent of the patients had adductor pain associated with their lower abdomen or inguinal pain. More patients had related adductor releases during the latter operative period. Examination unmasked 38 other abnormalities, including severe hip problems and malignancies. Ninety-seven percent of the athletes returned to previous levels of performance.

Conclusion.—This distinct syndrome of lower-abdominal/adductor pain in male athletes can apparently be corrected by a procedure designed to strengthen the anterior pelvic floor. The pain location and pattern and the operative success suggest that the cause is a combination of abdominal hyperextension and thigh hyperabduction, the pivot point being the pubic symphysis.

► To my knowledge, this article presents the largest series and the most comprehensive explanation for management of chronic inguinal or pubic area pain, exertional in nature and not explainable by a palpable hernia or other diagnosis. The authors define pelvic floor repair as a broad surgical reattachment of the inferior edge of the rectus abdominis muscle with its fascial investment to the pubis and adjacent anterior ligaments. Evaluation of the group revealed 38 other abnormalities, including hip problems and cancer, emphasizing the importance of a comprehensive evaluation of athletes with groin pain. This article is must reading for all those involved in the care of performance athletes.

J. S. Torg, MD

Is Diagnostic Arthroscopy of the Hip Worthwhile? A Prospective Review of 328 Adults Investigated for Hip Pain
Baber YF, Robinson AHN, Villar RN (Addenbrooke's Hosp, Cambridge, England)
J Bone Joint Surg Br 81-B:600-603, 1999   3–2

Objective.—The clinical indications for arthroscopy of the hip are not clear. The clinical and arthroscopic diagnoses were compared, and the effect of hip arthroscopy on the management of patients was assessed.

Methods.—Arthrography, CT, or MRI was performed when clinically indicated in 432 patients with hip pain. When a preoperative diagnosis could not be made, patients underwent diagnostic arthroscopy.

Results.—No cause for hip pain could be found for 154 (47%) patients. Arthroscopy revealed abnormalities in 124 patients including osteoarthritis in 48, osteochondral defects in 26, and torn labra in 17. In 174 patients with a preoperative diagnosis, arthroscopy revealed an abnormality different from the one diagnosed in 52 (30%) patients. The most common abnormality missed was osteoarthritis in 75 patients, osteochondral defects in 34, torn labra in 23, synovitis in 11, and loose bodies in 9. Operations performed in 172 (52%) patients included 70 procedures in the osteoarthritis group (47 chondroplasties, 17 labrectomies, 6 removals of foreign bodies). In 146 patients with preoperative and postoperative diagnoses that were the same, 69 had a procedure. Arthroscopy did not change the diagnosis in 77 patients, and these patients did not have operative treatment. Access failed in an additional 7 patients. Hip arthroscopy did not facilitate management of 84 (26%) patients. In comparative terms, if hip arthroscopy cost 1.0 unit, hip arthrography under general anesthesia cost 1.0, hip arthrotomy cost 1.8, and total hip arthroplasty cost 9.8 units. MRI costs 0.3 units.

Conclusion.—Hip arthroscopy facilitated the management of 74% of patients in this study.

▶ This article presents convincing evidence that arthroscopy of the hip joint is both safe and worthwhile. To my knowledge, this procedure is not performed with great frequency in the United States. The success that the English have had with this procedure may well be related to its being performed while the patient is under general anesthesia and in the lateral position, with leg traction and a padded peroneal bar to provide lateral thrust.

J. S. Torg, MD

Complications of Arthroscopy of the Hip

Griffin DR, Villar RN (Addenbrooke's NHS Trust, Cambridge, England; BUPA Cambridge Lea Hosp, England)

J Bone Joint Surg Br 81-B:604-606, 1999   3–3

Objective.—The rate and types of complications after arthroscopy of the hip are not known. The operative technique and complications encountered in the largest single series of arthroscopies of the hip ever reported were presented.

Methods.—Hip arthroscopy was performed on 253 males and 387 females, aged 6 to 78 years, between 1990 and 1997. Undiagnosed hip pain was present in 49% of patients. Preoperative history, clinical results, intraoperative findings, perioperative complications, and outcome were recorded.

Technique.—With patients under general anesthesia, traction were applied to the ipsilateral foot (Fig 1). A padded perineal bar was placed under the proximal hip and 200 to 300 N of traction was applied. The joint was distended with injected saline solution.

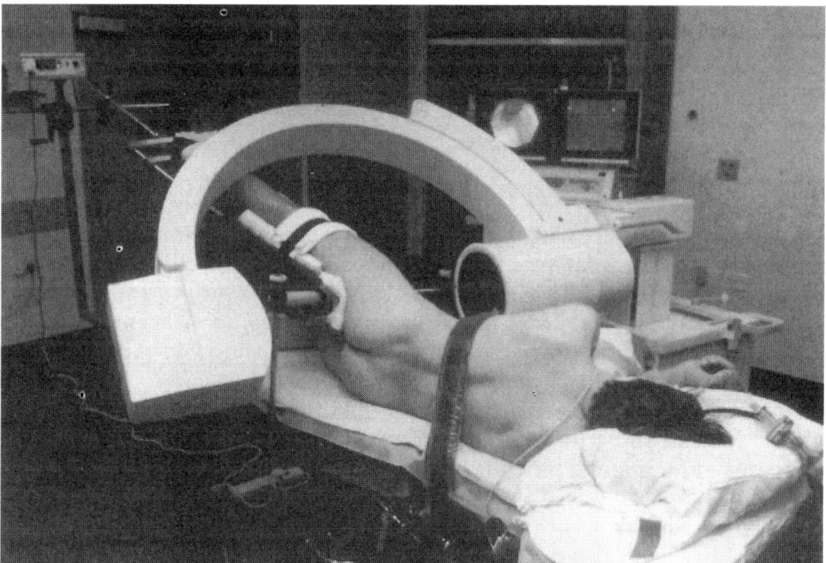

FIGURE 1.—Photograph of a patient lying in right lateral position with traction apparatus and image intensifier in place. The padded perineal bar provides lateral thrust. (Courtesy of Griffin DR, Villar RN: Complications of arthroscopy of the hip. *J Bone Joint Surg Br* 81-B:604-606, 1999.)

A spinal needle was inserted, and a flexible guidewire was inserted through the needle. The arthroscope cannula and trochars were inserted over the needle, and arthroscopy was performed with a 70-degree arthroscope. The joint was washed, and the wounds were covered. Each patient was discharged within 24 hours.

Results.—There were 10 complications from the procedures. These included 3 patients with transient palsy of the sciatic nerve (probably as a result of a technical error), 1 with transient palsy of the femoral nerve that resolved within 6 hours, and 1 with a small vaginal tear that healed spontaneously. Several weeks after surgery, trochanteric bursitis developed in 1 patient, and this was successfully treated with steroid injection. Another patient who bled from the arthroscope portal was successfully treated with superficial pressure. Another patient had a hematoma around the portal wound that resolved after 2 weeks. The tip of an arthroscope broke off in 1 patient but was immediately removed. An arthroscope forceps broke off in 1 patient, and a metal fragment lodged in the cotyloid fossa, where it remained. The minor complication rate was 1.6%.

Conclusion.—Arthroscopy of the hip has a low complication rate.

▶ As this study points out, complications resulting from arthroscopy of the hip joint fall into 2 groups: those associated with traction and those resulting from breakage of arthroscopic instruments. Although I have had minimal experience with this procedure, I would agree that, in competent hands, "it is possible to undertake this operation safely using the technique described."

J. S. Torg, MD

Sacral Stress Fractures in Long-Distance Runners
Major NM, Helms CA (Duke Univ, Durham, NC)
AJR 174:727-729, 2000   3–4

Introduction.—Sacral stress fractures in athletes are unusual, yet are important findings that often mimic sciatica. With missed diagnosis, appropriate treatment may be delayed. This article describes radiographic and clinical findings in 4 long-distance runners with sacral stress fractures.

Findings.—The mean age of 1 female and 3 male athletes was 34 years (range, 18-49 years). All were running more than 80 km/wk. All patients had complained of back pain and had been treated for disk disease. None improved with therapy. Patients underwent imaging. Three of 4 patients had normal findings on unenhanced radiographs. Three patients had CT, 2 had MRI, and 1 underwent radionuclide bone scanning. The CT images revealed unilateral vertical cortical disruption through the sacrum with sclerosis involving the region of the sacral foramina, compatible with a fracture. In the third patient, CT images demonstrated bilateral cortical disruption with increased sclerosis oriented vertically along the ala sacralis. These findings were diagnostic of bilateral stress fractures. The MRI results in 2 patients revealed unilateral low–signal intensity in a vertical and linear orientation in the lateral aspect of the sacrum on the T1-weighted image and high intensity on the T2-weighted image. Findings for both patients were compatible with a stress fracture. The bone scan revealed linear uptake in the sacrum consistent with a fracture; this was subsequently confirmed by MRI.

Conclusion.—Patients with sacral stress fractures recover within 4 to 6 weeks of rest. All patients in this series were able to continue running in 4 weeks. Gradual return to running is recommended. It is likely that sacral stress fractures are underreported. They should be suspected in long-distance runners with low back pain.

▶ This interesting article brings attention to an entity that probably goes unrecognized, is underreported, and infrequent in occurrence. I would imagine that most cases are found on bone scan and, perhaps, mistakenly diagnosed as sacroiliitis. The fact that the fractures heal within 4 to 6 weeks with rest and patients return to their activities in 4 weeks may account for the infrequent diagnosis.

J. S. Torg, MD

Increasing Hamstring Flexibility Decreases Lower Extremity Overuse Injuries in Military Basic Trainees
Hartig DE, Henderson JM (Hughston Clinic, PC, Columbus, Ga)
Am J Sports Med 27:173-176, 1999   3–5

Objective.—Most loss of training time in the military results from lower extremity overuse injuries. Tightness of hamstring muscles is a significant predictor of such injuries. Whether increasing hamstring musculotendinous flexibility decreases the risk of lower limb overuse injuries during basic training was studied.

Methods.—Hamstring flexibility was measured before and after basic training in 1 control company and 1 intervention company taking part in the 13-week infantry basic training course at Fort Benning, Georgia. The control company followed normal stretching routines. The intervention group added 3 hamstring stretching sessions.

Results.—Pretraining hamstring flexibility was 45.9 degrees in the control group and 41.7 degrees in the intervention group. The difference was significant. After training, hamstring flexibility was 42.9 degrees in the control group and 34.7 degrees. The difference was significant. The Seto hamstring flexibility score—which showed that hamstring flexibility less than 30 degrees short of neutral was unlikely to incur a lower extremity overuse injury—showed that both groups were inflexible at pretraining assessments. After training, the intervention group had significantly increased hamstring flexibility, with 48% of recruits flexible to less than 35 degrees and 6% of control recruits flexible to 35 degrees or less. The number of recruits with lower extremity overuse injuries was significantly lower in the intervention group than in the control group (29% vs 17%).

Conclusion.—Hamstring flexibility exercises significantly reduced the number of lower extremity overuse injuries in basic training recruits.

▶ The purpose of this study—to demonstrate that increased hamstring musculotendinous flexibility would decrease the number of lower extremity overuse injuries—was achieved. Although the authors have defined *injury* to include stress fractures, patellofemoral knee pain, muscle strains, tendinitis, plantar fasciitis, shin splints, and anterior compartment syndrome, there was no quantification in terms of severity. However, I believe the authors have made a very important observation with regard to a simple means of effecting injury prevention.

J. S. Torg, MD

Snapping Popliteus Tendon Syndrome: A Cause of Mechanical Knee Popping in Athletes

Cooper DE (Baylor Univ, Dallas)
Am J Sports Med 27:671-674, 1999   3–6

Objective.—The clinical findings, treatment options, and long-term results of treatment of traumatic or spontaneous snapping of the popliteus tendon are presented.

Methods.—Between 1990 and 1998, 6 patients (2 women), average age 27 years, were treated for snapping of the popliteus tendon. Three were professional or collegiate athletes, and 3 were recreational athletes. MRI scans were normal in 4 of 4 patients. Two patients had surgical exploration. Four were treated with rest and nonsteroidal antiinflammatory drugs. Lateral popping was exacerbated when the knee was loaded under varus stress and extended to 0 degrees. Popping was the result of trauma in 3 patients, spontaneous in 2, and surgically induced after osteochondral allograft transplantation in 1 patient. Follow-up averaged 4 years.

Results.—At last follow-up, a patient had persistent popping that did not warrant surgery. Both patients who had surgery were cured with no instability or loss of motion.

Conclusion.—Snapping popliteus tendon can be a cause of lateral knee popping. Although the condition is uncommon, it should be considered in the differential diagnosis of mechanical symptoms around the knee to avoid unnecessary diagnostic arthroscopy.

▶ This report by Cooper is the first comprehensive description of snapping popliteus tendon syndrome. The suggested surgical approach to the problem by resection of the snapping tendon is questioned in view of the recent interest in the role of the popliteus in knee joint mechanics. To be noted, in this small group treated both conservatively and surgically, no criteria are forthcoming with regard to these treatment options.

J. S. Torg, MD

Magnetic Resonance Imaging As a Tool to Predict Meniscal Reparability
Matava MJ, Eck K, Totty W, et al (Washington Univ, St Louis)
Am J Sports Med 27:436-443, 1999   3–7

Background.—Whether a meniscal injury can be repaired depends on several factors and can be difficult to predict preoperatively. The use of MRI for accurate prediction of whether such a repair would be successful was evaluated.

Methods.—Three examiners (a musculoskeletal radiologist, a senior orthopedic surgeon, and a general radiologist) evaluated the MR images obtained for 106 patients (115 tears). The tears were classified by morphologic type, maximum length, and minimum distance from the meniscosynovial junction, and predictions were made as to whether the repair would be successful. Arthroscopy of the knees was also performed.

Results.—Correct estimates were made in only 14% to 67% of the cases. There were no significant differences between the predictive accuracies of the three examiners. Average accuracy was 74%, sensitivity was 29%, specificity was 89%, positive predictive value was 50%, and negative predictive value was 80% for MRI. Predictions of meniscectomy had an average accuracy of 69%, a sensitivity of 68%, a specificity of 75%, a positive predictive value of 90%, and a negative predictive value of 43%.

Conclusions.—Training of the evaluator appeared to be insignificant with respect to ability to predict the reparability of meniscus injury. MRI evaluation of these injuries preoperatively to predict reparability yielded only moderate reliability.

▶ Why am I not surprised that MRI is only moderately reliable for the prediction of meniscal repairability? Geld et al[1] clearly showed both the shortcomings and the unreliability of MRI in the evaluation of internal derangements of the knee.

J. S. Torg, MD

Reference

1. Geld HJ, Glasgow SG, Sapega AA, et al: Magnetic resonance imaging of knee disorders: Clinical value and cost-effectiveness in a sports medicine practice. *Am J Sports Med* 24:99-103, 1996.

Silent Meniscal Abnormalities in Athletes: Magnetic Resonance Imaging of Asymptomatic Competitive Gymnasts

Ludman CN, Hough DO, Cooper TG, et al (Michigan State Univ, Lansing)
Br J Sports Med 33:414-416, 1999   3–8

Introduction.—MRI creates amazingly detailed images of the intra-articular structures of the knee. Recognizing the range of MRI appearances within a normal population is important to avoid attributing a greater significance than necessary to imaging abnormalities that may occur without clinically significant symptoms. In athletes, unnecessary treatment or intervention can be as damaging to their competitive future as failure to recognize a clinically significant injury. The MRI appearances in asymptomatic gymnasts were compared with those in a less active population to determine findings that may be observed in the absence of significant pathology.

Methods.—The MRI scans of 24 knees in asymptomatic competitive American collegiate gymnasts (age range, 18-22 years) were compared with those of a control group matched for age and sex. Established grading criteria were used to assess the menisci.

Results.—Six grade 3 intrameniscal signal changes were detected in 48 (13%) menisci evaluated in the gymnast group. All 3 abnormalities were within the lateral meniscus. In controls, 3 (6%) of 52 menisci had grade 3 signal changes, all located in the posterior horn of the medial meniscus. When compared with control subjects, the gymnast group had a significantly different distribution of grade 3 intrameniscal signal changes involving the lateral meniscus ($P < .001$).

Conclusion.—The incidence of asymptomatic grade 3 signal abnormalities in the gymnast group was comparable with that of controls. There was a significant difference in the location of these changes. Athletes had a 13% incidence of lateral meniscal changes, compared with a 6% rate of medial meniscal changes in controls.

▶ This article reiterates the basic principle that MRIs of the knee can be misleading and must necessarily be correlated with clinical signs and symptoms. As stated by Gelb et al,[1] "magnetic resonance imaging is overused in the evaluation of knee disorders and not a cost effective method for evaluating injuries when compared with a skilled examiner."

J. S. Torg, MD

Reference

1. Gelb HJ, Glasgow SG, Sapega GG, et al: Magnetic resonance imaging of knee disorders. Clinical value and cost-effectiveness in a sports medicine practice. *Am J Sports Med* 24:99-103, 1996.

Pull-Out Strength and Stiffness of Meniscal Repair Using Absorbable Arrows or Ti-Cron Vertical and Horizontal Loop Sutures

Boenisch UW, Faber KJ, Ciarelli M, et al (Steadman Hawkins Sport Medicine Found, Vail, Colo; Michigan State Univ, East Lansing)
Am J Sports Med 27:626-631, 1999   3–9

Background.—The all-inside meniscal repair with bioabsorbable polylactic acid arrows simplifies operative technique and minimizes neurovascular complications. The pull-out strength and linear stiffness of meniscal repair with the use of bioabsorbable arrows and vertical and horizontal loop sutures in fresh-frozen bovine lateral menisci were assessed.

Methods.—In phase I of the study, menisci repaired with 2-0 Ti-Cron vertical or horizontal loop suture or with 10-, 13-, or 16-mm Meniscus Arrows were loaded to failure at 12.5 mm/sec (Fig 1). In phase II of the study, the number of barbs engaged and the angle of insertion using 10- and 13-mm arrows were evaluated.

Findings.—Pull-out strengths in both suture repair groups significantly exceeded those of the arrow groups. The stiffness of vertical loop sutures was significantly greater than that of horizontal sutures and 10-mm arrows. Phase II of the study showed that the mean ultimate load to failure for the 10-mm arrows was 35.1 N, which was significantly stronger than in phase I. However, stiffness was still low. Five arrows in the 13-mm group inserted parallel to the tibial surface were not significantly different

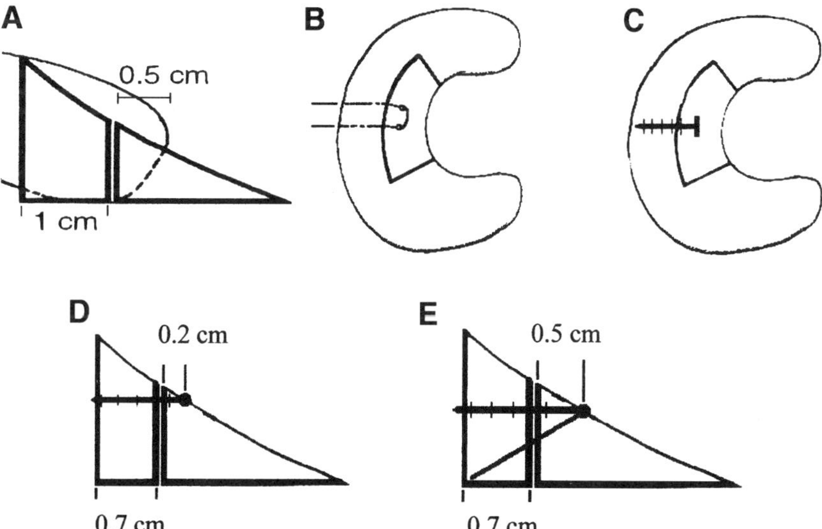

FIGURE 1.—In phase I, meniscal repair was performed with vertical suture loop (**A**), horizontal suture loop (**B**), or Meniscus Arrow (**C**). In phase II, the repair site was changed (**D**) and the angle of insertion was changed (**E**). (Courtesy of Boenisch UW, Faber KJ, Ciarelli M, et al: Pull-out strength and stiffness of meniscal repair using absorbable arrows or Ti-Cron vertical and horizontal loop sutures. *Am J Sports Med* 27:626-631, 1999.)

from in phase I. Five arrows inserted at more than a 30-degree angle were significantly weaker than in phase I.

Conclusion.—In this study, single vertical loop suture had the highest overall pull-out strength. Arrows are weaker than sutures but should provide enough stability for meniscal healing. The number of barbs engaged and angle of insertion are essential.

▶ The statement that "although weaker than sutures, arrows should provide sufficient stability for meniscal healing" is not supported by the data. However, our experience with the biodegradable arrow indicates 75% good and excellent results in the treatment of meniscal repairs primarily in the red red zone. Also, concomitant anterior cruciate ligament reconstruction appeared to facilitate meniscal healing.

J. S. Torg, MD

Osteochondritis Dissecans of the Patellofemoral Joint
Peters TA, McLean ID (Melbourne, Victoria, Australia)
Am J Sports Med 28:63-67, 2000   3–10

Introduction.—The cause of osteochondritis dissecans is unknown. It primarily affects the knee joint, with 85% of legions occurring in the medial femoral condyle and 15% in the lateral femoral condyle. The clinical features of 37 patients with osteochondritis dissecans of the patellofemoral joint are reported.

Clinical Features.—Twenty-four lesions were on the patella and 13 were on the trochlear groove. Two patients had medial trochlear lesions, which have not been previously reported. The osteochondral lesions involved the convex articular surfaces and were more common in males than females (4:1 ratio). Median patient age at initial evaluation was 15 years; 54% had open epiphyses. Osteochondritis dissecans of the patellofemoral joint can be missed unless quality radiographs are interpreted with care and, at arthroscopy, both the patella and trochlear groove are examined.

Treatment.—Treatment is dependent on symptoms, site, nature of the lesion, and patient age. Operative intervention is avoided in patients with open epiphyses unless symptoms indicate a loose fragment. Surgery is indicated for all patients with mechanical symptoms. Surgical approaches include arthroscopy with chondroplasty and removal of loose bodies and lateral retinacular release. Nonoperative treatment includes a modified McConnell program of lateral retinacular stretching, patellar taping, and eccentric vastus medialis oblique muscle exercises. Jumping, running, and twisting activities should be avoided, and patients should be encouraged to wear soft, well-cushioned shoes. Thirteen and 3 patients, respectively, with patellar and lateral trochlear groove lesions underwent nonoperative treatment; 11 and 8 patients, respectively, with these lesions were treated surgically. The 2 patients with medial trochlear groove lesions were treated arthroscopically. Most patients experienced symptom resolution with treatment. Some patients with articular cartilage damage had persistent patellofemoral crepitus and discomfort related to increased athletic activities or activities involving loads on the bent knee.

Conclusion.—Not all anterior knee pain is chondromalacia of the patella. Careful viewing of adequate radiographs, CT scans, and MRI are sufficient to make the diagnosis of osteochondritis dissecans.

▶ As pointed out by the authors, diagnosis of osteochondritis dissecans of the patellofemoral joint requires a high index of suspicion and careful radiographic analysis. I would agree with their criteria for surgery being mechanical symptoms such as locking, catching or giving way, effusion, and limitation of activity because of pain. I would further agree that surgical management necessarily involves a lateral retinacular release as well as debridement of the lesion. However, it should be emphasized that the results of surgical treatment are at all times guarded.

J. S. Torg, MD

An Outcome Study of Chronic Patellofemoral Pain Syndrome: Seven-Year Follow-up of Patients in a Randomized, Controlled Trial
Kannus P, Natri A, Paakkala T, et al (Tampere Univ Hosp, Finland)
J Bone Joint Surg Am 81-A:355-363, 1999   3–11

Objective.—The etiology, pathogenesis, and outcome of patellofemoral pain syndrome are not well understood. The long-term outcome and prognosis for patients who underwent nonoperative treatment for chronic patellofemoral pain syndrome were evaluated in a 7-year prospective, randomized, double-blind trial of the short-term (6-month) efficacy of glycosaminoglycan polysulfate, placebo, or quadriceps-muscle exercises.

Methods.—For 6 weeks, 53 patients (28 women; average age, 27 years) with unilateral patellofemoral pain syndrome received intensive isometric quadriceps exercises once daily and oral nonsteroidal anti-inflammatory medication for 20 days (group A), the same nonoperative treatment plus 5 intra-articular injections of lidocaine (group B), or the same nonoperative treatment plus 5 intra-articular injections of glycosaminoglycan polysulfate (group C). Patients were examined at baseline, after 6 months, and after 7 years. Pain and discomfort during activities, functional evaluation, clinical evaluation, and MRI and radiographic findings were recorded at each examination.

Results.—Functional, clinical, subjective, and radiographic findings were improved in all patients at 6 months. At 7 years, there was no significant change in functional evaluation for almost 75% of the patients. The number of patients with no symptoms on patellar compression and apprehension tests had decreased significantly from 93% and 89%, respectively, at 6 months to 67% and 69%, respectively, at 7 years. The proportion of patients with crepitation increased significantly from 58% at 6 months to 80% at 7 years. The physician's global assessment showed complete recovery in 76% of the patients at 6 months and in 67% at 7 years. Radiographic findings showed no progression of patellofemoral osteoarthritis in most patients. MRI findings at 7 years in 37 patients showed no abnormalities in 65% of the patients, mild abnormalities in 11%, moderate abnormalities in 19%, and severe abnormalities in 5%. At 7 years, there was a small but significant decrease in bone-mineral density of the affected knee.

Conclusion.—Nonoperative treatment was successful in maintaining function and in dealing with pain in most patients with chronic patellofemoral pain syndrome.

▶ The conclusions of the authors that nonoperative treatment of chronic patellofemoral pain syndrome yielded good results in approximately two thirds of the patients is in keeping with my own clinical experience.

J. S. Torg, MD

Patellar Tendinitis: The Significance of Magnetic Resonance Imaging Findings
Shalaby M, Almekinders LC (Univ of North Carolina, Chapel Hill)
Am J Sports Med 27:345-349, 1999   3–12

Objective.—Confirmation of patellar tendinitis sometimes requires radiologic evidence. Whether MRI or US is the better imaging modality is controversial. The use of MRI for confirming a diagnosis of patellar tendinitis was evaluated.

Methods.—T1- and T2-weighted midline sagittal MRI was performed in 10 patients (12 knees, 7 males) with a clinical diagnosis of patellar tendinitis and in 15 control patients (17 knees, 9 males) with diagnoses other than patellar tendinitis.

Results.—Seven (58%) patients' knees demonstrated intratendinitis on MRI, 3 (25%) showed no defect, and 2 (17%) had equivocal results (Fig 3). Four (24%) control knees had intratendinous lesions, 5 (29%) had no defect, and 8 (47%) had equivocal changes. The average tendon width was significantly larger in group 1 than in group 2 (5.0 vs 3.9 mm), and the average defect width was also significantly larger in group 1 than in group 2 (3.9 vs 2.4 mm). There were no significant differences between groups with respect to articular and nonarticular length. In knees with intratendinous changes, the average nonarticular surface/articular surface ratio (0.28) was significantly larger compared with the ratio for knees without changes (0.16). The sensitivity, specificity, and positive and negative predictive values of MRI were 75%, 29%, 43%, and 63%, respectively.

Conclusion.—Because of its low specificity, MRI is of limited value in detecting intratendinous changes, especially in mild cases of patellar tendinitis.

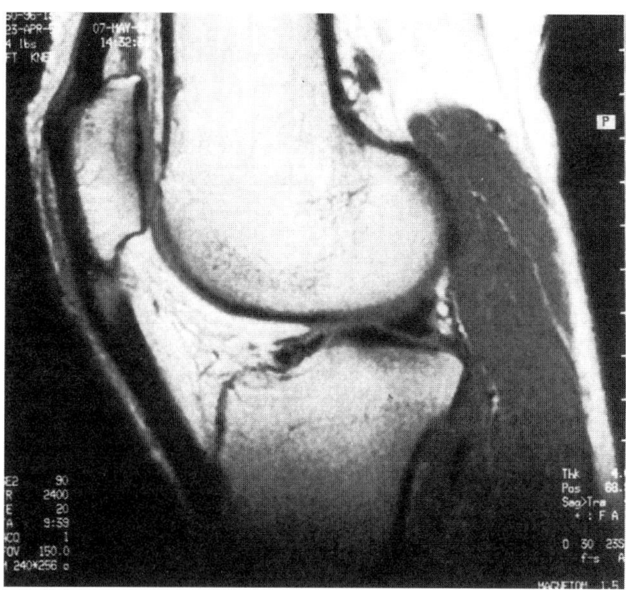

FIGURE 3.—MRI of the knee in a long-distance runner with patellar tendinitis and unequivocal tendon changes. (Courtesy of Shalaby M, Almekinders LC: Patellar tendinitis: The significance of magnetic resonance imaging findings. *Am J Sports Med* 27:345-349, 1999.)

▶ It appears to this observer that patellar tendinitis is a clinical diagnosis not requiring imaging substantiation. However, it would appear reasonable in those patients refractory to a conservative regimen that an MRI be ordered—both to substantiate an intertendinous lesion as well as to localize its position. Certainly, correlation of MRI and surgical findings would be helpful. Unfortunately, this was not done.

J. S. Torg, MD

Primary Repair of Patellar Tendon Rupture Without Augmentation

Marder RA, Timmerman LA (Univ of California at Davis, Sacramento)
Am J Sports Med 27:304-307, 1999   3–13

Introduction.—The traditional surgical management of an acute patellar tendon rupture is primary suture repair with cerclage augmentation, followed by up to 6 weeks of extension splinting. This method provides good results, but residual symptoms and other problems can occur. Results with a nonaugmented primary tendon repair, followed by early controlled knee motion, for patients with patellar tendon rupture, were reported.

Methods.—The experience included 15 consecutive patients with acute traumatic ruptures of the patellar tendon; all were men, with a mean age of 33 years. Most were recreational athletes. In 8 cases, the tendon was avulsed from the inferior pole of the patella, in 1 case it was avulsed from the tibial tubercle, and in 6 patients a midsubstance tendon tear was present. Both avulsions and ruptures were managed with primary suture repair, with no augmentation. The repairs permitted knee flexion of greater than 60°. The rehabilitation process started with heel slides, with flexion of up to 45° permitted for the first 3 weeks. Flexion increased to 90° between 3 and 6 weeks and was unrestricted thereafter. In addition, patients took part in an aggressive weight-bearing and muscle-strengthening program. Running was permitted at 16 to 20 weeks, proceeding to jumping and contact sports after 6 months. Fourteen patients were followed up at a mean of 2.6 months.

Results.—At follow-up, 12 of 14 patients had returned to their previous level of activity; the other 2 had reduced their activity level because of pain. The repaired knees showed no loss of extension or extensor lag, and a mean loss of 5° of flexion. Five patients had patellofemoral signs and symptoms, although this led to limitation of activity in only 2. Isokinetic testing in 11 patients revealed a mean peak torque of 92% at 60° per second. The average Lysholm-Gillquist functional score was 95.

Conclusions.—This experience shows excellent results in young patients with patellar tendon ruptures when nonaugmented primary repair was used with early, controlled motion. This technique allows most patients to return to their preinjury level of activity, without the need for prolonged immobilization, manipulation, or hardware removal.

▶ This is basically a techniques article without a control group for comparison. However, in addition to the surgical technique obviating internal fixating devices other than 2 No. 5 nonabsorbable sutures using a Krackow lip stitch in the medial and lateral halves of the patella tendon, an accelerated rehabilitation program was also implemented. Of note, the authors claim not to have observed any evidence of patella alta after repair.

J. S. Torg, MD

The Three-In-One Proximal and Distal Soft Tissue Patellar Realignment Procedure: Results, and Its Place in the Management of Patellofemoral Instability

Myers P, Williams A, Dodds R, et al (Brisbane Orthopaedic and Sports Medicine Centre, Queensland, Australia)

Am J Sports Med 27:575-579, 1999

3–14

Background.—There is ongoing debate as to the surgical management of patellar instability. Patients with patellofemoral chondral damage and ligament laxity may have poor results after extensor mechanism realignment surgery, and the surgical results may deteriorate over time. The technique and outcomes of a new "3-in-1" procedure for patellar realignment were reported.

Technique.—The procedure was performed in 48 knees with recurrent lateral dislocation of the patella after rehabilitation at-

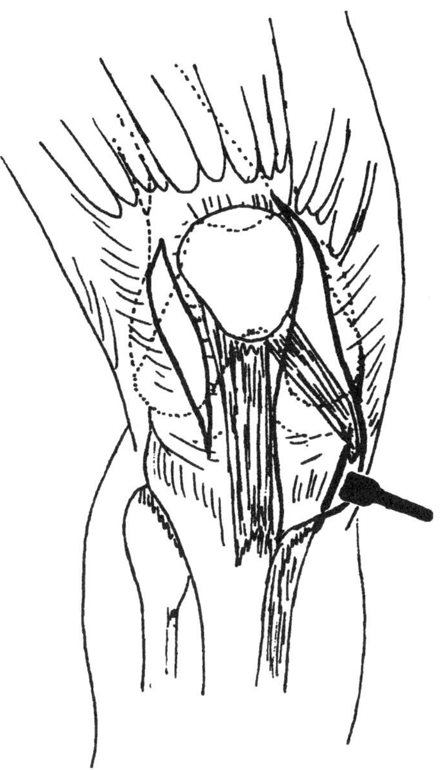

FIGURE 1.—Lateral release and transfer of the medial one third of the patellar tendon to the tibial collateral ligament in a right knee. (Courtesy of Myers P, Williams A, Dodds R, et al: The three-in-one proximal and distal soft tissue patellar realignment procedure: Results, and its place in the management of patellofemoral instability. *Am J Sports Med* 27:575-579, 1999.)

tempts had failed. After initial arthroscopic examination, the lateral and medial retinacula, patellar tendon, and superomedial patella were reached through a medial incision. The retinacula were divided, and a lateral release was performed, together with transfer of the patellar tendon to the tibial collateral ligament (Fig 1). The transferred portion of the patellar tendon formed an angle of 40 to 45 degrees with the intact tendon. Vastus medialis obliquus muscle advancement of 5 to 10 mm was performed with 3 or 4 interrupted plicating sutures (Fig 2). The retinaculum was then closed with a continuous suture.

Experience.—Forty-two knees of 37 patients were evaluated at a mean follow-up of 44 months. All knees had recurrent patellar dislocations preoperatively. The postoperative results were rated good or excellent in 76% of knees. Four knees had recurrent dislocation, a rate of 9.5%. The results were unaffected by skeletal immaturity, chondral damage, or gen-

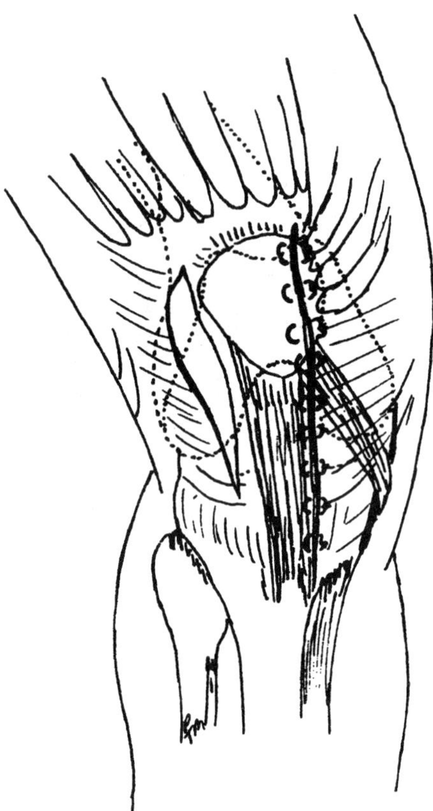

FIGURE 2.—Technique for advancement of the vastus medialis obliquus tendon insertion and closure of the medial retinaculum. (Courtesy of Myers P, Williams A, Dodds R, et al: The three-in-one proximal and distal soft tissue patellar realignment procedure: Results, and its place in the management of patellofemoral instability. *Am J Sports Med* 27:575-579, 1999.)

eralized ligamentous laxity. The results appeared to deteriorate significantly in from 2 to 4 years.

Conclusion.—In a combination procedure consisting of lateral release, vastus medialis obliquus transfer, and partial patellar tendon transfer for extensor mechanism realignment of the knee, the results are comparable to those achieved with other operative techniques. The surgical procedure for patellar instability should be selected according to the pathologic findings in the individual case. The 3-in-1 procedure described may be particularly appropriate for skeletally mature patients who have recurrent patellar instability with normal bony anatomy.

▶ As the article points out, this technique is a modification of the procedures described by Goldthwait,[1] Slocum et al,[2] and Mansat.[3] Of course, these 3 procedures, from a practical standpoint, are of only historical interest. Of concern is the fact that the results of this treatment deteriorated over time in the relatively short follow-up. Certainly, the indications and efficacy for the procedure described are not clear cut.

J. S. Torg, MD

References

1. Goldthwait JE: Slipping or recurrent dislocation of the patella, with the report of eleven cases. *Boston Med J* 150:169-174, 1904.
2. Slocum DB, Larson RL, James SL: Late reconstruction of ligamentous injuries of the medial compartment of the knee. *Clin Orthop* 100:23-55, 1974.
3. Mansat C: Déséquilibres rotuliens et instabilitiés rotatoires: Conceptions physio-pathologiques et thérapeutiques. Les stabilisations dynamiques internes (Symposium). *Rev Chir Orthop Reparatrice Appar Mot* 66:226-232, 1980.

Biomechanical Analysis of Flat and Oblique Tibial Tubercle Osteotomy for Recurrent Patellar Instability

Cosgarea AJ, Schatzke MD, Seth AK, et al (Johns Hopkins Univ, Baltimore, Md; Ohio State Univ, Columbus)
Am J Sports Med 27:507-512, 1999

3–15

Background.—Among the surgical procedures for treatment of patellar instability, the flat (Elmslie-Trillat) and oblique (Fulkerson) osteotomies are widely used to move the tibial tuberosity medially. In addition, the resultant anterior displacement that occurs in the oblique osteotomy decreases patellofemoral forces. However, there have been reports of proximal tibial fractures during early weight-bearing in patients who have undergone oblique osteotomy. The strength and failure mechanisms in the early postoperative phase after flat and oblique osteotomy were studied.

Methods.—Investigators obtained 13 pairs of matched, fresh-frozen cadaveric knees. The specimens were free of evidence of significant liga-

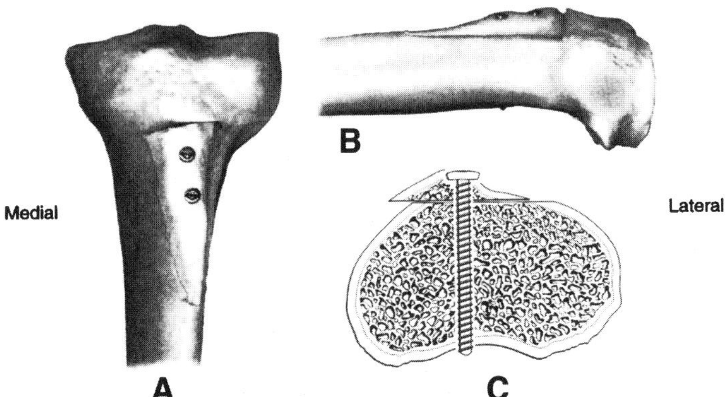

FIGURE 1.—The flat (modified Elmslie-Trillat) osteotomy. **A,** Anterior surface; **B,** lateral side; **C,** cross section at the level of the proximal screw. (Courtesy of Cosgarea AJ, Schatzke MD, Seth AK, et al: Biomechanical analysis of flat and oblique tibial tubercle osteotomy for recurrent patellar instability. *Am J Sports Med* 27:507-512, 1999.)

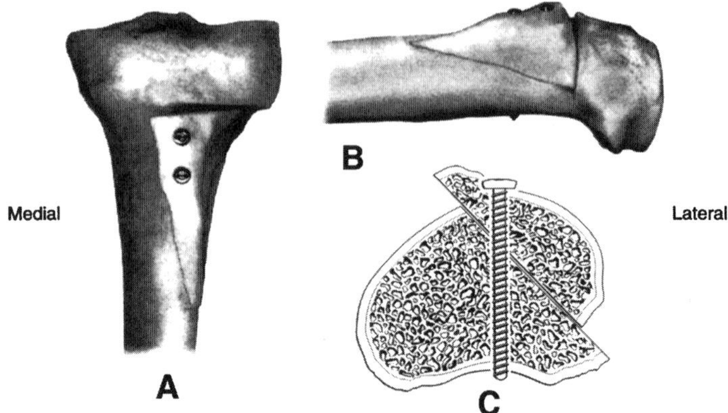

FIGURE 2.—The oblique (modified Fulkerson) osteotomy. **A,** Anterior surface; **B,** lateral side; **C,** cross section at the level of the proximal screw. (Courtesy of Cosgarea AJ, Schatzke MD, Seth AK, et al: Biomechanical analysis of flat and oblique tibial tubercle osteotomy for recurrent patellar instability. *Am J Sports Med* 27:507-512, 1999.)

ment damage or prior surgery. The mean age of the donors at death was 86 years. From each pair of specimens, investigators randomly assigned 1 knee to either the flat (Fig 1) or oblique (Fig 2) osteotomy. After surgery, the knees were tested to failure by loading through the quadriceps tendons at a rate of 1000 N/s. The aim of the test was to simulate an injury caused by stumbling. Comparisons between the 2 procedures were made by means of the Wilcoxon signed rank sum test for load to failure, total energy to failure, and stiffness.

Results.—There was a significantly higher mean load to fracture with the flat osteotomy (1639 N) as compared with the oblique osteotomy (1166 N). Total energy to failure was also higher in the flat osteotomy (224 N·m) as compared with the oblique osteotomy (127 N·m). However, the difference in stiffness between the 2 procedures was not significant (87 N/cm for the flat vs 74 N/cm for the oblique). In the flat osteotomies, the mechanism for failure was more likely to be tubercle "shingle" fracture. In the oblique osteotomies, the failure was more frequently by means of a tibial fracture or fixation failure in the posterior tibial cortex.

Conclusion.—The authors recommend use of the flat osteotomy in patients with isolated recurrent patellar instability. Use of the oblique technique is recommended for patients with concomitant patellofemoral pain or articular degenerative changes. When an oblique osteotomy is performed, the knee should be braced postoperatively and weight-bearing restricted until the osteomy is healed.

▶ As we recently reported,[1] a modified Elmslie-Trillat-Maquet procedure is indicated in patients with or without significant patellar or trochlear articular damage as well as in those with patellofemoral pain caused by degenerative changes. Because this study by Cosgarea et al did not include clinical correlation, their conclusion that the oblique osteotomy is indicated in patients with concomitant patellofemoral pain or articular degenerative changes and that the flat osteotomy is indicated in those without significant patellar or trochlear articular damage is not supported by the data.

J. S. Torg, MD

Reference

1. Naranja RJ Jr, Reilly PJ, Fuhlman JR, et al: Long-term evaluation of the Elmslie-Trillat-Maquet procedure for patello-femoral dysfunction. *Am J Sports Med* 924:679-784, 1996.

Comparison of Performance-based and Patient-reported Measures of Function in Anterior-Cruciate-Ligament-Deficient Individuals
Borsa PA, Lephart SM, Irrgang JJ (Oregon State Univ, Corvallis; Univ of Pittsburgh, Pa)
J Orthop Sports Phys Ther 28:392-399, 1998   3–16

Objective.—Because there are few objective measures of disability after anterior cruciate ligament (ACL) injury, disability is usually assessed based on performance-based measures or patient-reported disability. Whether performance-based or patient-reported measures of function are more effective in estimating disability in individuals with ACL-deficient knee was investigated.

Methods.—A regression equation model was used to estimate disability in 29 patients (14 women), aged 18 to 50 years, on average, 41.7 months after injury, and on average, 2.4 months of rehabilitation. Patients rated knee function on a scale of 0 to 100 with the Lysholm Knee Scale and a version of the Cincinnati Knee Scale. Performance-based measures used the proprioception index, the static balance index, the 1-leg hop index, and the quadriceps isometric strength index.

Results.—The Cincinnati Knee Scale was the best estimator of disability. Performance-based measures had a low correlation to patient disability.

Conclusion.—Patient-reported measures are the most reliable estimates of disability in ACL-deficient knees.

▶ The best method of evaluating the amount of disability a patient with an ACL-deficient knee experiences is addressed in this study. It appears that patient-reported measures are the best method of assessing function. The patient's satisfaction with level of function often determines whether he or she will elect to have surgery or continue with a more conservative approach.

F. J. George, ATC, PT

Rigorous Statistical Reliability, Validity, and Responsiveness Testing of the Cincinnati Knee Rating System in 350 Subjects With Uninjured, Injured, or Anterior Cruciate Ligament–Reconstructed Knees

Barber-Westin SD, Noyes FR, McCloskey JW (Deaconess Hosp, Cincinnati, Ohio; Univ of Dayton, Ohio)

Am J Sports Med 27:402-416, 1999   3–17

Background.—A variety of instruments have been developed over the past 20 years for the assessment of outcome after reconstructive surgery on knee ligaments. However, their is little documentation in the English-language literature regarding the reliability, validity, and responsiveness of these instruments. The reliability, validity, and responsiveness of 1 widely used instrument, the Cincinnati Knee Rating system were assessed.

Methods.—The study included 3 population groups. Group 1 consisted of 250 patients who were observed prospectively an average of 27 months after surgery by a single surgeon to reconstruct the anterior cruciate ligament. This group included 177 men and 73 women with a mean age of 29 years at surgery. Questionnaires for the Cincinnati Knee Rating System were completed by the patients both before surgery and at the most recent follow-up. Data from these questionnaires were used to test the validity and responsiveness of the instrument. Group 2 included 50 patients with chronic knee injuries or disorders. This group comprised 28 men and 22 women with a mean age of 36 years. Among the injuries and disorders in this group were meniscal and knee ligament tears, patellofemoral disorders, and degenerative joint disease. Group 3 consisted of 50 volunteers with no history of knee surgery and no current complaints of knee problems. The mean age of the 22 men and 28 women in this group was 34 years. Data gathered from groups 2 and 3 were used to determine test-retest reliability. The 100 subjects in these 2 groups completed questionnaires for the Cincinnati Knee Rating System an average of 7 days after their baseline evaluation.

Results.—High test-retest reliability for the Cincinnati Knee Rating System was demonstrated in this study. The questionnaire showed good content, construct, and item-discriminant validity. There were no "floor effects", or worst possible score, for the overall rating score demonstrated before or after surgery. No "ceiling effects," or the best score possible, were seen before surgery and were found in only 22 patients (9%) at follow-up.

Conclusion.—Results of data analysis indicate acceptable levels of reliability, validity, and responsiveness of the Cincinnati Knee Rating System for use in assessing the outcome of knee ligament reconstruction.

▶ In addition to the authors' failure to clearly define *statistical reliability*, *validity*, and *responsiveness*, as well as *acceptable levels* and *floor or ceiling effects*, the reader is further confused by several other issues. That is, reliability "was quantified with the interclass correlation coefficient rather than the more common Pearson product-moment correlation coefficient" to "provide a more sensitive assessment of variability within the data." Also, "the overall rating is assessed differently for knees with acute injuries." And modifications were required for assessment of symptoms and ligament function in those patients who have not attempted strenuous activities after ACL reconstruction.

J. S. Torg, MD

Knee Instability After Injury to the Anterior Cruciate Ligament: Quantification of the Lachman Test
Lerat JL, Moyen BL, Cladière F, et al (Centre Hospitalier Lyon-Sud, France)
J Bone Joint Surg Br 82-B:42-47, 2000   3–18

Background.—The primary restraint of anterior tibial translation is the anterior cruciate ligament (ACL). Measuring the translation of the tibia relative to the femur is not possible with clinical tests. The dynamic radiologic protocol for quantifying anterior and posterior displacements at an angle of 20 degrees of flexion using a load of 9 kg was described.

Methods and Findings.—Anterior and posterior displacements in 487 knees with chronic deficiency of the ACL and in 563 normal knees were measured. Stress radiography was done with a simple apparatus, which maintained the knee at 20 degrees of flexion while a 9-kg load was applied. Posterior translation in the 2 groups did not differ significantly. Measuring anterior translation was more reliable in the medial compartment than in the lateral compartment for diagnosing ACL rupture, with better specificity, sensitivity, and predictive values. The classification of anterior laxity based on the differential anterior translation of the medial compartment revealed 4 grades, each of which could be further classified into 4 subgroups for laxity of the lateral compartment. In each subgroup, either internal or external rotation may dominate. Sometimes major translation of both compartments is noted.

Conclusions.—Radiologic assessment of displacement of the knee in 20 degrees of flexion provides conclusive evidence of ACL rupture. With the use of laxity classification, surgical treatment specifically adapted for each type of laxity can be performed.

▶ It is certainly agreed that the Lachman test "has been shown to be the most reliable diagnostic sign of the ruptured ACL." To be questioned regarding this study is what advantages this radiographic method has when compared with the KT1000 device. Also to be questioned is the clinical relevance of the determinations.

J. S. Torg, MD

Eighteen- to Twenty-five-Year Follow-up After Acute Partial Anterior Cruciate Ligament Rupture

Messner K, Maletius W (Linköping Univ, Sweden)
Am J Sports Med 27:455-459, 1999　　　　　　　　　　　　　3–19

Introduction.—The term *partial anterior cruciate ligament (ACL) rupture* is used to describe varying degrees of initial damage to the ACL that may range from bleeding at 1 insertion point of the ligament to a rupture of 75% of the substance. Few patients with up to 50% ACL damage experience significant instability. Longitudinal data concerning knee function, activity, and radiographic osteoarthrosis in 22 consecutive patients with minor knee instability after a partial rupture of the ACL were reported.

Methods.—Data were available for all patients at 12-year follow-up. Twenty-year follow-up data were available for all except 1 patient, who died. Mean patient age at initial trauma was 29 years (range, 13-53 years). In all cases, diagnosis was based on stability testing with the patients under anesthesia, radiographic evaluation, and arthroscopy within 10 days of trauma. All patients experienced acute concomitant injuries in the injured knee. Nineteen patients were treated nonoperatively. Of the remaining 3 patients, 2 and 1, respectively, underwent surgical reattachment of complete rupture of the anteromedial and posterolateral bundle of the ACL. Patients were re-examined clinically and with weight-bearing radiographs after 9 to 16 years (mean, 12 years) and again at 18 to 25 years (mean, 20 years). The Lysholm score was used to assess knee function.

Results.—No patients needed to undergo ACL reconstruction during follow-up. Patients had excellent Lysholm knee function scores, which did not change between the 12- and 20-year follow-ups. At late follow-up, patients' activity level dropped from a median preinjury level of 7 (of a possible 10) to a median level of 6 after full rehabilitation. At 12-year follow-up, the median activity level was 5. This shows a change from recreational team sports (level 7) to physical fitness activities, including regular biking or jogging. At both the 12- and 20-year follow-up, 5 patients reported that they still performed at their preinjury levels. At 20-year follow-up, 12 patients were fully satisfied with knee function and 9 were partially satisfied. Eighteen reported that knee injury did not affect their work at all. Eight patients had a 1+ Lachman sign, 2 had a 2+ Lachman sign, and 1 had a 1+ positive pivot shift at 20-year follow-up. At late follow-up, 7 knees had no signs of radiographic osteoarthrosis, 10 had Fairbank's signs, and 3 had minor and 1 had major joint space reductions. Of 12 patients with a longitudinal radiographic observation, 3 knees had developed a greater degree of osteoarthritis and 9 remained unchanged. Mean patient age at follow-up was 48 years.

Conclusion.—This is the first 20-year follow-up report of patients with arthroscopically diagnosed partial ACL tears. Patients in this small series had a good 20-year prognosis, even in the presence of concomitant injuries. It is not likely that these findings will change with time, because activity demands will probably diminish. These results are regarded as the final outcome.

▶ The observation by the authors that these patients maintained good knee function and that major increase in knee laxity was the exception is in keeping with my own clinical experience.

J. S. Torg, MD

Arthroscopic Anterior Cruciate Ligament Reconstruction With Quadriceps Tendon–Patellar Bone Autograft
Chen C-H, Chen W-J, Shih C-H (Chang Gung Mem Hosp, Taoyuan, Taiwan)
J Trauma 46:678-682, 1999   3–20

Background.—The most common injury to knee ligaments is injury to the anterior cruciate ligament (ACL). Arthroscopic surgical reconstruction of the ACL is indicated for patients with ACL-deficient knees with symptomatic instability or patients with multiple ligament injuries. Generally, surgeons have used the bone–patellar tendon–bone autograft or hamstring or quadriceps tendons. An alternative technique for arthroscopic ACL reconstruction with the use of a quadriceps tendon–patellar bone autograft was reported.

Methods.—This alternative technique was used in 12 patients, 8 men and 4 women, requiring athroscopic surgery for ACL reconstruction. The mean age was 26 years, with a range of 20 to 39 years. Indications for surgery included acute ACL complete tear; tear of the ACL associated with meniscus or ligament injury; deficient ACL with anterior instability of grade 3 or greater and limitations in athletics and some activities of daily living; and symptomatic chronic anterior instability. Figure 1 illustrates the harvest of graft material from the proximal patella. Autologous bone from the bony tunnels was used to fill the bony defect in the patella. After debridement of the ACL remnant and location of the tibial footprint, the tibial tunnel was placed in the posterior half and medial-lateral center of the native ACL tibial footprint. This was done to minimize the risk of anterior graft impingement.

The femoral footprint was completely debrided and the femoral tunnel placed at the 11 o'clock position. The graft was fixed with a Beath pin at the patellar end of the quadriceps tendon–patella construct and an interference screw at the femoral bone plug. The tendon end of the graft was fixed to the anteromedial tibia with the knee in full extension with a bicortical screw and washer to which the sutures were tied. After stability testing and arthroscopic check for tension, a cold compression device was applied, and the knee braced and locked in full extension. One week after surgery, the patients were started on rehabilitation programs.

Results.—After a follow-up of 15 to 24 months, 10 of 12 patients returned to sports activity at the same or a higher level than before injury; 10 of 12 patients had ratings of normal or nearly normal based on the

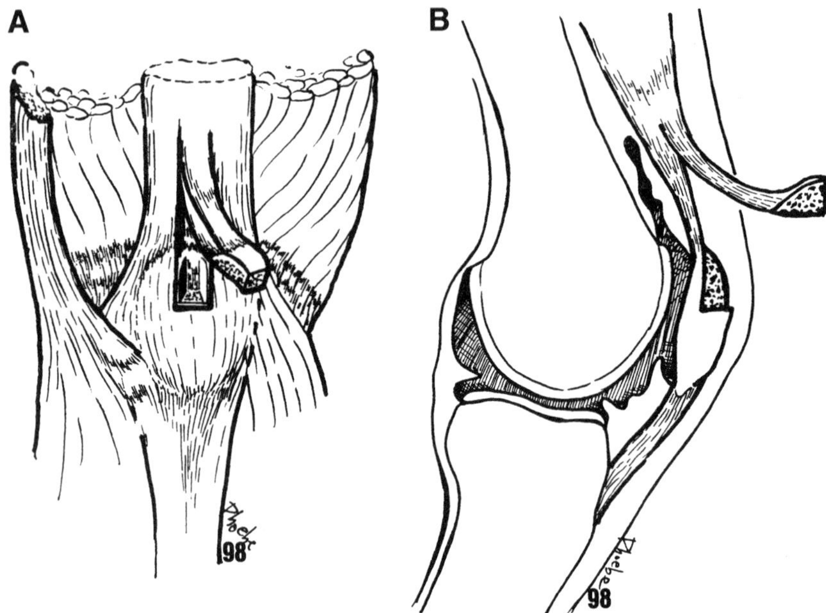

FIGURE 1.—**A** and **B**, Harvest of the combined rectus femoris and superior portion of the vastus intermedius with a bone plug from the proximal patella. (Courtesy of Chen C-H, Chen W-J, and Shih C-H: Arthroscopic anterior cruciate ligament reconstruction with quadriceps tendon-patellar bone autograft. *J Trauma* 46:678-682, 1999.)

International Knee Documentation Committee rating system. In 11 patients, quadriceps muscle strength returned to 80% of normal within 1 year.

Conclusion.—The quadriceps tendon–patellar bone autograft offers a number of advantages. The graft is larger and stronger than the patellar tendon, and morbidity with this harvest technique is lower than with the patellar tendon graft. There is minimal loss of strength in the quadriceps muscle after the procedure, and aggressive rehabilitation can provide a quicker return to athletic activity. This technique is an appropriate alternative for patients requiring ACL reconstruction but is not suited for either hamstring tendon autograft or bone–patellar tendon–bone autograft.

▶ Presented is a graft choice for ACL reconstruction with which I have not had experience. It should be noted that this is a small series with short follow-up that averaged 18 months (range, 15-24 months). However, the conclusion that the quadriceps tendon–patella autograft is "a reasonable alternative graft choice in primary revision ACL reconstruction when bone–patellar tendon–bone or hamstring tendons are not suitable for use" appears reasonable.

J. S. Torg, MD

The Effect of Cryotherapy on Intraarticular Temperature and Postoperative Care After Anterior Cruciate Ligament Reconstruction
Ohkoshi Y, Ohkoshi M, Nagasaki S, et al (Hakodate Central Gen Hosp, Japan)
Am J Sports Med 27:357-362, 1999   3–21

Background.—Cryotherapy was used to treat the pain and swelling that occurred after anterior cruciate ligament (ACL) reconstruction because of its ability to lower the temperature of tissue and thereby suppress metabolic activity. The effect of cryotherapy on intra-articular temperature and clinical results were studied.

Methods.—Isolated ACL reconstruction was performed on 21 knees; silicone balloon catheters were then implanted to measure intra-articular temperature while providing drainage. The knee was chilled, the air tourniquet was released, and the temperature of the knee was monitored for 48 hours. The patients were divided into 3 groups: a control group that was not exposed to cooling, a group exposed to 5°C of cooling, and 1 exposed to 10°C of cooling. The amount of blood loss, pain, and range of motion were evaluated to reveal the short-term clinical effects of cryotherapy.

Results.—Temperatures in the control group knees increased and then reached a thermostatic phase. Three phases were observed in the cooled knees: a low-temperature phase immediately after reconstruction, a temperature-rising phase, and a thermostatic phase. The suprapatellar pouch and the intercondylar notch temperatures were significantly lower than the body temperature during the low-temperature phase. In the 10°C group, both the pain score and the amount of analgesic required were less than in the control group, and blood loss in the 5°C group was significantly less than in the control group.

Conclusions.—Cryotherapy appears to reduce pain and temperature in knees that on which ACL reconstruction is performed. Thus, the patient may need fewer doses of analgesics for a level of comfort to be maintained.

▶ This study effectively demonstrates the effect of cryotherapy in the group of 21 patients who underwent ACL reconstruction. Specifically, both the pain score and the number of doses of analgesic required were significantly decreased in the cryotherapy groups. The study did not, however, clarify the optimal duration for cryotherapy or the effects of the anesthetic used.

J. S. Torg, MD

Absorbable and Metal Interference Screws: Comparison of Graft Security During Healing
Walton M (Univ of Otago, Dunedin, New Zealand)
Arthroscopy 15:818-826, 1999   3–22

Background.—To avoid the disadvantages of the use of metal interference screws, various screws are now made from absorbable polymers. The ability of an absorbable polyglyconate screw to hold a graft in position until healing after anterior cruciate ligament replacement was compared with the efficacy of a metal screw.

Methods.—Anterior cruciate ligament replacement surgery with the placement of a bone–patellar tendon–bone autograft was performed on 71 sheep. The sheep were fully bearing weight on the limb that was operated on within 5 days. Most of the specimens were retrieved within 12 weeks, except for 3 long-term specimens (1 was retrieved at 26 weeks and 2 were retrieved at 52 weeks). The specimens were then evaluated for mechanical and histological variables.

Results.—All of the grafts were successfully maintained in vivo. The failure strengths of the absorbable screws were initially lower but did not differ statistically from those of the metal screws. No difference was seen at 4 weeks. Histologic evaluation showed incorporation after 6 weeks, with a mild tissue reaction seen when the absorbable screw was used. Fibrous tissue almost completely replaced the screw in the specimens retrieved at 52 weeks.

Conclusions.—No significant differences were noted between the absorbable and the metal screws with respect to ability to hold the graft in position. The polyglyconate screw has the advantage of being absorbable when its supporting role is fulfilled.

▶ Several disadvantages of metal interference screws are recognized. Specifically, they may complicate subsequent surgery whether it is for graft failure or for total joint arthroplasty. This is a good study that clearly demonstrates that "although its performance was neither better nor worse, its greater value lies in its ability to [be absorbed] after having held the autograft sufficiently long for healing to have occurred."

J. S. Torg, MD

Outcomes of Postoperative Septic Arthritis After Anterior Cruciate Ligament Reconstruction

McAllister DR, Parker RD, Cooper AE, et al (Cleveland Clinic Found, Ohio)
Am J Sports Med 27:562-570, 1999   3–23

Objective.—Results of a retrospective review of septic arthritis after arthroscopically guided anterior cruciate ligament (ACL) reconstruction and its outcomes are reported.

Methods.—Between 1987 and 1998, arthroscopically guided ACL reconstruction was performed on 831 consecutive patients. Inpatient hospitalization costs were tallied and compared for patients with and without complications.

Results.—Postoperative septic arthritis developed in 4 (0.48%) male patients, aged 20 to 34 years. Three patients had chronic ACL deficiency and had had previous surgeries. All were treated with immediately arthroscopic lavage, incision, and drainage, extensive arthroscopic debridement of necrotic tissue, and partial synovectomy. All were given IV antibiotics for an average of 4.75 weeks and oral antibiotics for 3 weeks. All grafts were intact and all were retained. Aggressive deep wound debridement and extensive pulsatile lavage were performed. Loose packing and drains were inserted. Patients had an average of 2.75 procedures. The average inpatient hospital stay was 12.25 days. After the infection was controlled, patients participated in physical therapy. At an average of 36 months, patients completed the 36-item Short-Form Health Survey, the International Knee Documentation Committee score, the modified Lysholm knee scoring scale, the Tegner activity score, the KT-1000 arthrometry quantitative functional testing, isokinetic strength evaluation, plain radiographs, and MRI. Three patients with normal scores have minimal limitations and pain. One patient, with significantly lower physical functioning scores, has mild limiting pain that limits participation in vigorous activities. The inferior outcome was possibly the result of secondary damage to the articular cartilage as a result of the infection.

Conclusion.—The outcome in these patients was inferior to that in patients without complications.

▶ This article is noteworthy in that it justifies preservation of the ACL ligament graft in the face of postoperative septic arthritis. Also to be noted, the graft was not removed for an average of 11 months after the initial reconstruction. Actually, this is a good news/bad news report, in that although the infection can be successfully eradicated with stability of the joint maintained and near full range of motion achieved, as might be expected, the clinical outcomes of these patients were inferior to those of patients who had undergone an uncomplicated procedure. The authors assume that this is the result of secondary damage to the articular cartilage from the infection.

J. S. Torg, MD

Neuromuscular Electrical Stimulation After Anterior Cruciate Ligament Surgery

Paternostro-Sluga T, Fialka Ch, Alacamliogliu Y, et al (Univ of Vienna)
Clin Orthop 368:166-175, 1999   3–24

Objective.—Strengthening of the quadriceps femoris and hamstring muscles is a major clinical goal in patients who have undergone repair or reconstruction of the anterior cruciate ligament. Although neuromuscular electric stimulation is at least as effective as isometric exercise in increasing muscle strength, the value of electric stimulation plus exercise versus exercise therapy alone has been questioned. The efficacy of neuromuscular electric stimulation in addition to exercise after anterior cruciate ligament surgery was evaluated.

Methods.—The randomized controlled trial included 49 patients undergoing anterior cruciate ligament repair (24 knees) or reconstruction (25 knees). One group participated in neuromuscular stimulation plus exercise therapy; another participated in exercise plus transcutaneous electric nerve stimulation, used for its analgesic effect; and the third was consigned to exercise alone. Otherwise, all patients received a standardized rehabilitation program. The 2 types of electric stimulation were continued for 6 weeks after surgery. Isometric and isokinetic torque were measured in the knee extensor and flexor muscles at 6, 12, and 52 weeks postoperatively.

Results.—At no time during follow-up were the muscle strength values significantly different between groups. Regarding quadriceps isometric strength parameters, the descriptive evaluation showed a somewhat better tendency at 6 weeks in patients receiving neuromuscular electric stimulation. All patients complied with their rehabilitation regimen, including neuromuscular or transcutaneous electric stimulation.

Conclusion.—In patients undergoing anterior cruciate ligament repair or reconstruction, adding neuromuscular electric stimulation does not improve muscle strength more than an early exercise program alone. The good results achieved in this study are attributed to early and intensive exercise, a short period of knee immobilization, and the promptness of surgery after injury.

▶ Presented is a study with what may be defined as negative findings, with which I am in complete agreement.

J. S. Torg, MD

Operative Treatment of Arthrofibrosis of the Knee
Lindenfeld TN, Wojtys EM, Husain A (Deaconess Hosp, Cincinnati, Ohio; Univ of Michigan, Ann Arbor)
J Bone Joint Surg Am 81-A:1772-1784, 1999   3–25

Objective.—Arthrofibrosis encompasses a variety of knee conditions characterized by dense proliferative scar formation that progressively limits motion. Operative treatment and outcomes are discussed.

Characteristics.—Prevalence of complications after anterior cruciate ligament (ACL) reconstruction ranges from 4% to 35%. Diagnosis involves elimination of other causes of restricted activity and passive motion, including mechanical problems, neurologic deficit, acute injury, knee effusion, and joint immobilization. Unfortunately, arthrofibrosis can coexist with some of these conditions. Timing of reconstruction and its relationship to loss of motion is controversial. Poor rehabilitation is related to loss of motion. The cause is multifactorial and is typically related to injury or surgery. Clinical symptoms vary, but patients usually complain of stiffness, and a warm, swollen knee that is painful with motion, an antalgic, flexed-knee gait, atrophy of the quadriceps, and restricted flexion and extension. Articular cartilage degeneration, fibrous tissue formation, and soft-tissue chondrification and ossification are frequently seen. Patella infera is a severe complication that is found in 9% to 15% of patients. Scar formation and, less commonly, fibrosis, can cause loss of extension. Loss of flexion usually results from intraarticular fibrosis and scarring of the patellofemoral mechanism. Arthrofibrosis can result from aggressive inflammation. Intraarticular adhesions and capsular contracture, form early in the disease process. Synovial tissue contains dense fibrovascular tissue and chondrometaplasia.

Treatment.—Preventive measures should be instituted to control pain and inflammation after injury or surgery. Immobilization should be minimized, and physical therapy should be emphasized. Forced manipulation should be avoided. Arthroscopic treatment is the procedure of choice if surgical intervention is required.

Results.—Operative treatment usually improves knee motion, particularly if intervention takes place early. Functional outcome depends on the extent of arthrofibrosis.

> *Technique.*—Baseline muscle function, flexion, extension, and patellar mobility are documented and compared with the contralateral side. Articular cartilage is preserved. A lateral retinacular release is performed. A partial medial release may be necessary. The vastus lateralis and vastus medialis are not detached from the quadriceps tendon. All fibrous and scar tissue must be excised. The meniscus is displaced anteriorly, if possible. A posterior capsular release may be necessary. Once the normal volume of the suprapatellar pouch and the medial and lateral recesses have been restored, the knee is brought into gentle flexion.

Postoperative Care.—Pain relief is provided and continuous passive motion and heel hangs are started within 24 hours. The patients may require daily physical therapy for weeks.

Complications.—Failure to improve or loss of motion are common complications. Reoperation rates are as high as 43%. Other complications are related to the severity of the arthrofibrosis. These patients are also at risk of deep vein thrombosis and should receive mechanical and chemical prophylaxis.

▶ This is a comprehensive review of management of a very difficult post-surgical problem. Important principles presented are (1) arthroscopic treatment is the procedure of choice when limitation of motion is not progressive primarily because of a discreet intraarticular lesion, and (2) although the primary goal of operative treatment is restoration of joint motion, the important secondary goal is preservation of articular cartilage. The original article is recommended reading for all those dealing with surgical problems of the knee.

J. S. Torg, MD

The Natural History of Acute, Isolated, Nonoperatively Treated Posterior Cruciate Ligament Injuries: A Prospective Study
Shelbourne KD, Davis TJ, Patel DV (Methodist Sports Medicine Ctr, Indianapolis)
Am J Sports Med 27:276-283, 1999   3–26

Objective.—Previous reports suggest that patients with isolated tears of the posterior cruciate ligament (PCL) have good outcomes. The authors' experience suggests that the results achieved with surgical repair are similar to those of nonoperative treatment. There are few prospective data on the natural history of these injuries. A prospective study of the natural history of acute, isolated, nonoperatively treated PCL tears was reported.

Methods.—The study included 122 athletically active patients—110 males and 23 females; average age, 25 years—with acute isolated PCL injuries. Most of the injuries occurred as a result of low-velocity, sports-related trauma. All patients underwent nonoperative treatment, which included a home rehabilitation program to restore motion and strength. For an average of 5 years after injury, the patients completed an annual subjective questionnaire. In addition, long-term clinical follow-up, including posterior laxity testing, was available for 68 patients.

Results.—In 93% of the patients with clinical follow-up, the PCL laxity grade was essentially unchanged from the time of the initial injury to follow-up. The laxity grade was unrelated to radiographic joint space narrowing. At follow-up, the mean modified Noyes knee score was 84 points, the mean Lysholm score was 83, and the mean Tegner activity score was 6. These subjective knee scores were unrelated to the degree of posterior laxity or to time since injury. About one half of the patients were able to return to sports participation at the same level or higher, one third returned to sports at a lower level, and one sixth did not resume participation in the same sport. The likelihood of returning to sport was unrelated to the amount of posterior laxity.

Conclusions.—This prospective study suggests that isolated, nonoperatively treated PCL injuries generally heal with some degree of residual knee laxity, which does not increase during follow-up. Few patients have symptomatic meniscal tears; medial joint arthrosis develops in some, but this is unrelated to the degree of laxity. The amount of laxity is not correlated with objective or subjective knee function or with level of return to sports participation.

▶ The conclusion that "acute isolated posterior cruciate ligament tears treated nonoperatively achieved a level of objective and subjective knee function that was independent of the grade of laxity" is in keeping with the conclusions of our study on the natural history of the posterior cruciate ligament–deficient knee published in 1989.[1]

J. S. Torg, MD

Reference

1. Torg JS, Barton TM, Pavlov H, et al: Natural history of the posterior cruciate ligament–deficient knee. *Clin Orthop* 246:208-216, 1989.

Posterior Cruciate Ligament Injuries of the Knee Joint
Janousek AT, Jones DG, Clatworthy M, et al (Univ of Pittsburgh, Pa)
Sports Med 28:429-441, 1999

3–27

Objective.—There is no general agreement on how to treat posterior cruciate ligament (PCL) injuries. A review of PCL injuries and a treatment algorithm are presented.

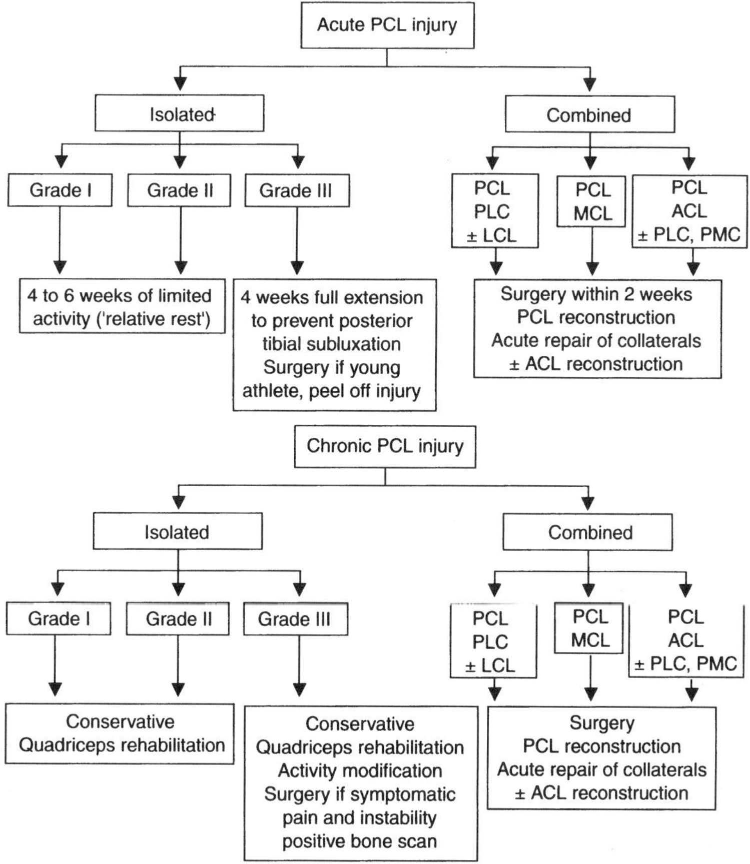

FIGURE 9.—Treatment algorithm for acute (*top*) and chronic (*bottom*) PCL injuries. *Abbreviations: ACL*, anterior cruciate ligament; LCL, lateral collateral ligament; MCL, medial collateral ligament; PLC, posterolateral corner; PMC, posteromedial corner. (Courtesy of Janousek AT, Jones DG, Clatworthy M, et al: Posterior cruciate ligament injuries of the knee joint. *Sports Med* 28:429-441, 1999.)

Anatomy and Biomechanics.—PCL restrains posterior tibial translation and external rotation and reduces articular contact pressures. The natural history has not been defined, but patients with isolated grade I or II PCL injuries do well in the short term. Degenerative changes will develop over time in the medial and patellofemoral compartment in some patients.

Incidence.—The reported incidence of PCL injuries varies from 3% to 38%.

Mechanism of Injury.—The 3 mechanisms proposed for PCL rupture are hyperflexion, prefibial trauma, and hyperextension.

Clinical Evaluation.—The clinical evaluation should include a thorough history, physical findings, and examination of all ligamentous structures of the ligamentous structures of the knee. Ancillary tests included radiographs and MRI.

Decision Making.—Treatment depends on the injury site and degree of laxity (Fig 9).

Nonoperative Treatment.—Nonoperative treatment is effective for patients with isolated grade I or II tears.

Operative Treatment.—Operative treatment is recommended for patients with symptomatic grade III and combined ligament injuries. Most injuries respond best to surgical management.

Postoperative Rehabilitation.—After 4 weeks of immobilization, patients are given active and passive range-of-motion exercise progressively over a period of 2 months.

Conclusion.—PCL injuries have a variety of causes. The type of injury determines the management. A skilled diagnosis is required to rule out neurologic injury. Extensive rehabilitation is required after repair.

▶ This comprehensive review is nicely illustrated and presents a workable algorithm for management of both acute and chronic PCL injuries. It is recommended reading for those involved in management of athletic injuries to the knee joint.

J. S. Torg, MD

Three-dimensional Knee Kinematics and Stability in Patients With a Posterior Cruciate Ligament Tear

Jonsson H, Kärrholm J (Univ Hosp in Northern Sweden, Umeå; Sahlgren Univ Hosp, Gothenburg, Sweden)
J Orthop Res 17:185-191, 1999   3–28

Background.—Conservative treatment is effective for isolated injuries to the posterior cruciate ligament. However, injuries to additional ligaments complicate the clinical picture and make conservative treatment less likely to achieve a favorable outcome. In recent studies, degenerative changes in the knee were seen over time in patients with isolated tears of the posterior cruciate. In addition, although instability is a major factor in development of osteoarthritis among patients with anterior cruciate ligament injuries, patients with injuries to the posterior cruciate ligament report knee instability, or "giving way" less frequently. The posterior cruciate ligament may be the most loaded ligament during walking, and climbing stairs places even greater loads on the ligament.

This study investigated the 3-dimensional kinematics and stability of the knee in a group of patients with tears of the posterior cruciate ligament. Specifically, investigators questioned whether climbing stairs affects knee kinematics in patients with an insufficient posterior cruciate ligament, whether a posterior cruciate ligament injury can be diagnosed with an instrumented anterior-posterior drawer test, and whether injury of the ligament altered coupled motions on the anterior-posterior drawer test.

Methods.—Eight patients, one woman and seven men, were studied. At the time of injury, the average age of the patients was 27 years, and they were examined at a mean of 4.4 years after injury (range, 5 months to 15 years). Six of the 8 patients had been injured during athletic activities, and 2 had sustained fractured femurs in conjunction with their ligament injury. Investigators performed several radiostereometric examinations while patients ascended a platform (the step-up test) as well as during instrumented anterior-posterior drawer tests, with the patient's knee placed in 30 degrees of flexion. The contralateral knee served as a control.

Results.—Although no changes in knee kinematics were demonstrated in the step-up test, investigators observed an increase in posterior laxity in all 8 patients. An increase of more than 2 mm in side-to-side laxity, both anteriorly and posteriorly, was noted in 4 patients.

Conclusion.—Results of the anterior-posterior drawer test indicated that it is possible to diagnose a rupture of the posterior cruciate ligament at 30 degrees of flexion; however, increased interior laxity can be misinterpreted as anterior cruciate ligament injury. The findings of unaffected knee kinematics during the step-up test suggest that during static examinations, joint load and congruity and muscle activity can compensate for an insufficient posterior cruciate ligament.

▶ This article corroborates our observations, published 11 years ago, that unidirectional posterior cruciate ligament (PCL) laxity behaves differently than multidirectional laxity.[1] The observation that "a rupture of the posterior cruciate ligament . . . can be erroneously interpreted as an injury to the anterior cruciate ligament" is well taken. To the experienced examiner, PCL laxity can be discerned by flexing both hips and both knees to 90 degrees and observing the posterior slope of the infrapatella tendon-proximal tibial metaphysis silhouette. With regard to manual stress examination, PCL laxity/instability presents with a negative Lachmans test and either anterior or posterior translation when a drawer examination is attempted.

J. S. Torg, MD

Reference

1. Torg JS, Barton TM, Pavlov H, et al: Natural history of the posterior cruciate ligament-deficient knee. *Clin Orthop* 246:208-216,1989.

Fasciotomy for Exertional Anterior Compartment Syndrome: Is Lateral Compartment Release Necessary?
Schepsis AA, Gill SS, Foster TA (Boston Med Ctr)
Am J Sports Med 27:430-435, 1999   3–29

Background.—Exercise-induced pain in the lower extremity can be caused by exertional or chronic compartment syndrome. An effective treatment for this condition involves surgical decompression with the release of both the anterior and the lateral compartments. The results when only anterior compartment release was performed were compared with those obtained with the use of the standard surgical approach.

Methods.—Thirty anterior compartment release procedures were performed on 20 patients, all of whom were athletes in running sports; 10 of the procedures were bilateral operations. The 10 patients who underwent bilateral surgery had an anterior and lateral compartment release on 1 leg and only an anterior release on the other leg; for the other 10 patients, both an anterior and lateral compartment release and only an anterior compartment release were alternately done. The results were measured with a subjective questionnaire and a visual analog pain scale. Excellent and good results were deemed satisfactory, whereas fair and poor were seen as unsatisfactory.

Results.—Twenty-seven of the 30 limbs (90%) were rated to have satisfactory outcomes. Fourteen of 15 (93%) of those who had anterior compartment release only and 13 of 15 (87%) of those who had both anterior and lateral releases had satisfactory outcomes. Athletes who underwent unilateral surgery fully returned to sports 8.1 weeks after anterior release only and 11.4 weeks after anterior and lateral release. Those with bilateral surgery required 12.1 weeks for a full recovery and return to sports participation, and they reported a quicker recovery for the leg that underwent only anterior release.

Conclusions.—Release of only the anterior chamber in patients who have exertional anterior compartment syndrome but no lateral involvement appears to be sufficient treatment. This limited approach may produce less morbidity potential and achieves comparable success to that seen with the release of both lateral and anterior compartments.

▶ This is an interesting article by experienced clinicians. It should be noted that patients suspected of having lateral compartment involvement were excluded from the study. However, the authors do not state what criteria was used. The authors do ". . . realize that the difference is small, the numbers are small, and the return to sport somewhat subjective, but the important point is that patients who had isolated anterior compartment fasciotomy enjoyed the same success level as patients who had release of both anterior and lateral compartments and less potential morbidity, such as that seen in dual-compartment release patients who had unsatisfactory results." They further conclude that anterior compartment release is not necessary in those that have only signs and symptoms consistent with exertional anterior compartment syndrome. Unfortunately, I often have difficulty in distinguishing between the two.

J. S. Torg, MD

Chronic Achilles Tendinopathy in Athletic Individuals: Results of Nonsurgical Treatment
Angermann P, Hovgaard D (Glostrup Hosp, Denmark)
Foot Ankle Int 20:304-306, 1999   3–30

Background.—Chronic Achilles tendinopathy is classified as either peritendinitis or tendinosis. Peritendinitis is characterized by inflammation of the tendon sheath and thickening and adhesion formations in the 2 layers of the sheath. Tendinosis commonly occurs in patients over 35 years of age and is characterized by intratendinous degeneration. A patient may have tendinosis for years before experiencing clinical symptoms. Although the nonsurgical treatment of chronic Achilles tendinopathy is considered very effective, there is little documentation in the literature for either its efficacy or long-term results. The long-term results of nonsurgical treatment of chronic Achilles tendinopathy in 22 patients were studied.

Methods.—The 22 consecutive patients with chronic Achilles peritendinitis were 18 men and 4 women. The mean age at treatment was 38.5 years; all the patients had been active in sports before the onset of symptoms, and in all patients, the onset of symptoms had caused them to stop their athletic activities. Ten of the patients were runners, 7 played soccer, 3 played badminton, 1 played handball, and 1 played basketball. None of them did heavy work as part of their occupations. The affected tendon was swollen in 11 patients and tender in all patients. All patients were given a diagnosis of peritendinitis. Hyperpronation was also seen in 3 patients, and 6 had cavovarus deformity. Treatment included elevation of the heel by 1 cm for 3 months, twice weekly massage and stretching of the triceps surae muscle for 3 weeks, and a graduated training program until the patient returned to athletic activity or for a maximum of 6 months.

Results.—Improvement or cure was seen in 70% of patients immediately after the treatment period. At follow-up, improvement or cure was seen in 65% of patients. Treatment failure or a poor long-term result was seen in 35% of patients. Early surgery may have been considered for the patients who experienced treatment failure or a poor outcome, but only 1 patient had peritendinitis surgery.

Conclusion.—Nonsurgical treatment, with an emphasis on active training, is recommended for active athletic patients with chronic Achilles tendinopathy. However, surgery should be considered if there is no progress after 3 to 6 months of nonsurgical treatment.

▶ Although I do not disagree with either the observations or the conclusions presented by the authors, it should be pointed out that there was no randomized, surgically managed control group.

J. S. Torg, MD

Chronic Achilles Tendinosis: Recommendations for Treatment and Prevention

Alfredson H, Lorentzon R (Umeå Univ, Sweden; Natl Inst for Working Life, Umeå, Sweden)
Sports Med 29:135-146, 2000
3–31

Objective.—Although the cause of chronic Achilles tendinosis is not known, changes in the collagen fiber structure and arrangement have been documented. Treatment of chronic injury and prevention of injury are reviewed.

Treatment.—Most clinicians recommend conservative treatment directed at etiologic factors, including biomechanical divergences (correction of excessive pronation, correction of underpronation, correction of forefoot or rearfoot varus, and heel lifts for relaxation of tight calf muscles), correction of training errors, stretching exercises, eccentric strength training to improve muscle weakness, and proper footwear. Other conservative methods include corticosteroid injections, nonsteroidal antiinflammatory drugs, local cold therapy, heat, massage, US, electrical stimulation, and laser therapy, or a combination of conservative therapies. One uncontrolled pilot study produced good results with a 12-week specially designed heavy-load eccentric calf muscle training program. Results with the eccentric program were significantly better than those with a concentric training regimen.

Surgical Treatment.—Surgery is necessary in about 25% of patients, and the frequency increases with age, duration of symptoms, and occurrence of tendinopathic changes. The technique most commonly used involved a straight longitudinal incision, followed by incision of the paratenon, excision of adhesions, and partial excision of the paratenon itself, if necessary.

Rehabilitation.—Although rehabilitative methods vary greatly, good short-term surgical results have been obtained in 80% to 100% of patients. There are few long-term studies.

Complications.—The reported surgical complication rates varies from 4.7% to 13%.

Prevention.—Chronic Achilles tendinosis is thought to be an overuse injury often combined with biomechanical abnormalities. Strength and flexibility training for calf muscles, avoiding overtraining. strengthening the tendon, and proper equipment are important prevention strategies.

Conclusion.—Tendinosis is a difficult condition to treat, and about 25% of patients will require surgery. Controlled treatment and rehabilitation studies need to be conducted. Long-term results are lacking. Prevention strategies are discussed.

▶ This article is a well-referenced comprehensive review of the problems related to chronic Achilles tendinosis. The original article is recommended for the interested reader.

J. S. Torg, MD

Surgical Decompression of Chronic Central Core Lesions of the Achilles Tendon
Maffulli N, Binfield PM, Moore D, et al (Univ of Aberdeen, Scotland; Warwick Gen Hosp, England; The London Hosp Med College)
Am J Sports Med 27:747-752, 1999   3–32

Objective.—Overtraining and poor technique can lead to Achilles tendinopathy, including chronically inflamed, thickened, and fibrotic paratenons, in runners. When conservative treatment fails, surgery is sometimes necessary to spur the tendon cell-matrix environment to begin the repair process. Results of surgical decompression and curettage of chronic degenerative central core lesions of the Achilles tendon were presented.

Methods.—Between 1987 and 1995, 14 patients (12 men and 2 women, aged 19-54 years) who had experienced symptoms for at least 24 months before surgery, who had undergone conservative management, and who had surgery for Achilles tendinopathy at least 24 months before entering the study, underwent US or MRI studies and outpatient surgery. Patient status was followed up for an average of 35 months, at which time 10 of 14 patients were interviewed.

> *Technique.*—The Achilles tendon was exposed. The paratenon was excised, preserving the anterior fat in Kager's triangle. Suspicious areas of the tendon were explored by 3 to 5 tenotomies, and areas of necrosis or mucinoid degeneration were excised. Tenotomies were not repaired. The wound was closed in 2 layers. Patients were mobilized with crutches immediately and discharged within 8 hours. Patients were evaluated at 2 and 6 weeks and then at 6 months. Patients were allowed gradual progression to full sports activity at 16 to 20 weeks but were discouraged from participation in competitive sports before 6 months.

Results.—All patients were fully weight-bearing by the end of postoperative week 1. Two patients' superficial wound infections were successfully treated with antibiotics. Hypersensitivity of the wound in 3 patients resolved by week 6. A hypertrophic scar in 1 patient was successfully treated with corticosteroid injections. Two patients were dissatisfied with the appearance of their scars. Six patients of the 14 underwent reoperation, but only 2 improved. Two patients had excellent results (complete relief of pain and return to the preinjury sport level), and 3 patients had good results (full return to preinjury sport level with mild or intermittent discomfort). Of these, 2 were reoperated for exploration. Five patients had fair results (unable to return to preinjury sport level because of discomfort), and 4 had poor results (unable to return to sport and discomfort in ADL). Older patients and patients with a longer duration of symptoms tended to have poorer results.

Conclusion.—Results after surgical decompression of chronic Achilles tendinopathy with central core degeneration are poor. Earlier surgery would probably improve the prognosis.

Chronic Achilles Tendon Overuse Injury: Complications After Surgical Treatment: An Analysis of 432 Consecutive Patients
Paavola M, Orava S, Leppilahti J, et al (Univ of Tampere, Finland; UKK Inst, Tampere, Finland; Tohtoritalo 41400 Hosp, Turku, Finland; et al)
Am J Sports Med 28:77-82, 2000   3–33

Objective.—About 25% of Achilles tendon overuse injuries require surgery. Complications are the most important causes of delayed healing and poor outcome. Complications after surgery for Achilles tendon overuse complaints were analyzed.

Methods.—Between April 1986 and December 1995, 432 patients (96 female), aged 13 to 67 years, with chronic Achilles tendon overuse injury had surgery performed by 1 surgeon after conservative treatment failed.

> *Technique.*—A longitudinal incision (or L-shaped incision for patients with insertional disorders) was made to the lateral side of the Achilles tendon, and the crural fascia was excised. Adhesions were cleaned, and any hypertrophic retrocalcanear bursa was removed. The posterior upper corner of the calcaneus was removed. Degenerated tissue was debrided, and the remaining tendon was reapproximated with side-to-side sutures. The ankle was mobilized immediately. For partial tendon rupture, the leg was immobilized for 2 weeks and then the ankle was mobilized. The patient returned to full sport training at 6 to 12 weeks. Patients were followed for at least 5 months. Complications and outcome were recorded.

Results.—There were 46 (11%) complications including 16 major complications: 14 skin edge necrosis, 1 new partial rupture, and 1 deep vein thrombosis. There were 30 minor complications including 11 superficial wound infections, 5 seromas, 5 hematomas, 5 fibrotic reactions or scar formation, and 4 sural nerve irritations. Fourteen patients were reoperated. The remaining patients were treated nonsurgically.

Conclusion.—Although surgical treatment of chronic Achilles tendon overuse injuries carries a high complication rate, most patients make a full recovery and return to their preinjury activities.

▶ These 2 articles (Abstracts 3–32 and 3–33) delineate 2 very important problems associated with Achilles tendon surgery: (1) poor outcome and (2) postoperative complications. Certainly, a word to the wise should be sufficient.

J. S. Torg, MD

The Strength of Percutaneous Methods of Repair of the Achilles Tendon: A Biomechanical Study

Čretnik A, Žlajpah L, Smrkolj V, et al (Teaching Hosp Maribor, Slovenia; Jožef Stefan Inst, Ljubljana, Slovenia; Univ Med Ctr, Ljubljana, Slovenia; et al)
Med Sci Sports Exerc 32:16-20, 2000   3–34

Background.—The best treatment for fresh Achilles tendon rupture has not been established. Although percutaneous suturing of the rupture tendon under local anesthesia appears to combine the advantages of surgical

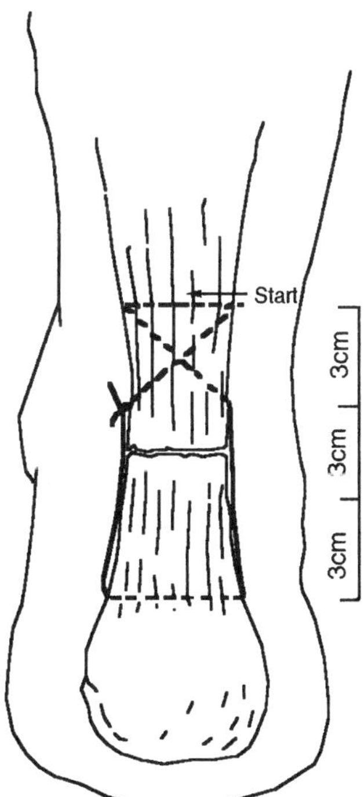

FIGURE 1.—Ma-Griffith repair configuration. (Courtesy of Čretnik A, Žlajpah L, Smrkolj V, et al: The strength of percutaneous methods of repair of the Achilles tendon: A biomechanical study. *Med Sci Sports Exerc* 32(1):16-20, 2000.)

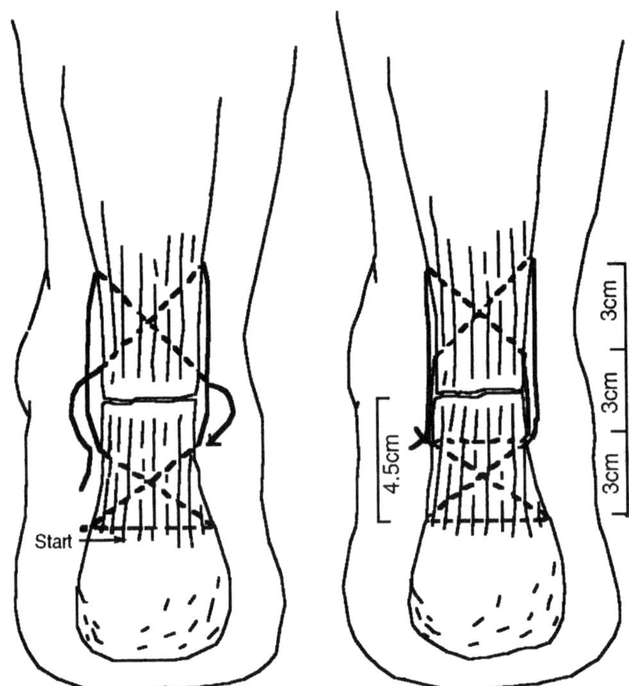

FIGURE 2.—The modified repair configuration. (Courtesy of Čretnik A, Žlajpah L, Smrokolj V, et al: The strength of percutaneous methods of repair of the Achilles tendon: A biomechanical study. *Med Sci Sports Exerc* 32(1):16-20, 2000.)

and conservative treatments, percutaneous suturing may be weaker than the open end-to-end repair. Whether a different percutaneous suturing technique can increase the strength of the repaired Achilles tendon was investigated.

Methods and Findings.—Thirty-six cadaveric Achilles tendons were used to compare different repairs. Repair strength and gapping resistance were assessed under different standardized experimental conditions. Each matched pair of cadaveric Achilles tendons was assigned randomly to repair by the original Ma-Griffith configuration (Fig 1) or to the new modified configuration (Fig 2). The tendons were then loaded to failure. The force displacement curve was measured by special equipment. The new modified technique resulted in significantly greater tensile strength and gapping resistance than did the Ma-Griffith repair configuration.

Conclusion.—These findings support the idea that stronger repairs can be achieved with new techniques for percutaneously suturing of the ruptured Achilles tendon. Under experimental conditions, the new modified technique nearly doubled the repair strength, compared with the Ma-Griffith repair.

▶ This well-designed in vitro study compares the strength of different Achilles tendon repairs. What is lacking, however, is clinical evidence that either repair would successfully withstand the stresses of currently employed early rehabilitation regimens.

J. S. Torg, MD

Percutaneous Tenodesis of the Achilles Tendon: A New Surgical Method for the Treatment of Acute Achilles Tendon Rupture Through Percutaneous Tenodesis
Gorschewsky O, Vogel U, Schweizer A, et al (Klink Permanece, Berne, Switzerland)
Injury 30:315-321, 1999   3–35

Objective.—Although Achilles tendon rupture is usually treated operatively, postoperative complications range from 11% to 29%. A cost-effective, reproducible, and simple percutaneous surgical procedure was developed that leads to good functional results and reduces the postoperative complication rate.

Methods.—The percutaneous tenodesis technique used 2 Lengemann extension wires to repair complete fresh Achilles tendon ruptures in 20 men, aged 28 to 58 years (Fig 4). Mobilization began on the day of surgery. Progressive rehabilitation exercises continued through the sixth postoperative week when the Lengemann wires were removed to beyond 3 months after surgery. Patients were evaluated at 2 and 6 weeks, 3 and 6 months, and 1 year for strength of calf muscle, range of ankle motion, calf circumference, and wound healing. Patients rated function, strength, and pain at 1 year.

Results.—Patients had surgery within 22 hours of injury. The operation lasted 20 minutes. The average hospital stay was 2.2 days (range, 1-5 days). Most patients were able to return to work at least part-time within 3 weeks. All patients were able to return to their sport after 4.2 months. One patient was injured at 3 weeks and reruptured the tendon. He was treated conservatively and had restricted mobility and ankle muscle strength at 8 months. His result was judged satisfactory. The remaining patients had very good results at 1 year.

Conclusion.—The outcome for percutaneous tenodesis was very good in 95% of patients. The complication rate was 5%.

▶ What is described as a percutaneous tenodesis certainly looks like an open procedure. Also, postoperative follow-up of 1 year was inadequate. However, from a technical standpoint, the procedure is interesting and longer follow-up is required.

J. S. Torg, MD

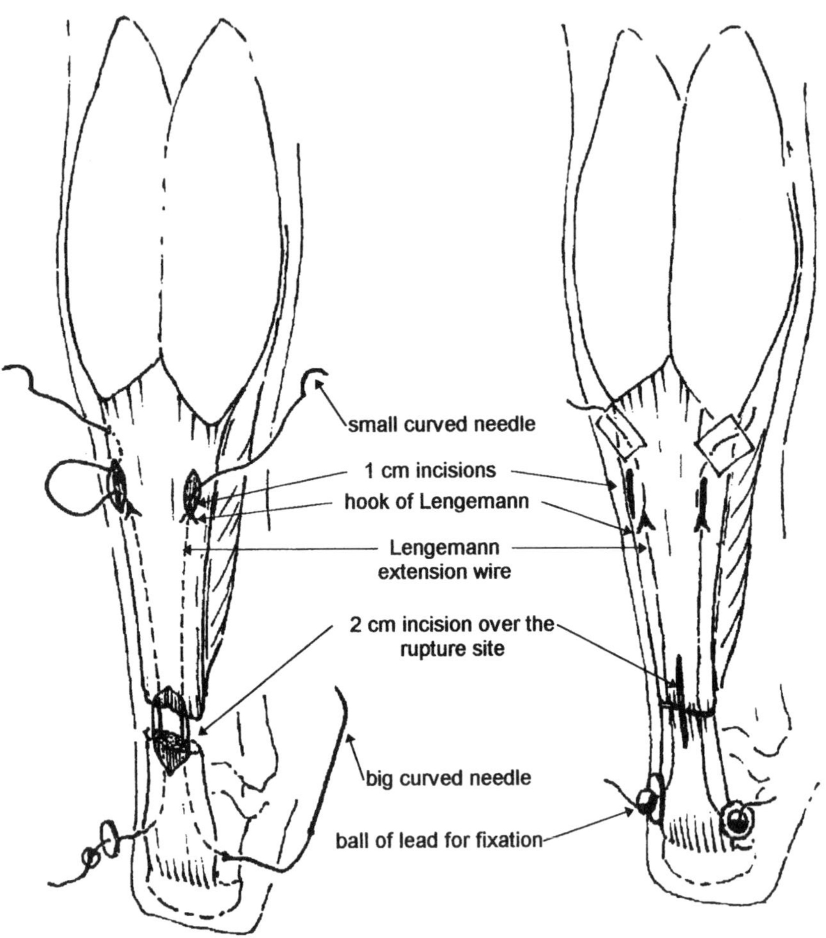

FIGURE 4.—The procedure of the percutaneous tenodesis of the ruptured Achilles tendon. (Reprinted from Gorschewsky O, Vogel U, Schweizer A, et al: Percutaneous tenodesis of the Achilles tendon: A new surgical method for the treatment of acute Achilles tendon rupture through percutaneous tenodesis. *Injury* 30:315-321, © 1999, with permission from Elsevier Science.)

Popliteal Fossa Neural Blockade as the Sole Anesthetic Technique for Outpatient Foot and Ankle Surgery

Hansen E, Eshelman MR, Cracchiolo A III (Univ of California Los Angeles)
Foot Ankle Int 21:38-44, 2000   3–36

Background.—The trend toward outpatient surgery continues as medical and surgical practice is increasingly influenced by economic pressures and the need for cost containment. One of the most important areas of outpatient surgery is anesthesia and the challenge of providing optimal pain control, rapid awakening, and minimization of postoperative nausea and vomiting. One approach to ambulatory anesthesia involves the use of regional nerve blocks. In surgery of the foot, midtarsal, and ankle, nerve blocks have been used with success. However, midtarsal and ankle blocks do not provide anesthesia to the calf and thus cannot be used for surgical procedures above the ankle or at the distal part of the calf. Intravenous regional anesthesia has been used, but it can be problematic, as can neuraxial regional blockade. The use of an anesthetic technique in which the sciatic nerve is blocked in the popliteal fossa and the saphenous nerve is blocked at the knee is described.

Methods.—The charts of patients operated on by a single orthopedic surgeon between November 1997 and May 1998 were reviewed. Figure 1A illustrates the anatomy of the popliteal fossa. Forty-eight patients underwent foot or ankle surgery with a popliteal fossa sciatic nerve block as the only anesthetic technique. The patient group consisted of 22 men and 26 women between the ages of 19 and 65 years, with an average age of 49 years. There were no contraindications for outpatient surgery, and all of the patients were in good health. In all 48 patients the operations were performed without complication. Figures 2A and 2B illustrate the procedure for identifying the needle-insertion site. After identification of the needle site, local anesthetic was administered in 5-ml increments for a total of 40 mL. A pneumatic tourniquet was placed around the proximal part of the calf, and IV midazolam or propofol was used at subhypnotic levels only to provide anxiolysis and patient comfort. A successful block

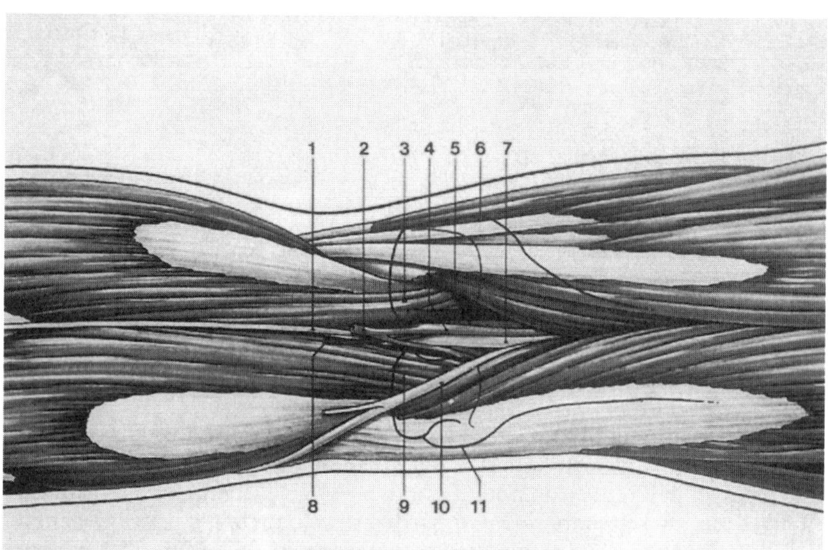

FIGURE 1A.—Posterior view of the popliteal fossa of a right knee. The sciatic nerve has divided into its 2 branches, the tibial nerve (7) and the common peroneal nerve (10). The boundaries of the popliteal fossa are as follows: proximally, the semimembranous and semitendinosus muscles medially (5 and 6), and the biceps femoris laterally (11). The inferior boundary is formed by the medial and lateral heads of the gastrocnemius muscles (3 and 9). (Courtesy of Hansen E, Eshelman MR, Cracchiolo A III: Popliteal fossa neural blockade as the sole anesthetic technique for outpatient foot and ankle surgery. *Foot Ankle Int* 21(1):38-44, 2000.)

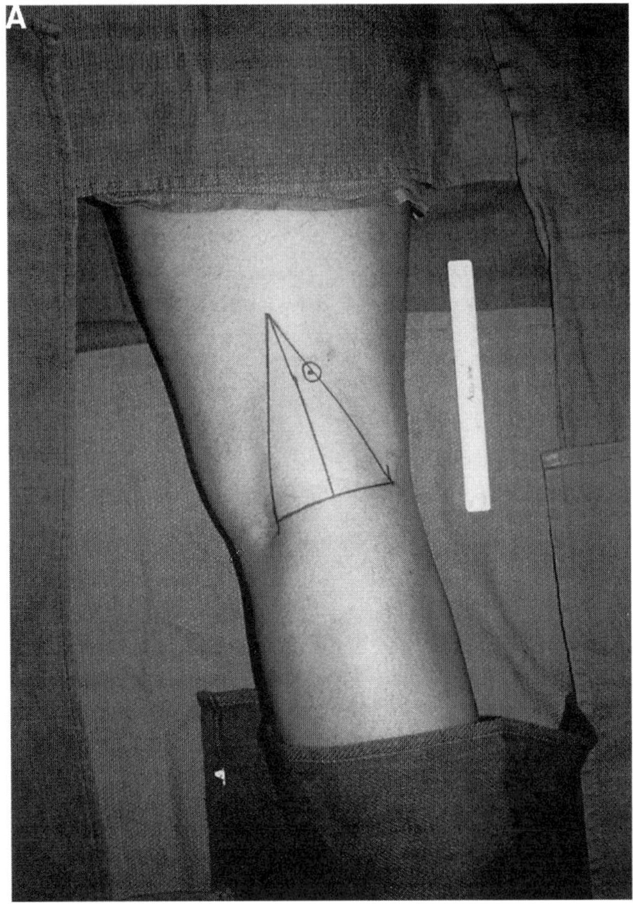

FIGURE 2A.—A posterior view of the politeal fossa of a right knee. A triangle is outlined; the base is a line drawn across the popliteal crease between the tendons of the semitendinosus and biceps femoris muscles. The tendons of these muscles form either side of the triangle. The midline axis of the triangle is marked with a vertical line; 7 cm cephalad along this line and 1 cm lateral locates the point of the needle puncture for the sciatic nerve block. (Courtesy of Hansen E, Eshelman MR, Cracchiolo A III: Popliteal fossa neural blockade as the sole anesthetic technique for outpatient foot and ankle surgery. *Foot Ankle Int* 21(1):38-44, 2000.)

was defined as needing no supplemental anesthesia or conversion to general anesthesia. Patients underwent a range of procedures, including bunionectomy, open reduction and internal fixation of fractures, ligament and Achilles tendon repair, removal of hardware, and arthroscopy of the ankle.

Results.—A successful block was achieved in 47 of the 48 patients (95%). In 1 patient, additional local anesthetic in the form of a saphenous nerve block at the ankle was required. Blocks were accomplished within 18 minutes for all patients. All 48 patients reported satisfaction with the popliteal fossa neural blockade. Seven patients reported that the technique was superior to their previous experiences with general anesthesia. Fol-

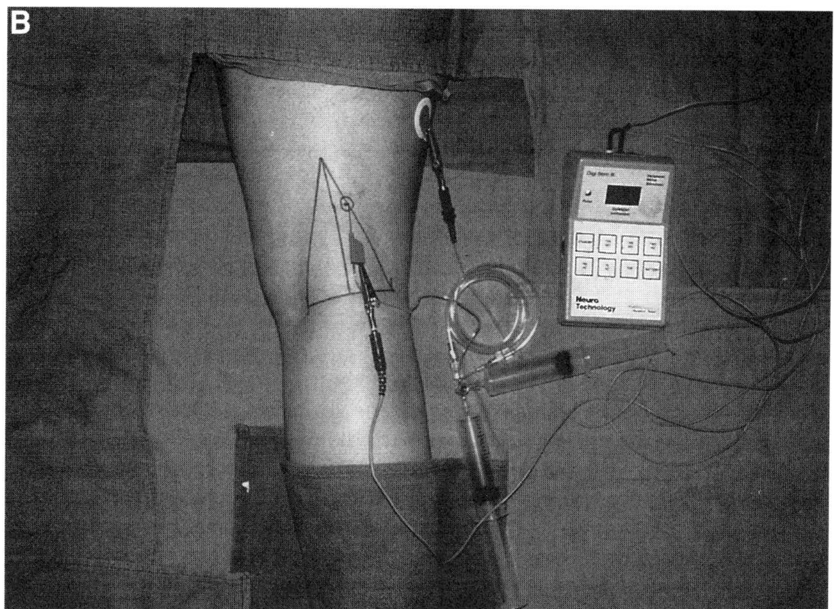

FIGURE 2B.—A 22-gauge Teflon-sheathed nerve stimulator needle has been introduced into the predetermined needle puncture site. The nerve stimulator is used to aid in locating the sciatic nerve. (Courtesy of Hansen E, Eshelman MR, Cracchiolo A III: Popliteal fossa neural blockade as the sole anesthetic technique for outpatient foot and ankle surgery. *Foot Ankle Int* 21(1):38-44, 2000.)

low-up indicated that the patients experienced excellent control of pain for an average of 10 hours after the procedure. There was no evidence of neurologic complications in any of the patients.

Conclusions.—Most surgery on the foot and ankle is now performed with the patient under regional anesthesia. The findings in this study indicate that the popliteal fossa block achieves excellent anesthetic results in the ambulatory surgery setting.

▶ An interesting article dealing with an innovative anesthetic technique for outpatient foot and ankle surgery. The authors state that "completion of the block was accomplished within 18 minutes and did not delay the start of the procedures." Because of this and the relative complexity of instilling the block, its advantage over an ankle block for foot and ankle surgical procedures is to be questioned.

J. S. Torg, MD

Talocrural and Subtalar Joint Instability After Lateral Ankle Sprain

Hertel J, Denegar CR, Monroe MM, et al (Pennsylvania State Univ, Univ Park)
Med Sci Sports Exerc 31:1501-1508, 1999   3–37

Objective.—Recurrent lateral ankle sprains (LAS) can lead to talocrural and subtalar joint instability. Assessment of subtalar joint injury when LAS is involved has not received much attention. The use of stress fluoroscopy and physical examination stress tests in the assessment of talocrural and subtalar joint instability was evaluated in individuals with and without a history of LAS.

Methods.—Twelve patients (3 men), average age 21.6 years, with a history of LAS and 8 healthy controls (5 women), average age 21.3 years, underwent anterior drawer (AD), talar tilt (TTPE), and medial subtalar glide (MSTG) tests for anterior displacement of the talus, excessive inversion of the talus, and excessive medial translation of the calcaneus on the talus, respectively. Ankles were graded on a 4-point laxity scale. Stress fluoroscopy, performed by a blinded examiner, was used for an anteroposterior view in subtalar neutral, an anteroposterior view with supination stress, a lateral modified Broden view in subtalar neutral, and a lateral modified Broden view with supination stress.

Results.—Imaging studies showed no significant laxity differences in either the anteroposterior or lateral views. Two controls and 9 patients showed subjective talocrural laxity differences between ankles on anteroposterior views. Two controls and 8 patients showed subjective laxity differences on Broden images. No controls and 7 patients showed anterior drawer laxity differences. One control and 7 patients showed TTPE laxity differences. One control and 7 patients showed medial subtalar glide laxity differences.

Conclusion.—Unilateral laxity differences were observed in 75% of patients during stress fluoroscopy, and 67% with talocrural laxity also had unilateral or bilateral laxity of the subtalar joint. Some patients with a history of LAS will have persistent talocrural and subtalar laxity.

▶ This is an excellent article emphasizing the role of subtalar joint instability in patients with chronic lateral ankle sprain. Nonoperative management is generally accepted as the treatment of choice for acute lateral ankle sprains. To be determined is what, if any, the role of lateral subtalar instability plays in those patients with chronic instability requiring surgery. Also to be answered is the question of whether the classic Brostrom procedure would be sufficient in those patients with chronic lateral talocrural and subtalar joint instability.

J. S. Torg, MD

Syndesmotic Ankle Sprains in Football: A Survey of National Football League Athletic Trainers

Doughtie M (Tufts Univ, Medford, Mass)
J Athletic Train 34:15-18, 1999

3–38

Background.—The most common ankle sprains among football players are injuries to the lateral ligamentous structures. These sprains are simple to treat and heal quickly, usually without any long-term adverse sequelae. However, the syndesmotic sprain is a unique injury involving the high ankle, both the anterior and posterior tibiofibular ligaments, and the interosseous membrane. All of these structures are located proximal to or above the level of the lateral ligaments. The syndesmotic sprain is commonly misdiagnosed, and the extended recovery period is a source of frustration to patients. Athletic trainers in the National Football League were surveyed to determine whether a specific treatment modality reduces recovery time for this unique type of ankle sprain.

Methods.—A survey consisting of 8 questions was mailed to head athletic trainers for all 30 National Football League teams. Responses were obtained from 23 of the trainers surveyed. Questions covered mechanism of injury, playing surface at time of injury, diagnostic tests, follow-up treatment modalities used, best treatment, taping procedure, and recovery time.

Results.—The responding trainers cited a number of causes for the syndesmotic sprains they treated, with a rotational component being the most frequently cited. Type of playing surface was not considered by these trainers to be a causative factor. Plain radiographs were used in the diagnostic process by 96% of the trainers, and 52% included MRI as well. Treatment modalities used most frequently during the acute phase of injury included ice; electrical stimulation of muscle; casting, bracing, or both; and administration of nonsteroidal antiinflammatory drugs. Follow-up treatment commonly included proprioception training, US, and taping. The best treatments for reducing recovery time were reported to be immobilization, injection of corticosteroids, use of ice, and exercise.

Conclusion.—No treatment modality or plan has been identified as clearly effective in enabling early and safe return to football for players with syndesmotic ankle sprains. Prospective studies are needed to compare treatment modalities and injury severity.

▶ As with most questionnaire surveys, this study lacks information about scientific format. However, I do not believe that anyone would take issue with the observation that there was "unanimous agreement that sprains of the syndesmosis require an extended period of recovery before the athlete can return to strenuous activity." The range of time loss is reported to be from 5 to 56 days. It is pointed out that the respondents were not asked to compare time loss with severity of injury. Also, with regard to rejection of the possible role of the playing surface in the incidence of these injuries, it should be noted that the respondents were not asked to specify the surface involved.

J. S. Torg, MD

Clinical Evaluation of the Modified Brostrom-Evans Procedure to Restore Ankle Stability

Girard P, Anderson RB, Davis WH, et al (Carolinas Med Ctr, Charlotte, NC; Miller Orthopaedic Clinic, Charlotte, NC; Carolinas Physical Therapy Network, Charlotte, NC)
Foot Ankle Int 20:246-252, 1999   3–39

Background.—Chronic lateral ankle instability has been repaired effectively with the use of the Brostrom procedure, but the usefulness of the Brostrom procedure may be questionable for overweight or hyperflexible patients and for those involved in heavy work or athletic activities. A modification of the Brostrom procedure with the use of part of the peroneus brevis tendon was tested to see if results were comparable to those achieved with the unmodified technique, specifically in relation to function, strength, and range of motion.

Methods.—Twenty patients underwent 21 lateral ankle reconstructions with the modified technique (Figs 1 to 3). The patients were then interviewed between 14 and 56 months after the surgery (average, 29.5 months). A physical therapist evaluated 14 of these patients. Activities of daily living and recreation were stressed.

Results.—The mean American Foot and Ankle Society ankle-hindfoot score was 98. 2; only one score was less than 95. Range of motion, strength, and function were highly acceptable to the patients.

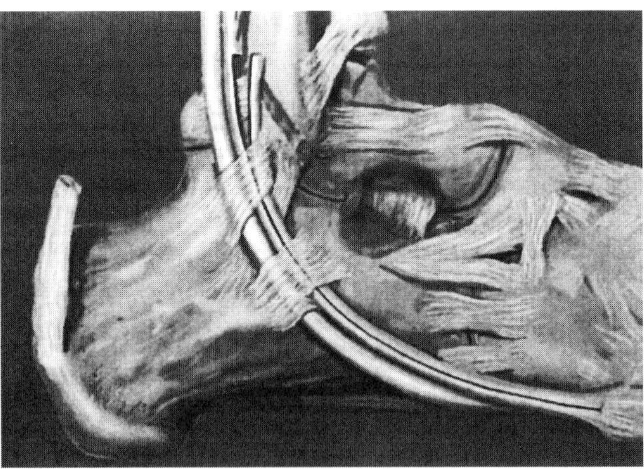

FIGURE 1.—Lateral aspect of the ankle. The anterior one third of the peroneus brevis tendon is harvested. The superior and, if possible, the inferior peroneal retinaculum is preserved. (Courtesy of Girard P, Anderson RB, Davis WH, et al: Clinical evaluation of the modified Brostrom-Evans procedure to restore ankle stability. *Foot Ankle Int* 20:246-252, 1999.)

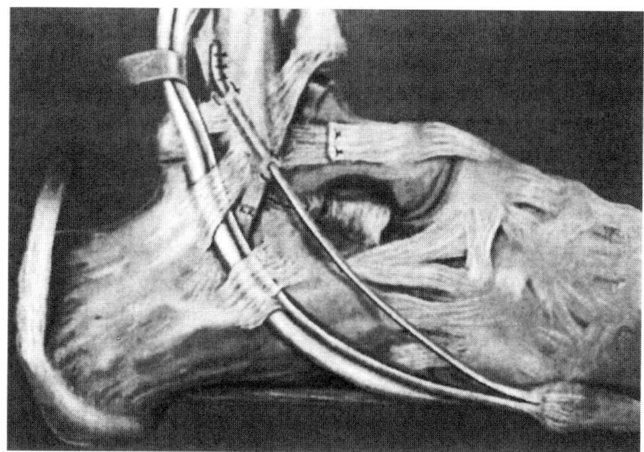

FIGURE 2.—The end-to-end repair of the calcaneofibular and anterior talofibular ligaments is achieved with nonabsorbable suture. The split tendon is rerouted through a drill hole in the distal fibula and is secured at both ends. (Courtesy of Girard P, Anderson RB, Davis WH, et al: Clinical evaluation of the modified Brostrom-Evans procedure to restore ankle stability. *Foot Ankle Int* 20:246-252, 1999.)

Conclusions.—The addition of the stability provided by the peroneal tendon to the Brostrom procedure did not appear to sacrifice peroneal strength as it augments static restraint.

▶ The authors infer that the modified Brostrom-Evans procedure is superior to the originally described Brostrom anatomical reconstruction because "this local tissue repair may fail eventually. . ." They have not compared these 2 procedures, and this inference is certainly not supported by their data. On

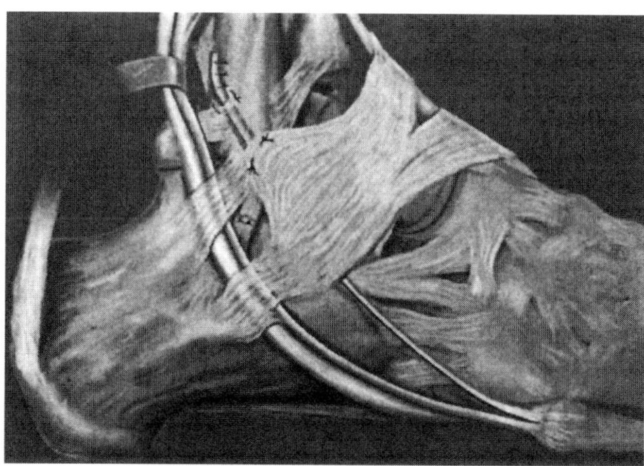

FIGURE 3.—Completion of the lateral repair includes an advancement of the extensor retinaculum to the distal fibula, as described by Gould et al. (Courtesy of Girard P, Anderson RB, Davis WH, et al: Clinical evaluation of the modified Brostrom-Evans procedure to restore ankle stability. *Foot Ankle Int* 20:246-252, 1999.)

the basis of my own clinical experience, I question whether the Brostrom procedure need be modified to obtain consistent acceptable results.

J. S. Torg, MD

Early Motion of the Ankle After Operative Treatment of a Rupture of the Achilles Tendon: A Prospective, Randomized Clinical and Radiographic Study
Mortensen NHM, Skov O, Jensen PE (Odense Univ, Denmark)
J Bone Joint Surg Am 81-A:983-990, 1999   3–40

Objective.—Studies of different early mobilization techniques after Achilles tendon repair have yielded variable results. Because many studies are not controlled, results cannot be compared. Outcomes of a prospective randomized clinical investigation after operative repair of a ruptured Achilles prospectively comparing early motion with 8 weeks of rigid immobilization in a below-the-knee cast are presented.

Methods.—Separation of metal markers, placed in the tendon, was observed on radiographs taken immediately after repair and at 6 and 12 weeks postoperatively in 71 patients (aged 20-73 years) with acute rupture of the Achilles tendon, who were randomly assigned to conventional immobilization in a plaster cast (n = 35, 10 women) for 8 weeks or to early restricted ankle motion in a below-the-knee brace (n = 36, 10 women) for 6 weeks. All patients had the same operation (Figs 1 and 2). Patients were evaluated at 12 weeks, when the cast or brace was removed, and at a median of 16 months.

Results.—At 12 weeks, median separation between markers was similar for the conventional (9 mm) and early mobilization (11.5 mm) groups and was correlated with tautness of repair. Patients who had early mobilization

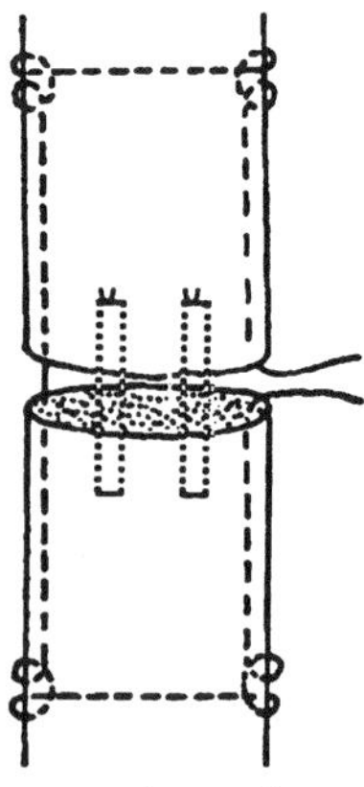

FIGURE 1.—The modified Kessler suture technique for repair of the Achilles tendon. (Courtesy of Mortensen NHM, Skov O, Jensen PE: Early motion of the ankle after operative treatment of a rupture of the Achilles tendon: A prospective, randomized clinical and radiographic study. *J Bone Joint Surg Am* 81-A:983-990, 1999.)

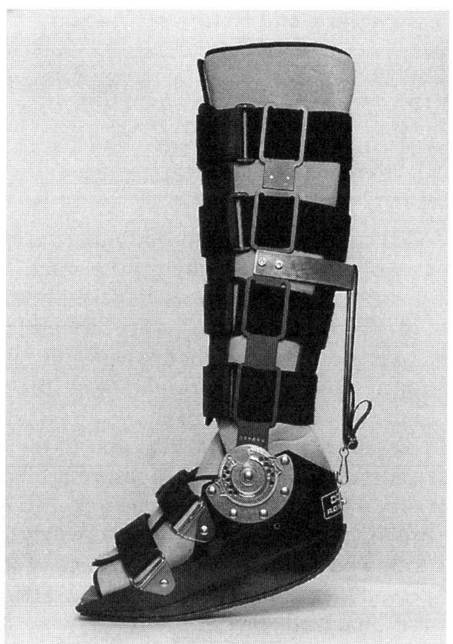

FIGURE 2.—Photograph of the modified DonJoy ROM-Walker brace. An elastic band pulls the ankle into 30 degrees of plantar flexion but allows active dorsiflexion to neutral. (Courtesy of Mortensen NHM, Skov O, Jensen PE: Early motion of the ankle after operative treatment of a rupture of the Achilles tendon: A prospective, randomized clinical and radiographic study. *J Bone Joint Surg Am* 81-A:983-990, 1999.)

returned to preinjury occupations and sports activities significantly sooner than patients who were treated conventionally and had significantly less decrease in range of motion and fewer adhesions. Achilles tendon thickness and atrophy of calf muscle were similar for both groups. No excessive lengthening of the tendon was observed in either group. The plantar flexion strength index was 0.89 with the ankle in 15 degrees of dorsiflexion and 0.75 with the ankle in 15 degrees of plantar flexion for both groups. The heel-rise index was 0.88 for early mobilization patients and 0.89 for patients treated conventionally.

Conclusion.—Although patients in the early-mobilization group re turned to work sooner and had fewer adhesions after Achilles tendon repair than did patients treated conventionally, Achilles' tendon thickness and calf muscle atrophy were similar for both groups.

▶ The observation that early restricted motion shortens rehabilitation time but does not necessarily prevent muscle atrophy after operative treatment of rupture of the Achilles tendon is in keeping with my own clinical experience.

J. S. Torg, MD

The Effect of Foot Structure and Range of Motion on Musculoskeletal Overuse Injuries

Kaufman KR, Brodine SK, Shaffer RA, et al (Mayo Clinic/Found, Rochester, Minn; Naval Health Research Ctr, San Diego, Calif; Naval Hosp, Camp Lejeune, NC)
Am J Sports Med 27:585-593, 1999   3–41

Objective.—Stress fractures are a common injury in runners. Feet can be classified on the basis of the medial longitudinal arch, with high-arched feet regarded as inflexible and flat feet as hypermobile. Previous studies have disagreed as to whether foot structure affects the risk of stress fractures and other overuse injuries. The association between foot structure and overuse injuries in military trainees was prospectively investigated.

Methods.—The 2-year study included 449 candidates undergoing highly rigorous Navy Sea, Air and Land (SEAL) training. Before the start of training, ankle and subtalar motion were measured and the characteristics of the foot arch were assessed under static and dynamic conditions. The subjects were then followed up for the development of injuries during the 25-week training period. Risk factors predisposing to lower extremity overuse injuries were analyzed. Stress fractures were diagnosed on the basis of clinical findings and positive results of a radiograph or bone scan.

Results.—About one third of the subjects experienced 1 or more lower extremity overuse injuries during training, most commonly stress fracture, iliotibial band syndrome, and patellofemoral syndrome. These injuries were most common in the initial phase of training. Subjects with pes planus or pes cavus were at nearly double the risk of stress fractures, compared with subjects with average arch height. Restricted ankle dorsiflexion and increased hindfoot eversion were also associated with increased risk of overuse injury. None of the foot structure factors identified increased the risk of iliotibial band syndrome or patellofemoral syndrome.

Conclusion.—Several foot structure variables are related to an increased risk of overuse injuries in the lower extremity. All of the risk factors identified are amenable to intervention through footwear or other approaches. The factors identified in Navy SEAL candidates may be applicable to civilian endurance athletes.

▶ This is an impressive, well-designed and controlled study that perhaps could be performed only in a military situation. Although its observations and conclusions are at variance with those in the literature, it is my belief that its design and implementation enhance its credibility. The authors' conclusion that the risk factors identified—pes planus, pes cavus, restricted ankle dorsiflexion, and increased hindfoot inversion—are all subject to intervention and injury prevention is not supported by their data. Clearly, their observations need be used to develop clinically applied strategies to prevent overuse injuries of the lower extremities.

J. S. Torg, MD

The Influence of Medial and Lateral Placement of Orthotic Wedges on Loading of the Plantar Aponeurosis: An *In Vitro* Study

Kogler GF, Veer FB, Solomonidis SE, et al (Southern Illinois Univ, Springfield)
J Bone Joint Surg Am 81-A:1403-1413, 1999   3–42

Background.—One of the most common disorders of the foot is plantar fasciitis, which in many cases is believed to be the result of repetitive trauma and overuse. The influence of an orthosis on loading of the plantar aponeurosis is critical in determining appropriate treatment for plantar fasciitis. The authors attempted to quantify the strain on the plantar aponeurosis resulting from a variety of combinations of orthotic wedges in cadaveric feet.

Methods.—The authors simulated the static stance using an in vitro test to characterize loading of the plantar aponeurosis. In 9 fresh-frozen cadaveric lower limbs, a differential variable reluctance transducer was implanted in the plantar aponeurosis. The limbs were mounted on a testing machine, and an axial load of up to 900 N was applied to the tibia. Wedges with a 6-degree incline were used to create 8 different combinations of test conditions. The wedges were placed or not placed, according to the various combinations, under the medial and lateral aspects of the forefoot and hindfoot and were then evaluated. The plantigrade foot provided a control.

Results.—In every case, the test combinations involving a wedge under the forefoot of the test limb produced a strain significantly different from the strain seen in the neutral control. Strain in the plantar aponeurosis was decreased when a wedge was placed under the lateral aspect of the forefoot. When a wedge was placed under the medial aspect, strain was increased. In the test combinations in which a wedge was placed under the hindfoot but not under the forefoot, the strain produced did not differ significantly from that seen in the neutral control.

Conclusion.—A wedge that is placed under the lateral aspect of the forefoot will transmit load through the foot's lateral support structures, locking the calcaneocuboid joint and, thus, diminishing the strain in the plantar aponeurosis. However, a wedge placed under the medial aspect of the forefoot results in a trusslike action by transmitting loads through the medial support structures of the forefoot. This increases strain in the plantar aponeurosis. It appears that orthotic wedges effectively control the load-path pattern in the foot, and offer the potential for reducing strain to the plantar aponeurosis. Data included in this study indicate that an orthotic wedge placed under the lateral aspect of the forefoot in patients with plantar aponeurosis may be an effective form of treatment.

▶ An interesting and creditable scientific study that demonstrates the clinical relevance of a wedge under the lateral aspect of the forefoot having the potential to reduce strain on the plantar aponeurosis, an effect not previously recognized. Of course, the next step is to correlate these findings with clinical observations.

J. S. Torg, MD

Subtalar Subluxation in Ballet Dancers
Ménétrey J, Fritschy D (Hôpitaux Universitaires de Genève, Switzerland)
Am J Sports Med 27:143-149, 1999   3–43

Purpose.—Ankle injuries account for up to one fourth of all injuries in dancers. Few studies have reported talar subluxation in dancers. An experience with subtalar joint subluxation is reported.

Patients.—Twenty-five cases of subtalar subluxation occurred over a 1-year period in 1 Swiss ballet company. These injuries, which occurred in 25 dancers out of a company of 60, accounted for 10.5% of all reported injuries and 58% of ankle injuries. Subtalar subluxations began appearing with the introduction of a grand plie on pointes or at the landing of a jump on demi-pointes (Fig 3). There was no apparent mechanism of ankle sprain. The subluxation was associated with a sudden, sharp pain in the talonavicular joint and hindfoot, along with a feeling of forward displacement of the foot. The talonavicular ligament, the anterior talofibular ligament, and the posteromedial portion of the subtalar joint were all painful to palpation. All affected dancers had limited ankle extension with obvious hypomobility of the subtalar joint. The mechanism of injury involved shearing forces on the midtarsal joint, resulting in posteromedial subtalar subluxation.

Treatment and Outcomes.—The subluxations were reduced by means of a 3-step manipulation with the patient in prone position and the knee flexed 90 degrees. The heel was immobilized with 1 hand, and the talar head was surrounded anteriorly with the other. A vertical upward force was applied with 1 hand holding the calcaneus to open the subtalar joint, while the other hand applied a posterior stress on the talar head. As the foot was progressively extended, the calcaneus was mobilized anteriorly, in eversion and abduction. Successful reduction was audible and was accompanied by instant pain relief. The reduction was maintained by taping around the midtarsal joint and ankle for 6 weeks. The patients resumed dancing in a swimming pool at 2 weeks and on the ground at 3 to 4 weeks. They were allowed to rejoin the company with protective taping to lock the talonavicular joint in the anterior direction. Subluxations recurred in many dancers and became more difficult to manage each time they occurred.

Conclusions.—A unique form of subluxation of the subtalar joint in dancers is described. The injury is commonly associated with ankle instability, hyperlaxity, or both. Treatment relies on reduction and maintenance of the reduction of the subtalar joint. More study of the biomechanics of this injury is required.

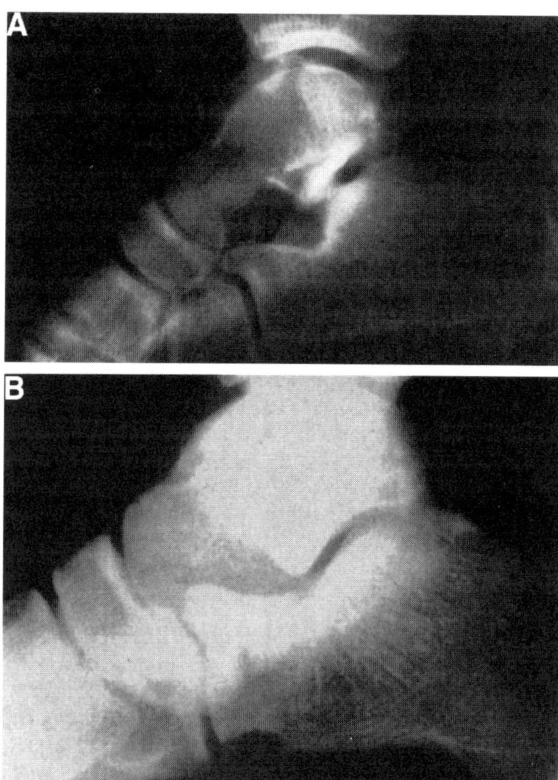

FIGURE 3.—A, Lateral radiographs of a dancer with a subtalar subluxation. B, Lateral ankle radiographs of the same dancer after reduction. (Courtesy of Ménétrey J, Fritschy D: Subtalar subluxation in ballet dancers. *Am J Sports Med* 27:143-149, 1999.)

▶ This interesting article describes a phenomenon that I am completely unfamiliar with. With regard to etiology, the authors hypothesize that when the dancer is on *pointes* or d*emi-pointes*, the interosseous ligament becomes horizontally oriented and is continuously stressed and sheared. Also, with the same mechanism, the anterior talar navicular ligament is permanently stretched because of the *coup de pied.* To be noted, the authors conclude that although their "approach is empirical, the findings suggest a distinct clinical entity."

J. S. Torg, MD

Plantar Fasciitis: How Successful Is Surgical Intervention?
Davies MS, Weiss GA, Saxby TS (Brisbane, Queensland, Australia)
Foot Ankle Int 20:803-807, 1999
3–44

Objective.—For the 5% of patients with plantar fasciitis who have persistent and disabling symptoms, surgery is an option. A retrospective review of results of partial plantar fascia release and decompression of the nerve to abductor digiti quinti minimi in patients with intractable plantar fasciitis was conducted.

Methods.—Surgery was performed on 47 heels in 43 patients between March 1992 and July 1996. All patients had symptoms for at least 12 months, and had not responded to conservative treatment. Sixty-six percent were overweight or obese. Patients were followed for an average of 31.4 months.

Results.—Follow-up was conducted in 41 patients (15 men, 45 heels), aged 23 to 79 years. Pain scores declined from 8.5 of 10 at baseline to 2.5. Walking distance improved for most patients with 95.6% of patients able to walk at least 500 m after surgery, compared with 31% before surgery. After surgery 24 patients had no limitation of activities, compared with 2 at baseline. Only 4 postsurgical patients had severe limitations, compared with 18 before surgery. The current level of symptoms was reached an average of 8 months after surgery. Thirteen patients had heel pain after surgery, and 14 required an orthosis. One patient had severe reflex sympathetic dystrophy after surgery, and another patient had a pulmonary embolus from which he recovered uneventfully. Six patients were dissatisfied with their results, and 5 of these were involved in worker's compensation claims.

Conclusion.—In the subgroup of patients with intractable plantar fasciitis, surgery is an option with imitations that should be thoroughly described to the patients before the operation.

▶ This article makes a salient point: persistent foot pain in patients who had plantar fasciotomy is multifactorial. It appears that this point is not well described in the literature. Clearly, patient selection is important and adequate informed consent is in order.

J. S. Torg, MD

4 Medical Problems

Athletes' View of the Preparticipation Physical Examination: Attitudes Toward Certain Health Screening Questions
Carek PJ, Futrell M (Med Univ of South Carolina, Charleston)
Arch Fam Med 8:307-312, 1999

4–1

Background.—Preparticipation physical examination (PPE) is the standard of care for athletes of all ages. The value that student athletes place on the PPE for ensuring safe sports participation was studied, as well as whether students would accept a station-based PPE with an emphasis on health-related issues.

Methods and Findings.—Seven hundred sixteen student athletes at 2 small colleges were surveyed. Sixty-six percent believed that they could safely participate in sports and avoid severe injury, minor injury, or death without undergoing a PPE. Most believed that the PPE prevents or helps prevent major (89%) and minor (76%) injuries. Although the respondents said that they would not be uncomfortable with a clinician asking questions about health-related issues, many students (especially women) believed that the PPE is not the place for specific questions related to sexual activity and health, eating disorders, smoking, or personal and family alcohol use.

Conclusions.—In this study, most student athletes did not see the benefit of the PPE in ensuring safe participation in athletics. With modifications to meet the needs and comfort level of student athletes, the PPE may be an opportunity to present health-related education and counseling.

▶ This study should be read in conjunction with Abstract 4–2. Perhaps the screening questions in the World Wide Web form would alleviate some of the concerns the athletes had answering questions about gynecologic health, eating disorders, and alcohol and nicotine use. It was interesting to note that a majority of the athletes believed they could participate safely in athletics without a PPE.

F. J. George ATC, PT

A Comprehensive and Cost-effective Preparticipation Exam Implemented on the World Wide Web

Peltz JE, Haskell WL, Matheson GO (Stanford Univ, Calif)
Med Sci Sports Exerc 31:1727-1740, 1999   4–2

Objective.—Although the preparticipation examination (PPE) medical assessment is commonly administered to college and high school athletes, its effectiveness in assessing risk factors for injury has not been confirmed. A comprehensive medical history PPE questionnaire, developed for the World Wide Web (WWW), was tested for its ability to improve medical care, improve ability to screen, and increase physician effectiveness.

Methods.—The content of the questionnaire was a composite of information gleaned from a literature review, previous PPE, and expert opinion and addressed medical, surgical, and musculoskeletal history, eating, menstrual and sleep disorders, stress, and risk behaviors. Sixteen physicians evaluated the PPE. Validity and accuracy were measured.

Results.—A total of 830 varsity athletes took the first year and returning year WWW version of the PPE. The sensitivities of the first year and returning year questionnaires were 0.97 and 0.97, respectively, for detecting positive responses. The specificity of the WWW PPE was 99.7%. Physicians (15 of 16) found that the PPE improved their ability to provide medical care, and 13 of 16 said the PPE reduced the time needed for each examination. Most (>90%) athletes said the PPE was "easy" or "moderately easy" to complete.

Conclusion.—There was good athlete compliance and acceptance of the new PPE. Physicians found that the PPE facilitated provision of medical care and shortened the time needed for the examination. The WWW form of the PPE had a high sensitivity and specificity.

▶ The PPE has become a problem for many large athletic programs. The authors have developed an excellent screening tool using the WWW. Programs such as these will certainly assist in alleviating most of the present inadequacies and problems in administering a PPE.

F. J. George ATC, PT

Prevalence of Sudden Cardiac Death During Competitive Sports Activities in Minnesota High School Athletes

Maron BJ, Gohman TE, Aeppli D (Univ of Minnesota, Minneapolis)
J Am Coll Cardiol 32:1881-1884, 1998   4–3

Introduction.—A variety of underlying and usually unsuspected structural cardiovascular diseases cause sudden deaths on the athletic field. The frequency of such deaths is still unknown, but such information would be useful in designing the most effective preparticipation screening strategies. A high school student population was studied to determine the number of

TABLE 1.—Profiles of Sudden Cardiac Deaths in Minnesota High School Athletes

No.	Age at Death (Years)	Year of Death	Race/ Gender	Sport	Circumstances of Collapse	Heart Weight (g)	Time of Day	Diagnosis
1	16	1990	W/M	Cross-country	During warm-up, stretching exercises	460	3 PM	Anomalous left main coronary artery
2	16	1993	W/M	Cross-country	Early during 5-K race	385	10 AM	Myocarditis
3	17	1996	W/M	Basketball	Minutes after entering game became fatigued; removed self from game; collapsed on bench	—	6 PM	Aortic valvular stenosis (bicuspid valve)

(Courtesy of Maron BJ, Gohman TE, Aeppli D: Prevalence of sudden cardiac death during competitive sports activities in Minnesota high school athletes. *J Am Coll Cardiol* 32:1881-1884, 1998. Reprinted with permission from the American College of Cardiology.)

deaths caused by cardiovascular disease and to establish reliable estimates of the frequency of these catastrophic events.

Methods.—In Minnesota, the precise number of sports participants and of deaths caused by cardiovascular disease was ascertained over a 12-year period on the basis of an insurance program for catastrophic injury or death. This insurance program was mandatory for all student athletes competing in interscholastic sports. There were 27 high school sports, 651,695 student athlete participants, and 1,453,280 overall sports participants.

Results.—There were 3 sudden deaths from cardiovascular disease in grades 10 to 12 over the 12-year period (Table 1). One death was from an anomalous origin of the left main coronary artery from the right sinus of Valsalva. Another was from congenital aortic valve stenosis with bicuspid valve, and the third was myocarditis. The athletes were male, white, and 16 or 17 years of age. One competed in basketball and the other 2 in cross-country/track. Per academic year, the calculated risk of sudden death was 1:500,000 participations and 1:217,400 participants. The estimated risk over a 3-year high school career for a student athlete was 1:72,500.

Conclusion.—In a population of high school student athletes, the risk of sudden cardiac death was small, in the range of 1 in 200,000 per year. In male athletes, this risk was higher. The limitations implicit in structuring productive and cost-effective, broad-based preparticipation screening strategies for high school athletes are underlined by the rare occurrence of sudden cardiac death in competitive sports.

▶ An average of 12 to 20 athletes, most of them high school students, die suddenly each year of congenital heart defects that are not detected during normal physical examinations. About one third of the cases of sudden cardiac death are caused by a congenital heart defect called hypertrophic cardiomyopathy (thickened heart muscle), with the next most frequent cause being congenital coronary anomalies.

The sudden death of a young athlete is tragic, but the financial, ethical, medical, and legal issues involved have created huge barriers to preparticipation screening. The American Heart Association holds that some form of preparticipation cardiovascular screening for high school and collegiate athletes is justifiable.[1]

In Minnesota, careful determination of the number of athletes participating in competitive interscholastic sports programs and the incidence of catastrophic injury and death allowed investigators to estimate prevalence rates (1 sudden death per 130,000 male athletes). Of the 3 deaths recorded over 12 years, only one might have been detected through preparticipation screening. Overall, this study indicates that death is extremely rare among high school athletes and that costly and extensive preparticipation screening is unwarranted.

D. C. Nieman, DrPH

Reference

1. American Heart Association: Cardiovascular preparticipation screening of competitive athletes. *Circulation* 94:850-856, 1996.

Sudden Death Due to Ischaemic Heart Disease in Young Aboriginal Sportsmen in the Northern Territory, 1982-1996

Young MC, Fricker PA, Thomson NJ, et al (Australian Inst of Sport, Canberra, ACT; Edith Cowan Univ, Perth, WA; Royal Darwin Hosp, NT)
Med J Aust 170:425-428, 1999   4–4

Objective.—As a result of the sudden death from occult ischemic heart disease (IHD) of several indigenous Australian footballers, the incidence of sports-related sudden cardiac death related to IHD among Aboriginal sportsmen in the Northern Territory was retrospectively compared with the incidence among the general population of sportsmen in Victoria. In addition, the possible risk factors for myocardial infarction and sudden cardiac death were identified, which could provide valuable information for indigenous sporting competitions.

Methods.—All sports-related sudden cardiac deaths in young competitive Aboriginal sportsmen between 1982 and 1996 were identified and compared with similar deaths in Australian footballers in Victoria.

Results.—There were 8 sports-related sudden cardiac deaths among Aboriginal sportsmen, aged 21 to 36 years. All deaths occurred in the north of the Northern Territory during the wet season, at or after half time. The average age at death was 29.4 years. There were 6 deaths in footballers, 1 in a soccer player, and 1 in a touch football player, all of whom had coronary artery disease and 4 of whom had myocardial abnormalities. The estimated incidence of IHD sudden cardiac death among Aboriginal footballers was 19 to 24 per 100,000 player-years. The estimated incidence of IHD sudden cardiac death in Australian footballers in Victoria was 0.54 per 100,000 player-years.

Conclusion.—There is a significant incidence of IHD in young Aboriginal Australian men. Specific interventions that are initiated, owned, and controlled by the community should be considered to reduce the incidence of sports-related IHD sudden cardiac death.

▶ Exercise-induced death in a group of Australian aborigenes might seem a rather eclectic topic for an article. However, the contribution of Young and associates is important in underlining the fact that the risk of sudden death during or immediately following physical activity is greatly increased by an adverse lifestyle. As with many indigenous groups, the Australian aboriginals have now developed a number of adverse behavior patterns and cardiac risk factors, including obesity, diabetes, cigarette smoking, and a high alcohol consumption. Young et al comment that 4 of the 8 cardiac incidents were associated with the drinking of alcohol or kava (an intoxicating drink peculiar to this region), and resulting dehydration. The depletion of body fluids is a particularly dangerous practice in the hot and humid environment of Australia's Northern Territory, where the wet bulb globe temperature is commonly in the extreme range (> 28°C). Unfortunately, no comment is made regarding obesity or smoking, but because the study included all deaths in organized sports teams, irrespective of the level of play, it is probable that some if not all of the 8 victims were both fat and smokers. The question arises as to the advice that should be given to players. Young et al propose cardiovascular screening, although most authorities now believe that anything more than a simple clinical examination is not cost-effective.[1] A violent, once-a-week burst of sport under extreme weather conditions is plainly undesirable, but regular and more moderate physical activity, coupled with the correction of other lifestyle problems, seems important to a reduction of long-term risk.

R. J. Shephard, MD, PhD, DPE

Reference

1. Shephard RJ: The athlete's heart: Is big beautiful? *Br J Sports Med* 30: 5-10, 1996.

Plaque Rupture and Sudden Death Related to Exertion in Men With Coronary Artery Disease

Burke AP, Farb A, Malcom GT, et al (Armed Forces Inst of Pathology, Washington, DC; Louisiana State Univ, New Orleans; Univ of Maryland, Baltimore)
JAMA 281:921-926, 1999   4–5

Objective.—Acute exertion and emotional and physical stress can precipitate sudden cardiac death. The association between acute plaque rupture and exertion-related sudden coronary death was prospectively investigated in a series of carefully studied autopsy hearts.

Methods.—Coronary artery fixation, cardiac dissection, and tissue sampling were performed on 141 hearts from men, average age 51 years, who died of sudden coronary death (natural death occurring without evidence of extracardiac cause of death and in which at least 1 epicardial coronary artery was more than 75% occluded by thrombus or plaque) between January 1994 and May 1997. Activity at time of death was reported where possible. Risk factors (total cholesterol [TC], high-density lipoprotein cholesterol [HDL-C], glycosylated hemoglobin, cigarette smoking) and presence of plaque rupture were subjected to multiple logistic regression. Association of risk factors was examined by multivariate analysis.

Results.—Deaths occurred at rest (n=116) or during exertion (n=25) and were witnessed in 90 cases. There was a significantly higher proportion of acute plaque rupture in the exertion group compared with the rest group (68% vs 23%). Cholesterol values were highest in the exertional plaque rupture group followed by the at rest plaque rupture group. Plaque rupture was significantly associated with exertion ($z=3.1$) and TC/HDL-C

(z=3.1). The latter ratio was significantly higher in the exertion group than in the rest group (8.2 vs 6.2). The average number of vulnerable plaques was 1.6 in the exertion group and 0.9 in the rest group. Plaque rupture occurred most commonly in the shoulder region or mid–fibrous cap. The degree of narrowing at these sites was 69% in the rest group and 70% in the exertion group. Both exertion and TC/HDL-C were significantly associated with plaque rupture and independent of age, body mass index, smoking, glycosylated hemoglobin level, and hypertension.

Conclusion.—Acute exertion is an independent risk factor for sudden cardiac death from acute plaque rupture in men with coronary artery disease.

▶ It has long been suspected that when a person dies during or shortly following vigorous exertion, the cause is bleeding into an atheromatous plaque, whereas the person who dies when sitting or sleeping has a thrombosis at the point of coronary vascular narrowing.[1] The article by Burke and associates provides confirmation of this hypothesis: 72% of exercisers show rupture, 26% of those sitting, and only 11% of those sleeping. Nevertheless, even with detailed postmortem evaluation of 141 cases of sudden death, the proof is relatively weak in statistical terms (P = .03). As in our earlier series,[1] a substantial range of physical activities was implicated, although with a tendency to dominance of "heavy" activities such as lifting and pushing; also in confirmation of our earlier report, emotional disturbances were responsible for seven of the 141 incidents. Although exercise can precipitate sudden death, the greatly reduced risk between exercise bouts leaves the exerciser better off than the person who remains sedentary.[1,2]

R. J. Shephard, MD, PhD, DPE

References

1. Shephard RJ: *Ischaemic Heart Disease and Exercise.* London: Croom Helm, 1981.
2. Siscovick DS, Weiss NS, Fletcher RH, et al: The incidence of primary cardiac arrest during vigorous exercise. *N Engl J Med* 311:874-877, 1984.

Cardiorespiratory Fitness, Body Composition, and All-Cause and Cardiovascular Disease Mortality in Men
Lee CD, Blair SN, Jackson AS (Univ of Houston)
Am J Clin Nutr 69:373-380, 1999   4–6

Objective.—The association between obesity and all-cause and cardiovascular disease (CVD) is not clear. The health consequences of body fatness and cardiorespiratory fitness in relation to all-cause and CVD mortality in men were examined in an observational cohort study, and the associations of fat mass, fat-free mass (FFM), and waist circumference to mortality were assessed after taking cardiovascular fitness into account.

Methods.—Preventive medical evaluations, including body composition analyses and treadmill testing, were performed in 21,925 men, aged 30 to

83, between 1971 and 1989. Patients followed up for an average of 8 years. The outcome measures were all-cause and CVD mortality.

Results.—There were 428 deaths, 144 from CVD, 143 from cancer, and 141 from other causes. After adjusting for possible confounders, the RR of all-cause mortality relative to fit lean men was 2.07 for lean unfit men. For normal, unfit men, relative to normal fit men, RR = 1.62 and for obese unfit men relative to fit obese, RR = 1.90. The corresponding multivariate cardiovascular disease mortality RRs were 3.16 for lean, unfit men, 2.94 for normal, unfit men, and 4.11 for obese, unfit men. Similar relationships were found for fat and fat-free mass. Fitness and fatness variables were significantly correlated, except for height and fatness. Body fatness was significantly correlated with both all-cause and CVD mortality. Fit men had a significantly lower risk for all-cause mortality in all waist circumference categories than did unfit men. Unfit men with the smallest waist circumferences had a higher risk for all-cause mortality than did fit men with large waist circumferences.

Conclusion.—Being lean is a health benefit only to fit men, and fitness may reduce the hazards of obesity.

▶ The 8-year follow-up data from the Cooper Clinic have seen numerous reincarnations during the past 11 years. One potential criticism of the data is that the classification of aerobic fitness (on the basis of treadmill endurance time) is influenced by both cardiovascular function and the obesity of the subjects. It is thus useful to see the data classified in terms of body fat content. The decrease in cardiovascular mortality associated with a high treadmill score seems to be lowest in those with 16.7% to 25.0% body fat but is rather similar in the lean (< 16.7% fat) and the obese (> 25% fat). One problem with the data is that even over 8 years, with a sample of 21,925, there were only 5 cardiovascular deaths in lean and unfit subjects, because almost all of the lean group were fit, at least in terms of the treadmill criterion; a still larger volume of data is required. There is also a need to extend these observations to women and to populations other than those men who are wealthy enough to attend the Cooper Clinic!

R. J. Shephard, MD, PhD, DPE

Safety of Medically Supervised Outpatient Cardiac Rehabilitation Exercise Therapy: A 16-Year Follow-up
Franklin BA, Bonzheim K, Gordon S, et al (William Beaumont Hosp, Royal Oak, Mich)
Chest 114:902-906, 1998   4–7

Objective.—Most of the information on the safety of physical training for coronary patients is based on two studies from 1960 and 1980. Results of a retrospective review of patient exercise hours and major cardiovascular complications was carried out to evaluate the safety of medically

TABLE 2.—Summary of Contemporary Exercise-based Cardiac Rehabilitation Complication Rates

Investigator	Year	Patient Exercise Hours	Cardiac Arrest	MI	Fatal Events	Major Complications*
Van Camp and Peterson[2]	1980-1984	2,351,916	1/111,996†	1/293,990	1/783,972	1/81,101
Digenio et al[14]	1982-1988	480,000	1/120,000‡		1/160,000	1/120,000
Vongvanich et al[13]	1986-1995	268,503	1/89,501§	1/268,503§	0/268,503	1/67,126
Beaumont data	1982-1998	292,254	1/146,127§	1/97,418§	0/292,254	1/58,451

MI, Myocardial infarction.
*MI and cardiac event.
†Fatal, 14%.
‡Fatal, 75%.
§Fatal, 0%.
(Courtesy of Franklin BA, Bonzheim K, Gordon S, et al: Safety of medically supervised outpatient cardiac rehabilitation exercise therapy: a 16-year follow-up. *Chest* 114:902-906, 1998.)

supervised outpatient cardiac rehabilitation therapy in a single center over 16 years, from 1982 through February 13, 1998.

Methods.—During a 16-year period, 3335 patients (70% men; average age, 61.6) took part in an exercise-based cardiac rehabilitation program that consisted initially of supervised low-level or symptom-limited exercise (phase 1) and progressed to supervised 50-minute aerobic exercise sessions at 50% to 80% of peak heart rate 3 times weekly for 4, 6, and 8 weeks for patients at low, moderate, and high risk (phase 2), and later to a variety of optional exercises with use of arm and leg ergometers, treadmills, automated step machines, cross-country skiing devices, progressive resistance equipment, and a swimming pool (phase 3).

Results.—During 292,254 patient exercise hours, there were 3 nonfatal myocardial infarctions and 2 cardiac arrests involving 4 men and 1 woman. One patient died. All complications occurred during phase 3 of rehabilitation. The overall rates of major cardiovascular complications per patient exercise hours were 1 in 49,315 for phase 1 and 1 in 58,451 for phases 2 and 3, lower than rates found in the literature (Table 2). The risk for cardiac arrest is significantly higher in individuals who violate the ceiling of their exercise prescription. Most patients (86% in one study[1]) experiencing cardiac arrest are successfully resuscitated.

Conclusion.—In medically supervised outpatients performing cardiac rehabilitation exercise therapy, the incidence of major cardiovascular complications is low.

▶ There have been previous reports showing the relative safety of cardiac rehabilitation programs, based on both questionnaires circulated to large numbers of centers[1,2] and analysis of data from a single large program.[3] There is some danger that centers with a poor record will not return questionnaires, and results from a single center thus seem more inherently reliable. Our early experience was a risk of about 1 cardiac event per 300,000 person-hours of supervised exercise and 1 episode per 100,000 hours of prescribed but unsupervised exercise. Franklin and colleagues argue that several factors suggest the need to update statistics: an increase in average age of the patients, the use of more aggressive therapies, risk stratification, and newer forms of pharmacotherapy. Although some centers have increased the intensity of their rehabilitation programs, a proportion of our patients were entering the Boston marathon as early as 1973. Other points of difference in current programs seem valid, but nevertheless the overall risk of a cardiac incident has not changed greatly from the 1 in 100,000 hours reported at a number of US centers. Much as in another study,[4] all of the cardiac incidents occurred in patients previously identified as a high-risk group, suggesting that stratification may be helpful in reducing the frequency of problems. It is also important to note that nursing and paramedical staff were able to resuscitate all patients without the intervention of a physician. Finally, although the difference was not statistically significant, as in other reports,[5] the incidence of problems was greater in the morning than in the afternoon (3 vs 2.4 per 100,000 cardiac complications of all types).

R. J. Shephard, MD, PhD, DPE

References

1. Van Camp SP, Peterson RA: Cardiovascular complications of outpatient cardiac rehabilitation programs. *JAMA* 256:1160-1163, 1986.
2. Haskell WL: Cardiovascular complications during exercise training of cardiac patients. *Circulation* 57:920-924, 1978.
3. Shephard RJ, Kavanagh T, Tuck J, et al: Marathon jogging in post–myocardial infarction patients. *J Cardiac Rehab* 3:321-329, 1983.
4. Van Camp SP, Peterson RA: Identification of the high risk cardiac rehabilitation patient. *J Cardiopulm Rehabil* 9:103-109, 1989.
5. Murray PM, Herrington DM, Pettus CW, et al: Should patients with heart disease exercise in the morning or afternoon? *Arch Intern Med* 153:833-836, 1993.

Results of a Multicenter Randomized Clinical Trial of Exercise and Long-term Survival in Myocardial Infarction Patients: The National Exercise and Heart Disease Project (NEHDP)

Dorn J, Naughton J, Imamura D, et al (State Univ of New York at Buffalo)
Circulation 100:1764-1769, 1999   4–8

Background.—Exercise programs are often recommended after myocardial infarction (MI) to return patients to a productive high-quality lifestyle and to decrease the risk for subsequent cardiac events or death. The effects of a supervised exercise program on 19-year survival among men after MI was investigated.

Methods.—The subjects were 651 men, aged 30 to 64 years, who had participated in the National Exercise and Heart Disease Project, a multicenter randomized clinical trial conducted between 1976 and 1979. The 315 men in the treatment group exercised in a laboratory for 8 weeks, after which they jogged, cycled, or swam guided by individualized target heart rate. The control group consisted of 319 men who engaged in normal

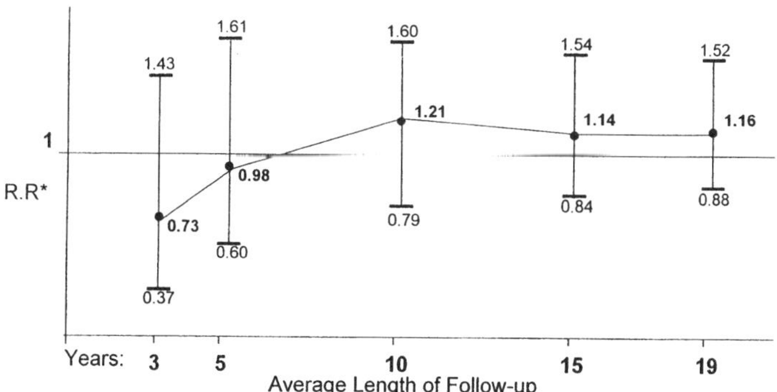

FIGURE 2.—Risk for cardiovascular disease mortality in exercise-treatment group compared with control subjects at various follow-up periods. *RR, relative risk; bars represent 95% confidence intervals. (Courtesy of Dorn J, Naughton J, Imamura D, et al: Results of a multicenter randomized clinical trial of exercise and long-term survival in myocardial infarction patients: The National Exercise and Heart Disease Project (NEHDP). *Circulation* 100:1764-1769, 1999.)

routines but who did not participate in any regular exercise program. The men were followed up until the end of 1995 or until they died.

Findings.—In a Cox proportional hazards analysis, the all-cause mortality risk estimates were 0.69 in the exercise group compared with the control group after a mean 3 years' follow-up. At 5 years, this risk was 0.84; at 10 years, 0.95; at 15 years, 1.02; and at 19 years, 1.09. Estimates for cardiovascular disease mortality for these periods were 0.73, 0.98, 1.21, 1.14, and 1.16, respectively (Fig 2). Each 1-MET increase in work capacity from baseline to the end of the original study resulted in consistent decreases in all-cause and cardiovascular disease mortality risk at each follow-up period, regardless of initial work capacity.

Conclusions.—Participating in an exercise program after MI nonsignificantly decreases mortality risk in the early follow-up period. Benefits declined with time. Contamination between groups over time may explain these diminished effects, as work capacity provided survival benefits for up to 19 years.

▶ This article is important mainly because of the length and completeness of follow-up. It is one of the first 2 or 3 randomized trials of coronary rehabilitation. At first inspection, the findings are disappointing. However, as in a trial conducted in southern Ontario, those who actually adopted an active lifestyle did gain considerable benefit relative to those who remained sedentary.[1] The main problem seems to have been that the lifestyle distinction between the original experimental and control groups became blurred over the years.

R. J. Shephard, MD, PhD, DPE

Reference

1. Cunningham DA, Rechnitzer PA, Andrew GM, et al: The issue of poor compliance in exercise trials: A place for post-hoc analyses? *Sports Training Med Rehab* 2:131-139, 1991.

Effects of Cardiac Rehabilitation and Exercise Training Programs on Coronary Patients With High Levels of Hostility
Lavie CJ, Milani RV (Ochsner Med Insts, New Orleans, La)
Mayo Clin Proc 74:959-966, 1999   4–9

Background.—Behavioral factors, such as depression, may be associated with coronary heart disease (CHD) events and with morbidity and mortality after such events. Previous studies have demonstrated a 7-fold increase in risk for CHD in persons with hostility, or unexpressed anger. The effects of cardiac rehabilitation interventions on patients with hostility were investigated.

Methods.—Five hundred consecutive patients were studied before and after cardiac rehabilitation. Sixty-five patients had high levels of hostility, assessed by validated questionnaires, and 435 had low levels of hostility.

TABLE 3.—Benefits of Cardiac Rehabilitation and Exercise Training in Patients With High Hostility Scores (n = 65)*

Characteristic	Before Rehabilitation	After Rehabilitation	% Change	P Value
Behavioral characteristics†				
Anxiety	11.2±4.8	6.1±5.2	−38	<.001
Depression	9.3±5.4	4.8±5.0	−48	<.001
Somatization	9.0±4.3	6.0±4.2	−33	<.001
Hostility	12.0±3.8	6.6±5.4	−45	<.001
Quality of life‡				
Mental health	19±5	21±5	+11	<.001
Energy	12±4	15±4	+25	<.001
General health	19±5	21±4	+11	<.01
Pain	7±2	9±2	+27	<.001
Function	32±8	40±8	+25	<.001
Well-being	38±9	45±9	+19	<.001
Total	88±17	106±18	+20	<.001

*Values are expressed in mean units ± SD, except as noted.
†A lower score indicates a more favorable behavioral trait.
‡A higher score indicates a more favorable quality-of-life trait.
(Courtesy of Lavie CJ, Milani RV: Effects of cardiac rehabilitation and exercise training programs on coronary patients with high levels of hostility. *Mayo Clin Proc* 74:959-966, 1999.)

Findings.—In the total cohort, scores for anxiety, depression, somatization, and total quality of life, but not for hostility, improved significantly after rehabilitation. Patients with high hostility levels had significant improvements in hostility scores and on the other measures. This subgroup also improved exercise capacity, percent body fat, body mass index, and total cholesterol and high-density lipoprotein cholesterol levels (Table 3). Compared with patients with low hostility levels, those with high hostility levels had greater relative improvement in scores on hostility, anxiety, general health, energy, mental health, and total quality of life. Improvements in exercise capacity, obesity indexes, lipid levels, and other behavioral characteristics and quality-of-life measures were similar between groups. The prevalence of high hostility levels after cardiac rehabilitation declined from 13% to 8%.

Conclusions.—Cardiac rehabilitation reduces hostility and significantly improves quality of life and other behavioral characteristics in patients with high levels of hostility. More attention to behavioral characteristics is needed in the primary and secondary prevention of CHD.

▶ Kavanagh et al[1] and others[2] have previously shown that a progressive exercise-centered program of cardiac rehabilitation is helpful in correcting the depression that is often initially associated with myocardial infarction. However, in terms of prognosis, the ability to modify the anger or hostility component of the disturbed personality is probably more important, because this is associated with up to a 7-fold increase in the risk for coronary events.[3] As in many studies of exercise and personality, benefit was largest in those individuals with the highest initial hostility scores; methodologists may object that a part of this apparent benefit is a "reversion toward the mean," because the effect on the group as a whole is not statistically significant.

R. J. Shephard, MD, PhD, DPE

References

1. Kavanagh T, Shephard RJ, Tuck JA: Depression after myocardial infarction. *Can Med Assoc J* 113:23-27, 1975.
2. Milani RV, Lavie CJ, Cassidy MM: Effects of cardiac rehabilitation and exercise training programs on depression in patients after major coronary events. *Am Heart J* 132:726-732, 1996.
3. Friedman M, Thiresen CE, Gill JJ, et al: Alteration of type A behavior and its effect on cardiac recurrences in post-myocardial infarction patients: Summary results of the recurrent coronary prevention project. *Am Heart J* 112:653-665, 1986.

Changes in Cardiorespiratory Fitness, Psychological Wellbeing, Quality of Life, and Vocational Status Following a 12 Month Cardiac Exercise Rehabilitation Programme

Dugmore LD, Tipson RJ, Phillips MH, et al (Cardiac Rehabilitation Centre, West Midlands, UK; Dudley Group of Hosps NHS Trust, West Midlands, UK; South Tyneside District Hosp, South Shields, UK; et al)

Heart 81:359-366, 1999   4–10

Background.—The value and benefit of cardiac rehabilitation are debated. Improvements in cardiorespiratory fitness, psychologic well-being, quality of life, and vocational status were assessed in patients during and after a comprehensive 12-month exercise rehabilitation program for recovery from myocardial infarction (MI).

Methods.—One hundred twenty-two men and 2 women with a clinical diagnosis of MI were assigned randomly to weekly aerobic training, 3 times a week for 12 months, or to no formal exercise program. At 5 years, a follow-up interview was conducted.

Findings.—Compared with the control group, the treatment group had significant improvement in cardiorespiratory fitness, psychologic profile, and quality of life scores (Table 6). Mortality did not differ significantly between groups. However, a larger proportion of patients in the treatment group resumed full-time employment and returned to work sooner than patients in the control group. Those in the control group tended to take lighter jobs, lost more time from work, and had more nonfatal reinfarctions.

Conclusions.—Regular, prolonged, supervised aerobic exercise training improves cardiorespiratory fitness, psychologic status, and quality of life in persons recovering from MI. In this study, the treatment group had a decrease in morbidity and significant improvement in vocational status compared with the control group in the 5 years since MI.

▶ In contrast with the article by Lavie et al, Dugmore and associates distributed their subjects in random fashion between an experimental and a

TABLE 6.—Selected Indices of Psychological Well-Being/Quality of Life: Exercisers vs Controls, 3 Weeks to 12 Months (Poor Prognosis Group)

	3 Weeks			4 Months			8 Months			12 Months		
	Exercisers	Controls	p	Exercisers	Controls	p	Exercisers	Controls	p	Exercisers	Controls	p
TAS depression "D" score	9.4 (0.8)	8.9 (0.6)	NS	8.0 (0.6)	8.7 (0.9)	NS	7.2 (0.6)	9.2 (0.9)	NS	6.6 (0.6)	9.9 (0.7)	< 0.001
POMS (1+4 only)												
1. Tension/anxiety	44.1 (1.5)	43.5 (1.7)	NS	42.3 (1.4)	43.0 (1.9)	NS	37.9 (1.2)	39.8 (1.6)	NS	37.4 (1.3)	42.0 (1.7)	< 0.05
4. Vigour/activity	53.5 (1.5)	51.0 (1.7)	NS	60.5 (1.6)	57.7 (1.5)	NS	62.1 (1.3)	57.5 (1.4)	< 0.05	64.0 (1.4)	57.3 (1.5)	< 0.01
Quality of life score	38.4 (3.7)	37.5 (3.0)	NS	76.3 (2.2)	57.7 (2.5)	< 0.001	78.9 (2.1)	58.0 (2.5)	< 0.001	80.8 (1.2)	59.4 (2.2)	< 0.001

Values are mean (SEM).
Abbreviations: POMS, Profile of Mood States; *TAS*, Toronto Attitude Scale.
(Courtesy of Dugmore LD, Tipson RJ, Phillips MH, et al: Changes in cardiorespiratory fitness, psychological wellbeing, quality of life, and vocational status following a 12 month cardiac exercise rehabilitation programme. *Heart* 81:359-366, 1999, with permission from the BMT Publishing Group.)

control group. They found that gains in mood-state and quality of life were seen only in subjects who had been allocated to the exercise regimen. Program compliance is not specifically mentioned, but the experimental subjects showed a large gain in maximal oxygen intake, while figures for the control group showed little change over the year of observation. The effect on mood state was demonstrated by 2 independent tests (the Toronto Attitude Scale and the Profile of Mood States [POMS]). As in our earlier study, the abnormal initial POMS values related to the anxiety rather than the depression scale. Benefit developed progressively over the 12 months of exercise, and contrary to one previous study,[2] near normal values had been restored by the end of the year. The correction of depression was associated with a greater quality of life, and (very important from the economic point of view) an earlier return to work.

R. J. Shephard, MD, PhD, DPE

References

1. Shephard RJ, Kavanagh T, Klavora P: Mood state during post-coronary cardiac rehabilitation. *J Cardiac Rehabil* 5:480-484, 1985.
2. Langosch W: Psychological effects of training in coronary patients: A critical review of the literature. *Eur Heart J* 9(suppl M):37-42, 1988.

Oxygen Uptake to Work Rate Relation Throughout Peak Exercise in Normal Subjects: Relevance for Rate Adaptive Pacemaker Programming
Lewalter T, Rickli H, Maccarter D, et al (Univ of Bonn, Germany; Univ of Zürich, Switzerland; ELA Med CA La Boursidière, Cedex, France; et al)
PACE 22:769-775, 1999   4–11

Objective.—Aerobic power or oxygen intake to work rate ratio is an important criterion for pacemaker functioning. The oxygen intake to work rate (VO_2/WR) relationship from rest to anaerobic threshold (AT) and from AT to peak exercise was measured separately in middle-aged individuals with pacemakers to detect relevant slope changes resulting from the shift in aerobic to anaerobic energy supply.

Methods.—Treadmill peak exercise testing was performed at different speeds in 78 healthy volunteers (34 women), average age 46 years. Breath-by-breath gas exchange was analyzed, and AT was calculated.

Results.—The slope of the oxygen intake to work rate relationship changed sharply and significantly at the AT (31%) for both men and women (Table 2). The slope change was more dramatic with women than with men, indicating that pacemakers for women should be programmed to generate a steeper VO_2/WR slope below AT with a sharper slope change at AT than for men. Otherwise, higher-than-necessary oxygen intake to work rate slopes at higher workload intensities can lead to overpacing.

TABLE 2.—Results of Slope Analysis for the Oxygen Uptake (VO_2 to Work Rate and Oxygen Uptake/kg to Work Rate Relationship from Rest to Peak Exercise, Rest to Anaerobic Threshold and Anaerobic Threshold to Peak

	$\dot{V}O_2$/WR (Rest-Peak) mL/Watt	$\dot{V}O_2$/WR (Rest-AT) mL/Watt	$\dot{V}O_2$/WR (AT-Peak) mL/Watt	$\dot{V}O_2$/kg/WR (Rest-Peak) mL/kg/Watt	$\dot{V}O_2$/kg/WR (Rest-AT) mL/kg/Watt	$\dot{V}O_2$/kg/WR (AT-Peak) mL/kg/Watt
Study Group (n = 78)	11.4 ± 2.7	14.4 ± 4.6	9.8 ± 4.0	0.17 ± 0.05	0.22 ± 0.09	0.15 ± 0.07
Women (n = 34)	11.1 ± 2.7	15.9 ± 5.7	9.1 ± 3.2	0.19 ± 0.05	0.27 ± 0.09	0.16 ± 0.06
Men (n = 44)	11.5 ± 2.7	13.3 ± 2.2	10.4 ± 4.5	0.15 ± 0.05	0.18 ± 0.05	0.14 ± 0.07

(Courtesy of Lewalter T, Rickli H, Maccarter D, et al: Oxygen uptake to work rate relation throughout peak exercise in normal subjects: Relevance for rate adaptive pacemaker programming. *PACE* 22:769-775, 1999.)

Conclusion.—Pacemakers for women should be programmed to generate a steeper VO_2/WR slope below AT with a sharper slope change at AT than for men to prevent overpacing.

▶ Pacemakers are now becoming sufficiently sophisticated that a ventilation or motion sensor can generate a nonlinear signal in relation to exercise intensity. Whether the signal operating the pacemaker is ventilation or oxygen consumption, the break point typically occurs at the AT. However, details of the signal/work-rate relationship differ between men and women and from individual to individual, and if a device is to function appropriately at higher work rates, individual laboratory adjustment seems a necessity.

R. J. Shephard, MD, PhD, DPE

Beneficial Effects of Exercise Training in Heart Failure Patients With Low Cardiac Output Response to Exercise—A Comparison of Two Training Models

Gordon A, Tyni-Lenné R, Jansson E, et al (Karolinska Inst, Huddinge, Sweden)

J Intern Med 246:175-182, 1999

4–12

Introduction.—In patients with chronic heart failure (CHF), cardiac function parameters do not necessarily reflect exercise capacity. However, previous studies have suggested that exercise training is advisable only for patients without severely reduced cardiac output (CO). For such patients, training of a small muscle mass might place a high local load on the working muscle without unduly straining the cardiovascular system. The responses to 2 different training models were compared in patients with CHF and a low CO response to exercise.

Methods.—The study sample comprised 16 patients with CHF (mean age, 63 years) and a mean resting left ventricular fraction of 30%. All patients were in clinically stable condition and had no other problems that would limit their exercise performance. At baseline, each patient under-

TABLE 4.—Exercise Capacity and Skeletal Muscle Oxidative Capacity in Different Training Groups

	Cycle Training Group ($n = 8$)			One-Legged Training Group ($n = 8$)		
	Before	After		Before	After	
Exercise capacity cycle ergometer (W)	105 ± 11	116 ± 11	†	94 ± 30	120 ± 34	**‡
VO_2 peak cycle ergometer (mL kg^{-1} min^{-1})	17.5 ± 2.7	17.8 ± 3.3	NS	16.0 ± 3.1	19.0 ± 3.0	**‡
VO_2 peak cycle ergometer (L min^{-1})	1.50 ± 0.28	1.52 ± 0.16	NS	1.31 ± 0.44	1.57 ± 0.55	**‡
Exercise capacity knee extension work (W)	29 ± 4	37 ± 6	†	28 ± 8	39 ± 11	†
VO_2 peak knee extension work (mL kg^{-1} min^{-1})	9.9 ± 1.4	10.7 ± 1.4	*	10.13 ± 1.4	11.16 ± 2.1	†
VO_2 peak knee extension work (L min^{-1})	0.82 ± 0.11	0.86 ± 0.09	*	0.77 ± 0.24	0.84 ± 0.28	*
Citrate synthase (μkat g^{-1} d w)	0.34 ± 0.10	0.43 ± 0.08	†	0.31 ± 0.06	0.45 ± 0.06	†

*$P < .05$ within groups.
†$P < .01$ within groups.
‡Two-way analysis of variance between groups, $P < .05$.
(Courtesy of Gordon A, Tyni-Lenné R, Jansson E, et al: Beneficial effects of exercise training in heart failure patients with low cardiac output response to exercise—a comparison of two training models. *J Intern Med* 246:175-182, 1999, Blackwell Science Ltd.)

went a cardiopulmonary exercise test, right heart catheterization, and a leg muscle biopsy. Their CO response to exercise was assessed, based on the CO response index: the ratio between the increase in CO and the increase in oxygen intake during exercise. After stratification for CO response index and other factors, patients were randomly assigned to 2 exercise programs, which differed in terms of active muscle mass: 20 minutes of a traditional cycle ergometer test or 1-legged knee extensor exercise for 16 to 18 minutes per leg, with a frequency of about 60 kicks per minute. The working muscle mass for these 2 types of exercise was about 10 kg for the former and 2 kg for the latter. Responses to the 2 training models were analyzed in terms of the CO response index.

Results.—The CO response index was significantly related to baseline exercise capacity. Both exercise programs improved exercise capacity, but 2-legged exercise brought a greater improvement: 28% versus 10% (Table 4). The exercise capacity response was unrelated to baseline exercise capacity; it was related to the CO response index in the training group performing 1-legged exercise but not in the training group performing 2-legged exercise. A negative correlation was noted between the CO response index and the peak exercise pulmonary capillary wedge pressure. Citrate synthase activity in the leg muscle increased after training in a way that was negatively correlated with the CO response index at baseline.

Conclusions.—In patients with CHF, the exercise response to 1-legged training is significantly related to the CO increase in relation to oxygen intake before training. Most patients will show an increase in exercise capacity in response to training, but the training model should be based on the patient's CO response to exercise. The authors call for further study of the benefits of training a limited muscle mass in patients with a low CO response to exercise.

▶ There is growing evidence that at least a part of the functional limitation in CHF is caused by an accumulation of "disuse" abnormalities in the skeletal muscles.[1-3] Attempts to restore the situation through an exercise regimen may founder because the cardiac condition will not support an exercise program of adequate intensity. The size of the present sample is small, and conclusions must be correspondingly cautious. Nevertheless, the idea that one can train the weak leg muscles and thus functional capacity 1 leg at a time is novel and may have therapeutic value.

R. J. Shephard, MD, PhD, DPE

References

1. Adamopoulos S, Coats AJS, Brunotte F: Physical training improves skeletal muscle metabolism in patients with chronic heart failure. *J Am Coll Cardiol* 21:1101-1106, 1993.
2. Gordon A, Tyni-Lenné R, Persson H, et al: Markedly improved skeletal muscle function with local muscle training in patients with chronic heart failure. *Clin Cardiol* 19:568-574, 1996.
3. Shephard RJ: Physical activity in the treatment of congestive heart failure. *Sports Med* 23:75-92, 1997.

Randomized, Controlled Trial of Long-term Moderate Exercise Training in Chronic Heart Failure: Effects of Functional Capacity, Quality of Life, and Clinical Outcome

Belardinelli R, Georgiou D, Cianci G, et al (Istituto Cardiologico "GM Lancisi," Ancona, Italy; Columbia Univ, New York)
Circulation 99:1173-1182, 1999

4–13

Background.—Whether exercise training (ET) is beneficial in the treatment of chronic heart failure (CHF) is unclear. The current study examined the effects of long-term moderate ET on functional capacity and quality of life in patients with CHF, as well as the associated outcomes.

Methods.—Ninety-nine patients with stable CHF were randomly assigned to ET at 60% of peak $\dot{V}O_2$ 3 times a week for 8 weeks followed by twice a week for 1 year (group T) or by no exercise (group NT). Cardiopulmonary exercise testing was done at baseline and at 2 and 14 months. In addition, 74 patients with ischemic heart disease underwent myocardial

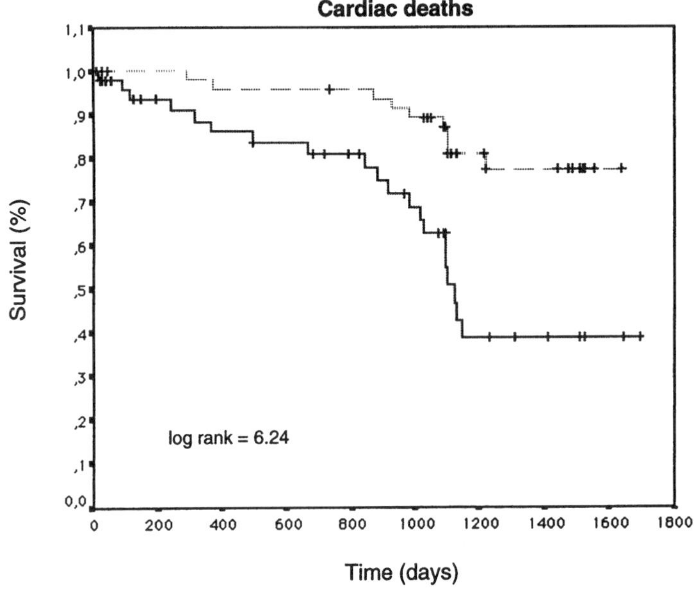

No. OF PATIENTS AT RISK

Untrained	49	46	43	42	41	37	29	29	29	29
Trained	50	50	48	48	48	45	42	41	41	41

FIGURE 4.—Kaplan-Meier survival curves of cardiac death in trained group (*broken line*) and untrained control group (*solid line*) during follow-up. *Plus sign* indicates censored cases. (Courtesy of Belardinelli R, Georgiou D, Cianci G, et al: Randomized, controlled trial of long-term moderate exercise training in chronic heart failure: Effects of functional capacity, quality of life, and clinical outcome. *Circulation* 99:1173-1182, 1999.)

scintigraphy. A questionnaire was administered to determine quality of life. Ninety-four patients finished the study.

Findings.—Changes occurred in group T patients only. Peak $\dot{V}O_2$ and thallium activity scores improved by 18% and 24%, respectively, at 2 months. These values did not change further after 1 year. In addition, quality of life improved, paralleling peak $\dot{V}O_2$. Exercise training was associated with lower mortality and hospital readmission rates for heart failure. Factors that independently predicted events were ventilatory threshold at baseline and posttraining thallium activity score. There was a significant difference between survival curves when separated by exercise training (Fig 4).

Conclusions.—Long-term moderate ET provides a sustained improvement in functional capacity and quality of life in patients with CHF. Favorable outcomes appear to be associated with this benefit.

▶ Previous research from the Toronto Rehabilitation Centre had rather similar findings.[1] Patients with congestive heart failure maintained their gains in aerobic power over a 1-year period, and an overall parallel was seen between gains in the quality of life and the increase of maximal oxygen intake. However, individual quality-of-life data did not show much correlation with physiologic variables.[2] The study of Belardinelli et al takes a relatively large (100 patients) randomized sample and shows that, in addition to early (2-month) gains in the quality of life (assessed by the disease-specific Minnesota "Living With Heart Failure" questionnaire,[3] there are convincing differences in clinical outcomes (hospitalizations, cardiac events, and cardiac deaths) between those who are exercised and those who are not.

R. J. Shephard, MD, PhD, DPE

References

1. Kavanagh T, Myers MG, Baigrie RS, et al: Quality of life and cardiorespiratory function in chronic heart failure: Effects of 12 months' aerobic training. *Heart* 76: 42-46, 1996.
2. Shephard RJ, Kavanagh T, Mertens DJ: On the prediction of physiological and psychological responses to aerobic training in patients with stable congestive heart failure. *J Cardiopulm Rehabil* 18:45-51, 1998.
3. Rector TS, Cohn JN: Assessment of patient outcomes with the Minnesota Living with Heart Failure questionnaire: Reliability and validity during a randomized, double blind, placebo-controlled trial of pimobendan. *Am Heart J* 1024:1017-1025, 1992.

Neuroendocrine Activation in Heart Failure Is Modified by Endurance Exercise Training

Braith RW, Welsch MA, Feigenbaum MS, et al (Univ of Florida, Gainesville; Louisiana State Univ, Baton Rouge; Furman Univ, Greenville, SC)
J Am Coll Cardiol 34:1170-1175, 1999   4–14

Background.—Patients with heart failure and neuroendocrine activation have poor long-term outcomes. It is generally agreed that exercise can improve the clinical outcome of chronic heart failure, although the mechanisms of this benefit are unclear. The effects of endurance exercise on neuroendocrine activity in patients with chronic heart failure were analyzed.

Methods.—The randomized trial included 19 patients with chronic but clinically stable coronary artery disease and New York Heart Association class II or III heart failure. One group was assigned to exercise, consisting of walking at 40% to 70% of maximum oxygen intake 3 times weekly for 16 weeks. The control group received no exercise training. Both groups continued taking their regular medications. The groups were compared on exercise tests and neurohormone assays.

Results.—At baseline, the 2 groups were comparable in terms of age, ejection fraction, and other characteristics. They were also similar in their resting and exercise levels of angiotensin II, aldosterone, vasopressin, and atrial natriuretic peptide. The control group showed no changes in any of these values, at rest or during exercise, after 16 weeks. The exercise group showed no change in peak neurohormone values during exercise. How-

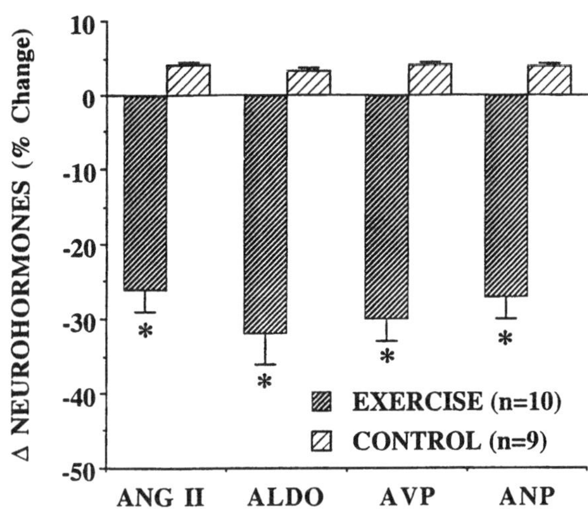

FIGURE 1.—Relative changes in angiotensin II (ANG II), aldosterone (ALDO), arginine vasopressin (AVP), and atrial natriuretic peptide (ANP) after 4 months of endurance exercise training or control period. Data are mean plus or minus SEM. *P .05 or less after training versus before training. (Reprinted with permission from the American College of Cardiology from Braith RW, Welsch MA, Feigenbaum MS, et al: Neuroendocrine activation in heart failure is modified by endurance exercise training. *J Am Coll Cardiol* 34:1170-1175, 1999.)

ever, exercise was associated with significant reductions in resting hormone levels, including a 26% decrease in angiotensin, a 32% decrease in aldosterone, a 30% decrease in vasopressin, and a 27% decrease in atrial natriuretic peptide (Fig 1).

Conclusions.—In patients with chronic heart failure, a 16-week program of endurance exercise can significantly reduce resting neurohormonal activation. This study documents reductions of 25% to 30% in angiotensin II, aldosterone, arginine vasopressin, and atrial natriuretic peptide. These reductions in circulating neurohormone levels might improve the long-term prognosis of heart failure.

▶ I am always in favor of natural rather than pharmacologic treatment where possible. The benefits of suppressing neurohormonal activity by angiotensin-converting enzyme inhibitors in congestive heart failure is well-established,[1] but it is encouraging to find some evidence that a similar pattern of response can be obtained by a regimen of progressive endurance training, beginning at quite a modest intensity of effort. Although the resting levels of angiotensin, aldosterone, vasopressin, and atrial natriuretic peptide were reduced, the peak exercise levels were unchanged at the end of the 16 weeks of training. This reflects the fact that the program increased the peak intensity of exercise by 25%.

R. J. Shephard, MD, PhD, DPE

Reference

1. Grassi G, Cattaneo BM, Servavalle G, et al: Effects of chronic ACE inhibition on sympathetic nerve traffic and baroreflex control of the circulation. *Circulation* 96:1173-1179, 1997.

Exaggerated Blood Pressure Response to Dynamic Exercise and Risk of Future Hypertension
Matthews CE, Pate RR, Jackson KL, et al (Univ of South Carolina, Columbia; Cooper Inst for Aerobics Research, Dallas, Texas)
J Clin Epidemiol 51:29-35, 1998   4–15

Objective.—Normotensive individuals who have an exaggerated blood pressure response to exercise testing are at two to three times the risk for development of hypertension. Studies, however, have not always controlled for confounders. The association between future hypertension and an exaggerated blood pressure response to exercise, the latter defined by taking resting blood pressure into account, and controlling for potential confounders, was examined in a prospective and retrospective nested case-control study.

Methods.—Between 1971 and 1982, baseline clinical examinations, resting blood pressure measurements, and exercise testing results were obtained in 5,386 healthy, normotensive men. Participants (73%) completed a questionnaire. Follow-up questionnaires mailed in 1986 solicited

TABLE 5.—Sensitivity, Specificity, and Predictive Values for Variables Found to Be Significantly Associated With Future Hypertension

Variable	Cases ($n = 151$)	Controls ($n = 201$)	Sensitivity	Specificity	Predictive Value
EBPR[a]					
Yes	36	23	23.8	88.6	8.0
No	115	178			
Weight gain[b]					
>10 kg	35	29	23.2	85.6	6.3
<9.9 kg	116	172			
SBP					
<131	34	24	22.5	88.1	7.3
≥131	117	177			
DBP					
<86	56	47	37.1	76.6	6.2
≥86	95	154			

(Reprinted from Matthews CE, Pate RR, Jackson KL, et al: Exaggerated blood pressure response to dynamic exercise and risk of future hypertension. *J Clin Epidemiol* 51:29-35, copyright 1998, with permission from Elsevier Science.)

information on individuals with diagnosed hypertension, cardiovascular disease, and other major medical conditions.

Results.—Compared with normotensive individuals, those who had been diagnosed with hypertension at follow-up had significantly higher body mass at baseline and follow-up, greater body mass change from age 21 years to follow-up, and higher body mass index, percent body fat, and plasma glucose levels. History of smoking and family history of hypertension were similar for cases and controls. Those who were diagnosed with hypertension were 2.4 times more likely to have had an exaggerated blood pressure response. According to multivariate analysis, an exaggerated blood pressure response, sitting systolic and diastolic blood pressure, weight change from age 21 to follow-up, age at entry, and body mass index were significantly associated with hypertension outcome (Table 5).

Conclusion.—An exaggerated blood pressure response to exercise was significantly associated with development of hypertension, accounting for 33% of the overall risk after controlling for confounding factors.

▶ The association between an exaggerated blood pressure response to exercise and subsequent hypertension has been recognized for a number of years.[1] The present set of data confirms this finding on a substantial longitudinal study of individuals attending the Cooper Clinic, basing the diagnosis on the *change* from rest to exercise blood pressures, and adding the information that the odds ratio is increased slightly (3.0 vs 2.4) after controlling for a substantial number of covariates. The problem is that although statistically significant, the sensitivity of the exaggerated blood pressure (like other predictors such as weight gain and resting blood pressure) is low. Thus, predictions are not very successful in individual patients. The problem is compounded by a low prevalence of exaggerated blood pressure responses in apparently healthy individuals.[2,3] Given that hypertension is a more frequent problem in female patients, it will be important to repeat these observations in women.

R. J. Shephard, MD, PhD, DPE

References

1. Benbassat J, Froom P: Blood pressure response to exercise as a predictor of hypertension. *Arch Intern Med* 146:2053-2055, 1986.
2. Jackson AS, Squires WG, Grimes G, et al: Prediction of future resting hypertension from exercise blood pressure. *J Cardiopulm Rehabil* 3:263-268, 1983.
3. Wilson NV, Meyer BM: Early prediction of hypertension using exercise blood pressure. *Prev Med* 10:62-68, 1981.

Effects of Leisure-Time Physical Activity and Ventilatory Function on Risk for Stroke in Men: The Reykjavík Study
Agnarsson U, Thorgeirsson G, Sigvaldason H, et al (Natl Univ Hosp, Reykjavík, Iceland)
Ann Intern Med 130:987-990, 1999   4–16

Objective.—Physical activity reduces cardiovascular risk factors. The risk for stroke and its association with leisure-time physical activity and ventilatory function was evaluated in men in a long-term, prospective, population-based cohort study.

Methods.—A total of 4484 men, aged 45 to 80 years, were followed up on average for 10.6 years. Patients completed a health and social factor questionnaire at study entry and underwent a physical examination, including blood analysis, and spirometry. The outcome measure was the number of strokes. Risk factors for stroke were investigated with multivariate analysis.

Results.—During the study period, 249 men (5.6%), average age 70.1, had a stroke (44 hemorrhagic, 205 ischemic), 62 of them fatal. Leisuretime physical activity after age 40 was associated with reduced total risk (relative risk [RR], 0.69) and ischemic stroke risk (RR, 0.62) (Table 2). Univariate analysis found that risk for stroke increased with older age, current smoking, hypertension, high body mass index, and lowest pulmonary function quintile compared with the highest quintile (RR, 1.85).

Conclusion.—Regular leisure-time activity may protect men older than age 40 against stroke. Decreased FEV_1 is an independent predictor of stroke.

▶ Given that regular physical activity can reduce systemic blood pressure, it seems logical that it should also reduce the risk of stroke, and there is growing evidence in support of such a hypothesis. The present report is based on a substantial sample, followed up for an average of more than 10 years, and the multivariate analysis includes a variety of other important risk factors; the main limitation was the distant recall of physical activity patterns. Age and hypertension are plainly the dominant influences for both total and ischemic stroke, but nevertheless there is substantial protection

TABLE 2.—Multivariate Analysis of Risk for Stroke in 4,484 Men

Variable	Relative Risk (95% CI)	P Value
Total stroke		
Age	1.09 (1.06-1.11)	0.001
Fasting blood glucose level	1.15 (1.04-1.28)	0.007
Smoking		
Former	0.73 (0.51-1.04)	0.08
Current	1.43 (1.04-1.96)	0.03
Hypertension	2.14 (1.66-2.77)	0.001
Leisure-time physical activity after age 40	0.69 (0.47-1.01)	0.06
FEV_1		
2.54 L	1.57 0.94-4.64)	0.09
2.55-2.95 L	1.36 (0.83-2.24)	>0.2
2.96-3.32 L	0.97 (0.57-1.65)	>0.2
3.33-3.70 L	0.99 (0.57-1.70)	>0.2
Ischemic stroke		
Age	1.09 (1.06-1.11)	<0.001
Body mass index	1.04 (1.00-1.08)	0.03
Smoking		
Former	0.64 (0.43-0.95)	0.03
Current	1.41 (1.00-1.99)	0.05
Hypertension	1.99 (1.49-2.66)	<0.001
Leisure-time physical activity after age 40	0.62 (0.40-0.97)	0.03
FEV_1		
2.54 L	1.85 (1.06-3.25)	0.03
2.55-2.95 L	1.38 (0.79-2.38)	>0.2
2.96-3.32 L	0.95 (0.53-1.71)	>0.2
3.33-3.70 L	0.86 (0.46-1.60)	>0.2

(Courtesy of Agnarsson U, Thorgeirsson G, Sigvaldason H, et al: Effects of leisure-time physical activity and ventilatory function on risk for stroke in men: The Reykjavík study. *Ann Intern Med* 130:987-990, 1999.)

from regular physical activity after allowing for these factors. In contrast with the Honolulu Heart Program study,[1] no protection was found for hemorrhagic stroke, but this may be because there were relatively small numbers with a hemorrhagic etiology. Moreover, the type of stroke was verified by CT in only 77.5% of cases. The favorable impact on ischemic stroke may come from changes in lipoprotein profile[2] or changes in fibrinolysis and platelet adhesiveness.[3] The type of physical activity that was most beneficial appeared to be of fairly low intensity (walking and swimming), although the data were insufficient to be conclusive in this regard.

R. J. Shephard, MD, PhD, DPE

References

1. Abbott RD, Rodriguez BL, Burchfield CM, et al: Physical activity in older middle-aged men and reduced risk of stroke: The Honolulu Heart Program. *Am J Epidemiol* 139:881-893, 1994.
2. Bronner LL, Kanter DS, Manson JE: Primary prevention of stroke. *N Engl J Med* 333:1392-1400, 1995.
3. Eliasson M, Asplund K, Evrin P: Regular leisure time physical activity predicts high activity of tissue plasminogen activator: The Northern Sweden MONICA Study. *Int J Epidemiol* 25:1182-1188, 1996.

Exercise and Risk of Stroke in Male Physicians

Lee I-M, Hennekens CH, Berger K, et al (Harvard Med School, Boston; Univ of Muenster, Germany)
Stroke 30:1-6, 1999   4–17

Objective.—Studies of the association between exercise and stroke have yielded disparate results. The Physicians' Health Study investigated the association between risk of stroke and age, cigarette smoking, and hypertension.

Methods.—The effect of low-dose aspirin and β-carotene was investigated in 21,823 men, aged 40 to 84 years, in a randomized, double-blind, placebo-controlled trial. Participants filled out a questionnaire at baseline, at 6 and 12 months, and annually thereafter, that included information on physical activity. The first occurrence of stroke was analyzed, the association between physical activity was assessed at baseline, total stroke incidence was calculated, the number of ischemic and hemorrhagic strokes was determined, and the effects of age, cigarette smoking, and history of hypertension on the association between physical activity at baseline and total stroke incidence was investigated.

Results.—There were 437 ischemic strokes, 84 hemorrhagic, and 12 of unknown type. The risk of stroke declined significantly with increasing physical activity, with the most active men having a 26% lower risk than the least active men. When adjusted for age (Table 2) the relative risk of stroke was 1.00 for an exercise frequency of less than 1 time per week, 0.80 for 1 time per week, 0.74 for 2 to 4 times per week, and 0.74 for 5 or more times per week. When history of hypertension, body mass index, high cholesterol, and diabetes mellitus were factored into the analysis, the relation between physical activity and stroke incidence was no longer significant. Physical activity was inversely related to risk of stroke, but the relationship attained borderline significance only for hemorrhagic stroke when adjusted for age. Age, cigarette smoking, or history of hypertension

TABLE 2.—Relative Risks of Total Stroke, According to Physical Activity

Frequency of Vigorous Exercise	No. of Events	RR* (95% CI)	Multivariate RR1† (95% CI)	Multivariate RR2‡ (95% CI)
<1 time/wk	189	1.00 (referent)	1.00 (referent)	1.00 (referent)
1 time/wk	87	0.80 (0.62-1.03)	0.79 (0.61-1.03)	0.81 (0.61-1.07)
2-4 times/wk	172	0.74 (0.61-0.92)	0.80 (0.65-0.99)	0.88 (0.70-1.10)
≥5 times/wk	85	0.74 (0.57-0.95)	0.79 (0.61-1.03)	0.86 (0.65-1.13)
P for trend		0.004	0.04	0.25

*Adjusted for age and treatment assignment.

†Additionally adjusted for cigarette smoking, alcohol consumption, history of angina, and parental history of myocardial infarction at age less than 60 years.

‡Adjusted for all the variables above, plus body mass index, history of hypertension, history of high cholesterol, and history of diabetes mellitus.

Abbreviations: RR, relative risk; *CI,* confidence interval.

(Courtesy of Lee I-M, Hennekens CH, Berger K, et al: Exercise and risk of stroke in male physicians. *Stroke* 30:1-6, 1999. Reproduced with permission, copyright 1999, American Heart Association.)

did not modify the association between physical activity and stroke incidence.

Conclusion.—Although physical activity reduces stroke incidence in men, exercise was not significantly associated with reduced risk but appeared to mediate its effect through controlling weight, blood pressure, cholesterol, and glucose tolerance.

▶ This study suggests that exercise that is sufficient to work up a sweat offers a 20% protection against stroke, even if it is performed only once per week, and that little additional protection is gained from more regular exercise sessions. However, it would be wrong to use this finding as a pretext for advocating infrequent exercise. The offsetting risks of vigorous physical activity—musculoskeletal injuries, immunosuppression and exercise-induced sudden death—become more likely if the exercise is taken infrequently. Multiple regression analysis of the present data indicated that the main mediators of the exercise response were a reduction in body mass, the control of hypertension, and improved glucose tolerance and serum lipids. In such an analysis, the number of contributing variables that can be identified depends in part on the sample size. The subject numbers were large (21,823 men, followed-up over 11.1 years), but nevertheless, an even larger study might have revealed some additional mechanisms whereby exercise was helpful. The present data should not be interpreted as showing that equivalent benefit could be obtained simply from dieting and the use of antihypertensive medication, because exercise also has a major influence on overall prognosis by preventing many conditions other than stroke.[1]

R. J. Shephard, MD, PhD, DPE

Reference

1. Bouchard C, Shephard RJ, Stephens T: *Physical Activity, Fitness and Health.* Champaign, Illinois, Human Kinetics, 1994.

Physical Activity and Ischemic Stroke Risk: The Atherosclerosis Risk in Communities Study
Evenson KR, for the Atherosclerosis Risk in Communities (ARIC) Study Investigators (Univ of North Carolina, Chapel Hill)
Stroke 30:1333-1339, 1999   4–18

Introduction.—Even though physical activity is known to affect risk factors for stroke, such as hypertension, the link between physical activity and stroke remains unclear. The relationship between physical activity and risk of ischemic stroke was analyzed in a large cohort from the Atherosclerosis Risk in Communities Study.

Methods.—The cohort included 14,575 men and women, age 45 to 64 years at baseline, at which time they had no self-reported history of stroke or coronary heart disease. Surveillance and patient reports were used to identify possible hospitalizations for stroke, which were validated with the use of hospital records. Physical activity, including sport, leisure, and work activity, was assessed by means of the Baecke questionnaire. Cardiovascular and demographic factors were assessed as well. Multivariate analyses were performed to assess the association between level of physical activity and incidence of ischemic stroke.

Results.—A total of 189 incident ischemic strokes occurred over an average follow-up of 7.2 years. Patients with the lowest levels of physical activity in all categories had the highest incidence of ischemic stroke. The hazard rate ratio for subjects in the highest quartile of sport physical activity, compared with the lowest quartile, was 0.83 (95% CI, 0.52-1.32), after adjustment for age, sex, race, education, and smoking. The ratio for leisure physical activity was 0.89 (95% confidence interval, 0.57-1.37), and that for work physical activity was 0.69 (95% confidence interval, 0.47-1.00). These associations were significantly reduced by adjustment for likely intermediate variables, such as hypertension, diabetes, fibrinogen, and body mass index.

Conclusions.—A high level of physical activity is associated with some reduction in the risk of ischemic stroke among middle-aged adults. The findings may reflect the effects of physical activity on known risk factors for stroke, although a chance association cannot be excluded. The use of a clinically defined, validated diagnosis of stroke is a major strength of the new study.

▶ This article illustrates the problems of determining the value of regular physical activity in prevention of ischemic stroke. A large sample of 14,575 older adults were followed prospectively for 7.2 years, and interesting apparent benefits were demonstrated for sport, leisure activity, and work (the last yielding a risk ratio [RR] of 0.69 when the top and bottom quartiles of trial participants were compared). A careful, clinically validated diagnosis of stroke was used, and the activity questionnaire that was selected (that of Baecke[1]) is one of the more reliable instruments. Nevertheless, the effects were only at the borderline of statistical significance. Surprisingly, the effect of occupation (RR, 0.69) seems greater than that of sport (RR, 0.83) or leisure activity (RR, 0.89); the authors suggest that this may be because of the healthy worker effect (those workers with various cardiovascular problems tend to drop out of physically demanding work).

R. J. Shephard, MD, PhD, DPE

Reference

1. Baecke J, Burema J, Fritjers J: A short questionnaire for the measurement of habitual physical activity in epidemiological studies. *Am J Clin Nutr* 36:936-942, 1982.

Intensity of Leg and Arm Training After Primary Middle-Cerebral-Artery Stroke: A Randomised Trial

Kwakkel G, Wagenaar RC, Twisk JWR, et al (Univ Hosp Vrije Universiteit, Amsterdam; Boston Univ)
Lancet 354:191-196, 1999
4–19

Background.—Differences in the efficacy of 3 stroke rehabilitation programs were studied. The effects of different intensities of arm and leg rehabilitation training on the functional recovery of activities of daily living (ADL), walking ability, and dexterity in the affected arm were determined.

Methods.—Participants met the following eligibility criteria: primary stroke of the middle cerebral artery, with no prior history of stroke; age between 30 and 80 years; impaired motor function of the arm and leg; inability to walk at the initial assessment; absence of other complicating factors in the medical history; absence of significant impairment of memory, communication, or comprehension; and ability to give informed consent, either orally or in writing. Participants also had to possess sufficient motivation to take part in the study. Within 14 days of their stroke, 101 patients with severe impairments were randomly assigned to 1 of 3 rehabilitation programs: (1) immobilization of the paretic arm and leg with an inflatable pressure splint (control group); (2) a rehabilitation program that emphasized arm training; (3) a program that emphasized leg training. The

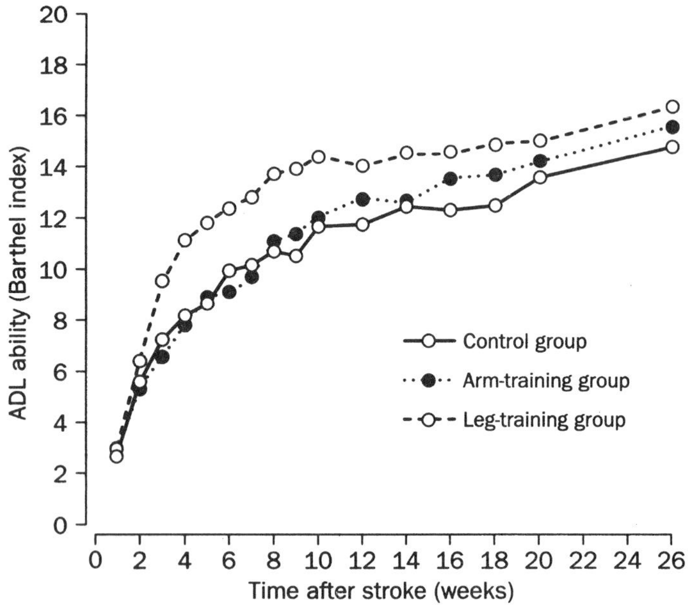

FIGURE 2.—Mean recovery patterns of Barthel index. *Abbreviation: ADL,* activities of daily living. (Courtesy of Kwakkel G, Wagenaar RC, Twisk JWR, et al: Intensity of leg and arm training after primary middle-cerebral-artery stroke: A randomised trial. *Lancet* 354:191-196. Copyright 1999, The Lancet Ltd.)

TABLE 4.—Secondary Outcomes

| | Mean (SD) Value | | |
	Control Group	Arm-Training Group	Leg-Training Group
Comfortable walking speed (m/s)			
Week 6*	0·17 (0·37)	0·21 (0·39)	0·40 (0·45)†
Week 12*	0·31 (0·39)	0·46 (0·47)	0·58 (0·50)†
Week 20*	0·37 (0·41)	0·55 (0·46)	0·65 (0·46)†
Week 26	0·44 (0·44)	0·55 (0·44)	0·63 (0·47)
Maximum walking speed (m/s)			
Week 6*	0·22 (0·50)	0·33 (0·60)	0·55 (0·65)†
Week 12*	0·41 (0·55)	0·55 (0·63	0·79 (0·65)†
Week 20*	0·52 (0·58)	0·76 (0·64)	0·88 (0·66)†
Week 26	0·57 (0·60)	0·73 (0·62)	0·85 (0·65)
Used walking aids			
Week 6	6 (16%)	11 (36%)	10 (32%)
Week 12	14 (40%)	12 (40%)	12 (47%)
Week 20	17 (49%)	14 (47%)	12 (47%)
Week 26	17 (49%)	17 (57%)	14 (53%)
Sickness impact profile‡			
Week 12§	36·8 (11·7)	31·1 (11·4)	26·9 (12·5)‖
Week 26	32·9 (12·0)	27·9 (13·1)	25·7 (12·7)
Nottingham health profile‡			
Week 12	14·5 (5·6)	10·4 (7·3)	9·4 (6·1)
Week 26	11·6 (7·9)	9·5 (5·9)	9·8 (8·1)
Frenchay activities index			
Week 26	8·2 (7·8)	10·9 (8·3)	13·7 (9·5)

*P less than .05 for difference among groups.
†P less than .05 for difference from control group.
‡High scores indicate poor status.
§P less than .05 for difference in improvement among groups.
‖P less than .05 for difference in improvement from control group.
(Courtesy of Kwakkel G, Wagenaar RC, Twisk JWR, et al: Intensity of leg and arm training after primary middle-cerebral-artery stroke: A randomised trial. *Lancet* 354:191-196. Copyright 1999, The Lancet Ltd.)

training for groups 2 and 3 was given by occupational therapists 5 days a week for 30 minutes per day, for 20 weeks after the stroke. All groups received 15 minutes of leg rehabilitation and 15 minutes of arm rehabilitation every day, as well as 1.5 hours per week of ADL training. The Barthel index, functional ambulation categories, and Action Research arm test were used to measure the 3 major outcomes of ADL, walking ability, and dexterity of the paretic arm, respectively.

Results.—There were significant differences among the 3 groups at 6, 12, and 20 weeks after the stroke (Fig 2). Table 4 shows the secondary outcomes. The leg-training group scored higher than the control group in all 3 categories of ADL ability, walking ability, and dexterity. The arm-training group scored significantly higher than the control group in only 1 category, dexterity. At 20 weeks, there were no significant differences in the end points of these measures between the arm-training and leg-training groups.

Conclusions.—The degree of functional recovery and health status overall is greater with greater intensity of leg rehabilitation as compared with greater intensity of arm rehabilitation, which benefits primarily the dexterity in the affected arm. In addition, degree-of-disability measurements at

26 weeks after stroke showed no significant follow-up effects. This suggests that, for patients who are severely disabled by their stroke, intense arm and leg rehabilitation should continue for a longer period.

▶ The residual effects of stroke can have a devastating impact on quality of life, and traditional stroke rehabilitation programs have proved less than optimal in restoring functional capacity. The results of this study suggest that early initiation of an intensive stroke therapy program focused on the lower extremities accelerates the return of ability to perform activities of daily living. However, although improvements in function of patients in the leg-training program were superior to those of patients in either the arm-training program or the control group for the first 12 weeks of therapy, this superiority was not sustained through the remaining 14 weeks of the study. In this regard, it is not clear whether the plateau in improvement represented an inability of patients to achieve further gains, or whether the rehabilitation program was inappropriately designed to continue to induce adaptations. A plateau would be expected to occur if the stimulus (ie, the exercise prescription) remained constant rather than being progressively incremented throughout the period of treatment. The encouraging findings suggest that further studies of intensive, progressive exercise training of the lower extremities subsequent to stroke should be carried out to determine the extent to which functional capacity can be restored.

W. M. Kohrt, PhD

Oxygen Uptake Kinetics During Exercise Are Slowed In Patients With Peripheral Arterial Disease
Bauer TA, Regensteiner JG, Brass EP, et al (Univ of Colorado, Denver; Harbor-UCLA, Los Angeles, Calif)
J Appl Physiol 87:809-816, 1999   4–20

Objective.—Oxygen intake during exercise is impaired in patients with cardiovascular disease. Patients with peripheral arterial disease (PAD) have a diminished ability to adapt the rate of oxygen uptake in response to exercise, possibly as a result of increase of VO_{2max}. Oxygen intake was compared in patients with PAD and healthy, age-matched, nonsmoking controls, oxygen intake kinetics were characterized, and the role of hemodynamic severity in altering oxygen intake kinetics was investigated.

Methods.—Oxygen intake and VO_{2peak} were measured in 8 patients with bilateral PAD, 7 patients with unilateral PAD, 9 healthy nonsmoking controls, and 7 smoking, healthy controls during multiple treadmill exercise tests and constant-load exercise tests at 3.2 km per hour at 0% and 4% grade (Fig 1). Oxygen intake was calculated and compared for all groups.

Results.—VO_{2peak} values for patients with unilateral and bilateral PAD were 51% and 55% lower than for the control groups. Although resting VO_2 levels were similar for all groups, overall phase 2 VO_2 kinetics at 0%

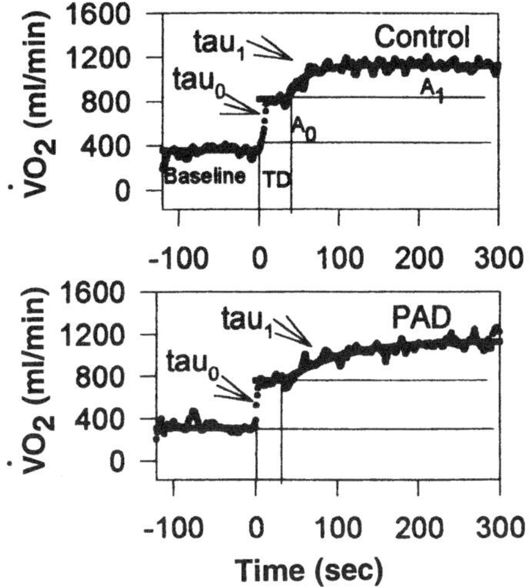

FIGURE 1.—Representative oxygen uptake ($\dot{V}o_{2max}$) kinetic response curves for 2.0 miles per hour, 4% grade treadmill exercise transitions from rest to exercise. *Top*, Time-aligned averaged data and curve fit of a representative nonsmoking control subject (*Control*). *Bottom*, Exercise data from patient with bilateral peripheral arterial disease (*PAD*). Both demonstrate a stable resting baseline $\dot{V}o_{2max}$. Transition from rest to exercise is marked by a rapid increase in $\dot{V}o_2$ to an early plateau of phase 1 response. *Tau$_0$*, Time constant for phase 1; A_0, change in $\dot{V}o_2$ from rest to the end of phase 1. After a time delay (*TD*) that encompasses phase 1, phase 2 is characterized by a tau$_1$ (phase 2), time constant, and A_1, change in $\dot{V}o_2$ to the new steady state. (Courtesy of Bauer TA, Regensteiner JG, Brass EP, et al: Oxygen uptake kinetics during exercise are slowed in patients with peripheral arterial disease. *J Appl Physiol* 87:809-816, 1999.)

grade for patients with unilateral and bilateral PAD were slower than for controls groups, and at 4% grade were significantly slower for patients with unilateral or bilateral PAD (60.1 and 58.7 s, respectively) than for the smoking and nonsmoking control groups (27.9 and 28.4 s, respectively). Attenuated oxygen intake kinetics were associated with the presence of PAD but not with severity of disease. Impaired kinetics was observed only during phase 2.

Conclusion.—Oxygen intake is significantly impaired during exercise in patients with PAD. The degree of impairment is not related to smoking status or disease severity, but may reflect peripheral flow limitations or alterations in skeletal muscle metabolism.

▶ The on-transient of oxygen consumption is slowed by both aging and a variety of cardiovascular and muscular disorders. In some cases, such as orthotopic cardiac transplantation, a specific factor (the absence of cardiac sympathetic innervation) is responsible for the slow increase in oxygen consumption as exercise begins.[1] However, in most cases, the major explanation is probably loss of physical condition secondary to a disease-related reduction in habitual physical activity. This possibility needs to be considered in relation to the slow on-transient of patients with peripheral vascular disease. In support of my suggestion, there is now good evidence that a normal, youthful on-transient can be restored in an elderly patient through participation in a systematic program of aerobic training.[2]

R. J. Shephard, MD, PhD, DPE

References

1. Shephard RJ, Kavanagh T, Mertens DJ, et al: Kinetics of the transplanted heart. *J Cardiopulm Rehabil* 15:288-296, 1995.
2. Babcock MA, Paterson DH, Cunningham DA: Effects of aerobic endurance training on gas exchange kinetics of older men. *Med Sci Sports Exerc* 26:447-452, 1994.

Smoking History Is Related to Free-living Daily Physical Activity in Claudicants

Gardner AW, Montgomery PS, Womack CJ, et al (Univ of Maryland, Baltimore; Maryland Veterans Affairs Health Care System, Baltimore)
Med Sci Sports Exerc 31:980-986, 1999   4–21

Objective.—Because cigarette smoking is a primary risk factor for cardiovascular disease as well as peripheral arterial occlusive disease (PAOD), many patients with PAOD also have coronary and cerebrovascular disease. Patients with intermittent claudication tend to have a sedentary lifestyle, which is also a risk factor for cardiovascular mortality. The authors believe that smoking may also be associated with a reduction in free-living physical activity. The effects of smoking history on daily physical activity among patients with PAOD were examined.

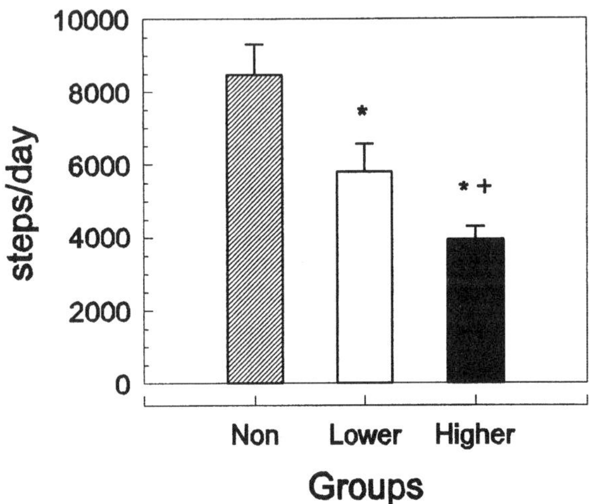

FIGURE 2.—Free-living daily physical activity measured with a pedometer in smokers with a higher and lower pack-year history of smoking and in nonsmoking patients with intermittent claudication. Values are mean plus or minus SE. *Significantly lower than the nonsmoking group ($P < .05$). +Significantly lower than the lower pack-year group ($P < .05$). (Courtesy of Gardner AW, Montgomery PS, Womack CJ, et al: Smoking history is related to free-living daily physical activity in claudicants. *Med Sci Sports Exerc* 31(7):980-986, 1999.)

Methods.—The study included 98 patients with PAOD and intermittent claudication: 35 who had never smoked, 33 with a smoking history of 40 pack-years or less, and 30 with a smoking history of more than 40 pack-years. On 2 consecutive study days, the patients' level of physical activity was monitored using an accelerometer and a pedometer. The relationship between smoking history and physical activity level was assessed. Adjustment was made for other factors related to physical activity: ambulatory function, peripheral circulation, and body composition.

Results.—Based on accelerometer data, the mean daily physical activity level was 2020 kJ/d in those who had never smoked versus 1520 kJ/d in patients with a lower pack-year history versus 950 kJ/d in those with a higher pack-year history. Physical activity also declined with increasing smoking history on analysis of the pedometer data (Fig 2). The differences in physical activity level among the smoking groups became nonsignificant after adjustment for differences in 6-minute walking distance and calf transcutaneous heating power.

Conclusions.—Among PAOD patients with intermittent claudication, the level of free-living daily physical activity decreases at greater levels of cigarette smoking. These differences result mainly from smoking-related reductions in ambulatory function and peripheral circulation. For patients at the highest level of smoking exposure, the daily activity level is about half that of nonsmokers.

▶ The observations presented in this article are based on a small-scale retrospective trial. One potential weakness is a reliance on self-reported cigarette consumption, which is notoriously unreliable. On the other hand, the accelerometer and pedometer measurements of current habitual energy expenditures are likely to be more precise than the usual self-reported amounts of exercise. The inverse association between the reported cigarette consumption and habitual daily activity has been reported previously.[1] Because the study demonstrates an association rather than cause and effect, it is still unclear whether smoking leads to a reduction in physical activity in this population or whether sedentary habits encourage smoking. The disappearance of the smoking effect after adjustment for disease severity in terms of the 6-minute walk distance and calf transcutaneous heating power supports the first of these explanations, although there is also some evidence that, even in the absence of peripheral vascular disease, smokers have less interest in a healthy lifestyle, including physical activity.[2,3]

R. J. Shephard, MD, PhD, DPE

References

1. Gardner AW, Sieminski DJ, Killewich LA: The effect of cigarette smoking on free-living daily physical activity in older claudication patients. *Angiology* 48:947-955, 1997.
2. Shephard RJ: Exercise and lifestyle change. *Br J Sports Med* 23:11-22, 1989.
3. Gardner AW, Sieminski DJ, Montgomery PS: Physical activity is related to ankle/brachial index in subjects without peripheral vascular arterial occlusive disease. *Angiology* 48:883-891, 1997.

Physical Activity and Risk of Lung Cancer

Lee I-M, Sesso HD, Paffenbarger RS Jr (Harvard School of Public Health, Boston; Harvard Med School, Boston; Stanford Univ, Calif)
Int J Epidemiol 28:620-625, 1999   4–22

Background.—Although physical activity has been shown to have beneficial effects on the risk for some types of cancer, it has been unclear whether lung cancer risk could be affected. In addition, no studies have noted the influence of specific types or levels of intensity of activity with respect to the development of lung cancer. Whether physical activity would decrease the risk for lung cancer was studied, and the types and intensity of activities involved were examined.

Methods.—Health questionnaires given out in 1977 were used to enroll 13,905 male Harvard University alumni in this prospective cohort study. Participants listed the number of blocks walked daily, flights of stairs climbed daily, and all sports or recreation in which they actively partici-

TABLE 3.—Incidence Rates and Relative Risks of Lung Cancer Among Harvard Alumni, 1977-1993, According to Different Physical Activity Components in 1977

Physical Activity Component	No. of Events	Incidence Rate* (Per 10 000)	Relative Risk† (95% CI)
Distance walked (km/week)			
<5	101	16.5	1.00 (referent)
5 to <10	49	12.0	0.76 (0.54-1.07)
10 to <20	55	10.7	0.71 (0.51-0.99)
≥20	40	9.2	0.65 (0.45-0.94)
			P trend = 0.01
Stairs climbed (storeys/week)			
<10	86	17.4	1.00 (referent)
10 to <20	43	10.7	0.63 (0.44-0.92)
20 to <35	43	10.6	0.64 (0.44-0.93)
≥35	73	11.0	0.74 (0.54-1.02)
			P trend = 0.08
Activities at <4.5 MET‡ (kJ/week)			
None	152	12.5	1.00 (referent)
1 to <1050	26	13.8	1.20 (0.79-1.83)
1050 to <2520	19	11.6	0.92 (0.57-1.48)
2520 to <5880	19	10.3	0.81 (0.50-1.32)
≥5880	29	13.3	0.99 (0.66-1.48)
			P trend = 0.62
Activities at ≥4.5 MET‡ (kJ/week)			
None	133	16.0	1.00 (referent)
1 to <1050	38	12.2	0.84 (0.58-1.22)
1050 to <2520	19	8.3	0.64 (0.39-1.04)
2520 to <5880	33	11.4	0.93 (0.62-1.39)
≥5880	22	7.2	0.60 (0.38-0.96)
			P trend = 0.046

*Age-adjusted.

†Adjusted for age (single years), cigarette smoking (nonsmoker, smoker of ≤20 cigarettes per day, smoker of >20 cigarettes per day, or smoker of unknown amount, assessed in 1977), body mass index (<22.5, 22.5-<23.5, 23.5-<24.5, 24.5-<26.0, or ≤26.0 kg/m^2), and the other 3 components of physical activity (categorized as in the Table).

‡Multiples of resting metabolic rate.

(From Lee I-M, Sesso HD, Paffenbarger RS Jr: Physical activity and risk of lung cancer. *Int J Epidemiol* 28:620-625, 1999. Reproduced by permission of Oxford University Press.)

pated during the previous year. The mean age of participants was 58.3 years. Total energy expended per week was estimated from the data obtained by questionnaire. On follow-up questionnaires in 1988 and 1993 the men reported whether lung cancer had occurred. Death certificates for those who died through 1992 were used to screen for lung cancers not reported earlier.

Results.—Lung cancer was found in 245 men. Data were adjusted for age, whether the man smoked cigarettes, and body mass index, and these were related to estimated weekly energy expenditure, yielding relative risks for lung cancer. Men who expended more weekly total energy had lower lung cancer incidence rates, and these rates were similar whether the men were smokers, nonsmokers, or former smokers. Data on types and intensity of exercise revealed that lung cancer risk fell with greater distance walked, more stairs climbed (up to 19 storeys a week), and at least moderate intensity sports and recreational activities (Table 3).

Conclusions.—Lung cancer risk appears to decline in men who engage in physical activity weekly. Risk could be significantly cut by an energy expenditure of 12,600 kJ/wk, requiring about 6 to 8 hours of at least moderate intensity physical activity.

▶ The beneficial effects of physical activity on the risk for colonic, breast, and reproductive tract cancers are now fairly well established, but there is much less evidence concerning habitual physical activity and lung cancers.[1] The obvious problems when studying pulmonary and bronchial tumors are that the adverse effects of smoking on risk levels far outweigh any possible beneficial influence of physical activity, and smoking tends to be associated with other adverse health habits, such as lack of physical activity. In theory, an epidemiologist could get around the confounding influence of smoking by including this as a covariate in a multiple regression analysis. However, this is difficult to do in practice, because people's recollections of smoking habits are unreliable, and information on smoking behavior tends to be collected in a "yes or no" fashion only once or twice in the life spectrum. In 1 study, it was also possible to show that the effects of physical activity were greatest in types of lung cancer (adenocarcinomas and small cell carcinomas) that are largely unrelated to smoking[2] and that benefit was seen in both nonsmokers and heavy smokers when these 2 groups were considered separately. In the present study, the demonstration of a dose-response relationship for distance walked also points to a true beneficial effect of physical activity.

Mechanisms for any protective effect of regular exercise remain unclear. Suggestions to date include effects from enhanced immune function and enhanced pulmonary function, but these possibilities still require critical evaluation.

R. J. Shephard, MD, PhD, DPE

References

1. Shephard RJ, Futcher R: Physical activity and cancer: How may protection be maximized? *Crit Rev Oncogenesis* 8:219-272, 1997.

2. Thune I, Lund E: The influence of physical activity on lung cancer risk: A prospective study of 81,516 men and women. *Int J Cancer* 70:57-62, 1997.

Aerobic and Strength Training in Patients With Chronic Obstructive Pulmonary Disease

Bernard S, Whittom F, LeBlanc P, et al (Université Laval, Ste-Foy, Québec)
Am J Respir Crit Care Med 159:896-901, 1999   4–23

Objective.—Although lower-extremity aerobic training is known to improve exercise tolerance in patients with chronic obstructive pulmonary disease (COPD), strength training in these patients has not been studied. Whether strength training would provide any additional benefits in patients with COPD who are involved in an aerobic training program was investigated. The effects of aerobic training alone and in combination with strength training were compared for gains in peripheral muscle mass and strength, exercise tolerance, and quality of life in patients with COPD.

Methods.—COPD patients (n = 45, 12 women) participated in a 12-week aerobic training program including a 45-minute period of relaxation

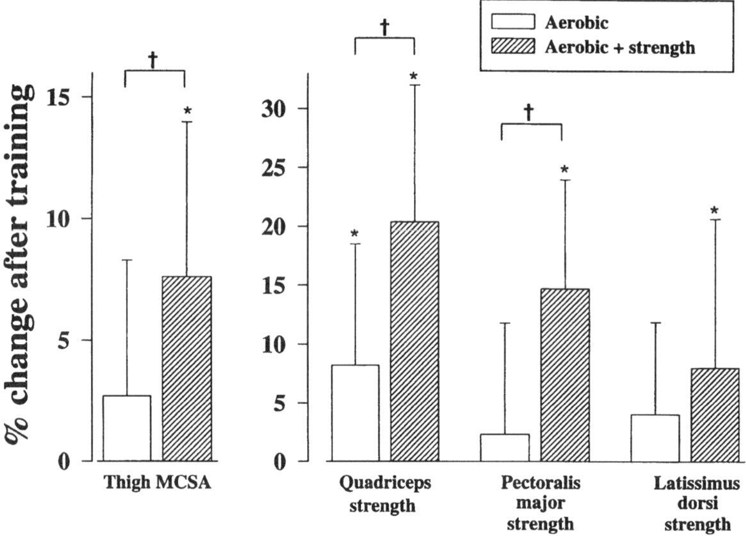

FIGURE 1.—Mean ± SD percent change in bilateral thigh MCSA and in the strength of the quadriceps, pectoralis major, and latissimus dorsi muscles before and after training in the AERO and AERO + ST groups. *Note:* The improvement in bilateral thigh MCSA and in the strength of the 3 muscle groups was statistically significant in the AERO + ST group. Quadriceps strength also showed a significant increase in the AERO group. As can be seen, the magnitude of the changes in thigh MCSA and in the strength of the quadriceps and pectoralis major muscles was significantly greater in the AERO + ST group than in the AERO group. *$P < .05$ for pretraining versus posttraining within each study group. †$P < .05$ for the AERO group versus the AERO + ST group. (Courtesy of Bernard S, Whittom F, LeBlanc P, et al: Aerobic and strength training in patients with chronic obstructive pulmonary disease. *Am J Respir Crit Care Med* 159:896-901, 1999. Official Journal of the American Thoracic Society. Copyright American Lung Association.)

and breathing exercises for the aerobic training alone (AERO) group (n = 19) and a 45-minute period of strength training for the AERO + strength training (ST) group (n = 26). Participants were evaluated at baseline and at the end of the program. Thigh muscle cross-sectional area (MCSA) was determined by computed tomography (CT), and strength was measured during dynamic contractions against hydraulic resistance. An exercise test was performed on an electrically braked ergocycle. Participants performed a 6-minute walking distance test (6MWD). Quality of life was assessed using the Chronic Respiratory Questionnaire. Differences between groups were analyzed statistically.

Results.—There were 15 (4 women) patients in the AERO group and 21 (4 women) in the AERO + ST group who completed the program. The average absolute training intensity was significantly higher in the AERO + ST group than in the AERO group. The strength of all 4 muscle groups increased significantly in the AERO + ST group. Quadriceps strength increased significantly in both groups, with the greatest gain in the AERO + ST group (Fig 1). The increase in thigh MCSA and strength of the pectoralis major muscle was significant only in the AERO + ST group. Peak exercise work rate, 6MWD, and quality of life increased a comparable amount for both groups.

Conclusion.—Including strength training in rehabilitation of COPD patients increases muscle mass and strength but does improve peak exercise, work rate, 6MWD, or quality of life relative to aerobic training alone.

▶ The exercise tolerance of patients with COPD can certainly be enhanced by a program of progressive physical activity, but reasons for this response remain unclear. One suggestion was that lack of physical activity led to muscular weakness, and because of muscular weakness, an increased accumulation of lactate led to a vicious cycle of ever-increasing breathlessness and diminishing habitual physical activity.[1] At first inspection, the present study seems to run counter to such an explanation. However, further trials are required before such a conclusion can be endorsed. The period of training was relatively short, and the difference in strength gains between AERO and AERO + ST programs was small. Further, the strength training was concentrated on 4 muscle groups (pectoralis major, latissimus dorsi, gluteus maximus, and vastus lateralis). A longer and more broadly based program might still support the earlier hypothesis.

R. J. Shephard, MD, PhD, DPE

Reference

1. Mertens DJ, Shephard RJ, Kavanagh T: Long-term exercise for chronic obstructive lung disease. *Respiration* 35:96-107, 1978.

Asthma in United States Olympic Athletes Who Participated in the 1996 Summer Games

Weiler JM, Layton T, Hunt M (Univ of Iowa, Iowa City; United States Olympic Committee, Colorado Springs, Colo)
J Allergy Clin Immunol 102:722-726, 1998   4–24

Objective.—It is believed that 10% of competitive American athletes have exercise-induced asthma. The number of US athletes at the 1996 Atlanta Summer Olympic Games with exercise-induced asthma was determined, and their performance was compared with that of athletes participating in the 1984 Games. Whether the prevalence of asthma varied among sports and whether a history of asthma affected performance were also evaluated.

Methods.—Responses to questionnaires completed by US athletes at the 1996 Summer Olympic Games were analyzed for a history or symptoms of asthma.

Results.—The questionnaire was completed by 699 athletes, 107 (15.3%) of whom had a history of asthma and 97 (13.9%) of whom had taken asthma medications at some time. There were 117 (16.7%) who had been diagnosed with asthma or had taken asthma medication, and 73 (10.4%) were taking asthma medication on a permanent or semipermanent basis. Half of the cyclists and mountain bikers, 29.6% of synchronized swimmers and swimmers, and 25.3% of canoers/kayakers, rowers, and sailors/yachters had a history of asthma or had taken asthma medications. In addition, 18.2% of athletes who participated in track and field, and pentathlon and 15.6% who participated in boxing, wrestling, and judo had asthma. Active asthma was present in 45% of cyclists and mountain bikers. No divers or weight lifters reported problems with asthma. A significantly higher percentage of female than male athletes reported problems with asthma; active asthma was present in 11.6% of female athletes and 9.5% of male athletes. Of 117 athletes with asthma or taking asthma medications, 35 (29.9%) won medals. Of 73 athletes with active asthma, 24 (32.9%) won 31 medals. Of 582 athletes without asthma, 167 (28.7%) won medals.

Conclusion.—The prevalence of asthma in Olympic athletes is higher than the prevalence in the general population. The presence of asthma may affect the sport an athlete selects.

▶ The prevalence of asthma in the general population is between 4% and 7%, although this figure may be rising. Previous reports from the mid-1980s have suggested the incidence is about twice as great among international athletes as in the general population.[1,2] However, the present report from the Atlanta Olympic Games suggests that there may have been a further increase among athletes, to 15% to 20% of all participants, and up to 45% of cyclists and mountain bikers. The article does not speculate on reasons for this apparent change, but a number of factors may be at work. The diagnostic criteria in most of the studies of athletes have been weak: in this case, a reported diagnosis of asthma or the use of an asthma medication. There is now a greater awareness of both the condition and potential remedies, so that diagnoses and supposed diagnoses would likely be more frequent. Some athletes may also have perceived the medication as enhancing their performance. Further, the range of competition has increased, and some sports such as mountain biking may have exposed participants to cold dry air. The key issue is the success rate: 29.9% of the supposed asthmatics won medals, as compared with 28.7% of nonasthmatics. Plainly, performance is not endangered in the typical international athlete who complains of asthma.

R. J. Shephard, MD, PhD, DPE

References

1. Voy RO: The U.S. Olympic Committee experience with exercise-induced bronchospasm, 1984. *Med Sci Sports Exerc* 18:328-330, 1986.
2. Fitch KD: Management of allergic athletes: Management of allergic Olympic athletes. *J Allergy Clin Immunol* 73:722-777, 1984.

High-Intensity Physical Training in Adults With Asthma: A Comparison Between Training on Land and in Water
Emtner M, Finne M, Stålenheim G (Univ Hosp, Uppsala, Sweden)
Scand J Rehabil Med 30:201-209, 1998   4–25

Objective.—Many persons with asthma avoid physical activity. Although adults with asthma can exercise at maximal intensity in water without experiencing exercise-induced asthma, many patients do not have access to a swimming pool. Whether patients with inactive asthma can perform high-intensity exercise as well on land as in water was tested during a 10-week randomized rehabilitation study.

Methods.—After attending a hospital 5 days a week for 2 weeks, 32 asthma patients (14 women) were randomly allocated to 45 minutes of either land (n=14) or water (n=18) exercise twice weekly for 8 weeks. Patients underwent a submaximal 6-minute ergometry test, a 12-minute walking test, and spirometry, peak expiratory flow rate, and a methacholine provocation tests 10 weeks before the start of the program, at baseline, and after 2 and 10 weeks. Patients completed questionnaires concerning physical exercise, effects of asthma on everyday life, and experiences during the 10-week rehabilitation period. Patients kept a training log and a diary; emergency room visits were recorded; and a maximal exercise test was performed.

Results.—During the 2-week training period, all patients were able to maintain the high-intensity training without having an asthma attack (Table 3). There were no cardiovascular or respiratory changes. Whereas before the rehabilitation program questionnaire responses indicated that patients were unfamiliar with and anxious about training, felt limitations in their daily lives, and were inhibited about joining activities, after reha-

TABLE 3.—Perceived Exertion According to the 10-Graded Borg Scale, the PEFR (L/min), and the Training Intensity as Indicated by Heart Rate in % of Predicted Maximal Heart Rate; Mean (SD)

	After Warming-Up			After Interval Training			After Cooling-Down		
	Borg	PEFR	HR (%)	Borg	PEFR	HR (%)	Borg	PEFR	HR (%)
Land group	2.9 (1.4)	484 (123)	77 (18)	7.2 (1.5)	481 (97)	96 (10)	4.8 (2.0)	457 (104)	73 (12)
Water group	4.2 (1.6)	536 (81)*	79 (14)	8.0 (1.0)	532 (85)*	91 (10)	4.3 (1.1)	483 (93)	70 (9)

The presession peak expiratory flow rate values were 464 (90) L/min in the land group and 489 (87) in the water group (NS).
*$P<.05$ compared with presession values.
(Courtesy of Emtner M, Finne M, Stålenheim G: High-intensity physical training in adults with asthma: A comparison between training on land and in water. *Scand J Rehabil Med* 30:201-209, 1998.)

bilitation all of these feelings improved. Emergency room visits declined in both groups, and no changes in medication were reported.

Conclusion.—Rehabilitation reduced exercise anxiety in asthma patients and improved their cardiovascular and respiratory condition and their ability to carry out everyday activities, responses being very similar for land-based and pool exercises.

▶ Popular wisdom is that patients with asthma should undertake swimming or pool exercises, because this type of activity is less likely to induce bronchospasm than land-based training.[1,2] The greater humidity of the pool is usually advanced as the explanation of any observed difference. In some countries, access to a swimming pool is limited, and, in addition, not everyone enjoys swimming. Emtner and colleagues thus undertook a small-scale randomized trial to show that, under some conditions at least, land-based training can be equally effective. Notice that the study used the newer form of the Borg scale, so that the intensity of both water-based and land-based exercise was very high, yet the perceived effort was similar under the 2 conditions. The air in the gymnasium was colder (22° vs 24°C), and the relative humidity was also substantially lower (20%-30% vs 60%) than in the pool area. The reasons why land-based training was successful seem to be extensive premedication[3] (corticosteroids, often supplemented by β_2 agonists and theophylline), a good warm-up,[4] and adoption of an interval training regimen.[5] Favorable outcomes included a reduction in anxiety about exercise, alleviation of asthma symptoms, and a reduction in emergency room visits.

R. J. Shephard, MD, PhD, DPE

References

1. Fitch K, Morton A: Specificity of exercise-induced asthma. *Br Med J* 4:577-581, 1971.
2. Schnall R, Ford P, Gilliam I, et al: Swimming and dry land exercises in children with asthma. *Austr Pediatr J* 18:23-27, 1982.
3. Cochrane L, Clark C: Benefits of a physical training programme for asthmatic patients. *Thorax* 45:345-351, 1990.
4. Garfinkel S, Kesten S, Chapman K, et al: Physiologic and non-physiologic determinants of aerobic fitness in mild to moderate asthma. *Am Rev Respir Dis* 145:741-745, 1992.
5. Morton A, Fitch K, Hahn A: Physical activity and the asthmatic. *Physician Sports Med* 9:51-64, 1981.

Heart Attacks and Lower-Limb Function in Master Endurance Athletes
Kujala UM, Sarna S, Kaprio J, et al (Univ of Helsinki; Natl Public Health Inst, Helsinki; Univ of Turku, Finland; et al)
Med Sci Sports Exerc 31:1041-1046, 1999   4–26

Objective.—Whether exercising frequently at great intensity confers more benefits than detriments is not clear. The risks of heart attacks and

TABLE 3.—Prevalence of Self-reported Physician Diagnosed Hip and Knee Osteoarthritis as Well as Hip and Knee Pain and Disability Among Orienteering Runners and Controls, and Their Age-adjusted Odds Ratios in Runners Compared With Controls*

	Orienteering Runners (N = 264)	Controls (N = 179)	Odds Ratio†	P
	N (%)		OR (95% CI)	
Osteoarthritis				
Hip	14 (5.3)	13 (7.3)	0.78 (0.35 to 1.73)	0.55
Knee	45 (17.0)	19 (10.6)	1.79 (1.10 to 3.54)	0.025
Weekly pain				
Hip	19 (7.2)	18 (10.1)	0.74 (0.37 to 1.46)	0.38
Knee	40 (15.2)	18 (10.1)	1.75 (0.96 to 3.18)	0.071
Disability index >1				
Hip	14 (5.3)	21 (11.7)	0.46 (0.22 to 0.93)	0.030
Knee	30 (11.4)	29 (16.2)	0.69 (0.39 to 1.21)	0.20
Pain or discomfort in going up or down stairs				
Hip	10 (3.8)	15 (8.4)	0.47 (0.20 to 1.08)	0.046
Knee	27 (10.2)	24 (13.4)	0.78 (0.43 to 1.41)	0.40

*Data from 1995 follow-up questionnaire.
†By logistic regression analysis compared with controls and adjusted for age.
(Courtesy of Kujala UM, Sarna S, Kaprio J, et al: Heart attacks and lower-limb function in master endurance athletes. *Med Sci Sports Exerc* 31(7):1041-1046, 1999.)

lower-limb osteoarthritis and disability were investigated in middle-aged and older master endurance athletes participating in very vigorous competitions.

Methods.—In 1995, questionnaires assessing diagnosed illnesses and disabilities were sent to the 269 top Finnish orienteers of 1984, who were stratified by age into 5 groups: 35 to 39 years, 40 to 44 years, 45 to 49 years, 50 to 54 years, and 55 to 59 years. Questionnaires were also sent to a control group consisting of 188 men from an earlier study born in 1925 or later who were healthy at age 20 years and had responded to a health questionnaire in 1985. Smokers, obese individuals, and those with coronary heart disease (CHD) were excluded from the control group. Orienteering involves running, usually for an hour, at maximal physical effort through rough and hilly terrain. Mortality was tracked.

Results.—There were 5 deaths in the running group, none from CHD, and 9 in the control group, 3 from CHD. More orienteers than controls reported knee osteoarthritis and knee pain, although pain and disability during exercise were lower in the orienteers than in the control group (Table 3). The prevalences of hip osteoarthritis and hip pain were similar for both groups.

Conclusion.—The risk of heart attack and lower-limb disability is low in middle-aged and older orienteers.

▶ One of the unresolved questions in sports medicine is how regular exercise affects the risk of osteoarthritis. Studies of distance runners during a 5-year interval have suggested little or no risk relative to controls.[1] In this study, a comparison of risk in orienteers with healthy Finns of similar age suggests a doubling of risk of osteoarthritis in the knee. The difference in this study was that subjects were running over rough terrain rather than on tracks or roads, and were thus relatively vulnerable to acute injuries of the knee. In other sports, the main factors predisposing to subsequent osteoarthritis seem to be contact injury, overloading, and a high body mass.[2,3]

At first inspection, the 6-fold difference in risk of myocardial infarction seems an important benefit of orienteering. However, we must be cautious in attributing all of this benefit to the activity; a selection bias leads those with a high percentage of slow-twitch muscle fibers to engage in distance running, and the percentage of slow-twitch fibers is also correlated with increased high-density lipoprotein (HDL) cholesterol levels.[4]

R. J. Shephard, MD, PhD, DPE

References

1. Lane NE, Michel B, Björkengren A, et al: The risk of osteoarthritis with running and aging: A 5-year longitudinal study. *J Rheumatol* 20:461-468, 1993.
2. Kujala UM, Kettunen J, Paananen H, et al: Knee osteoarthritis in former runners, soccer players, weight lifters and shooters. *Arthritis Rheum* 38:539-546, 1995.
3. Spector TD, Harris PA, Hart DJ, et al: Risk of osteoarthritis associated with long-term weight bearing sports: A radiological survey of the hips and knees in female ex-athletes and population controls. *Arthritis Rheum* 39:988-995, 1996.
4. Tikkanen HO, Härkönen M, Näveri H, et al: Relationship of skeletal muscle fiber type to serum HDL cholesterol and apolipoprotein A-I levels. *Atherosclerosis* 90:49-57, 1991.

Effects of Exercise Training on Oxygen Uptake Kinetic Responses in Women With Type 2 Diabetes

Brandenburg SL, Jeffers BW, Reusch JEB, et al (Univ of Colorado, Denver)
Diabetes Care 22:1640-1646, 1999   4–27

Background.—Type 2 diabetes is associated with a reduction in VO_{2max}, even when there is no cardiovascular disease. Women with type 2 diabetes also show impairment of VO_2 kinetics. This study examined the effects of exercise training on VO_{2max} and VO_2 kinetics in women with type 2 diabetes.

Methods.—The study included 8 premenopausal women with diabetes but no complications or co-morbidity. All were sedentary and moderately overweight. Also included were 2 groups of nondiabetic women: 9 overweight and 9 lean. All groups were of similar age and activity level. The subjects took part in a 3-month exercise training program. Before and after exercise training, the women underwent a bicycle ergometer test to measure VO_{2max} and VO_2 kinetics.

Results.—At baseline, the diabetic women had the lowest VO_{2max} and the slowest VO_2 kinetics of any of the 3 groups. Both the diabetic group and the overweight controls showed significant improvement in VO_{2max} after exercise training. The degree of improvement was 28% in the diabetic group and 8% in the overweight control group, compared with a nonsignificant 5% improvement in the lean control group. Exercise improved VO_2 kinetics in the diabetic group by 39% at 20 W and 22% at 30 W. Neither of the control groups had any significant change in VO_2 kinetics.

Conclusions.—Moderate-intensity exercise can significantly improve VO_{2max} and VO_2 kinetics in women with type 2 diabetes. This is so despite initial impairment of maximal and submaximal cardiovascular responses to exercise. The exercise-related improvements in VO_{2max} and VO_2 kinetics appear to arise from improvements in conditioning as well as in some diabetes-related defect in oxygen delivery, oxygen use, or both.

▶ Exercise is a cornerstone of the treatment of type 2 diabetes mellitus. The results of this study emphasize the importance of exercise, as they demonstrate that moderate-intensity exercise training can markedly enhance cardiovascular function in women with type 2 diabetes who are otherwise healthy. Since cardiovascular events are the leading cause of death among individuals with type 2 diabetes, it will be important to determine whether habitual exercise, when initiated early in the disease process, can diminish the morbidity and mortality of type 2 diabetes mellitus.

W. M. Kohrt, PhD

Effects of Diabetes Mellitus on the Biomechanical Properties of Human Ankle Cartilage
Anthanasiou KA, Fleischli JG, Bosma J, et al (Univ of Texas, San Antonio)
Clin Orthop 368:182-189, 1999   4–28

Background.—Metabolic changes from diabetes mellitus affect many of the body's organ systems. Patients with diabetes have more musculoskeletal injuries and also have more morbidity associated with injury and treatment than do persons without diabetes. The intrinsic material properties of human ankle articular cartilage from persons with and without diabetes were compared.

Methods and Findings.—Fifteen specimen ankles were obtained from persons who had had diabetes, and 15 from persons who had not had diabetes (Fig 1). Aggregate modulus, Poisson ratio, shear modulus, and permeability differed significantly between specimen groups. Cartilage from diabetic persons was significantly softer and more permeable than that from nondiabetic persons. In the central part of the talus, cartilage from the diabetic group had a 38% smaller aggregate modulus, 37% smaller shear modulus, and 111% larger permeability than tissue from nondiabetic persons.

Conclusions.—In this study, ankle cartilage from diabetic persons had biomechanical properties inferior to those of nondiabetic persons. Pathologic processes in the joint in diabetic patients may be associated with compromised structural integrity of articular cartilage.

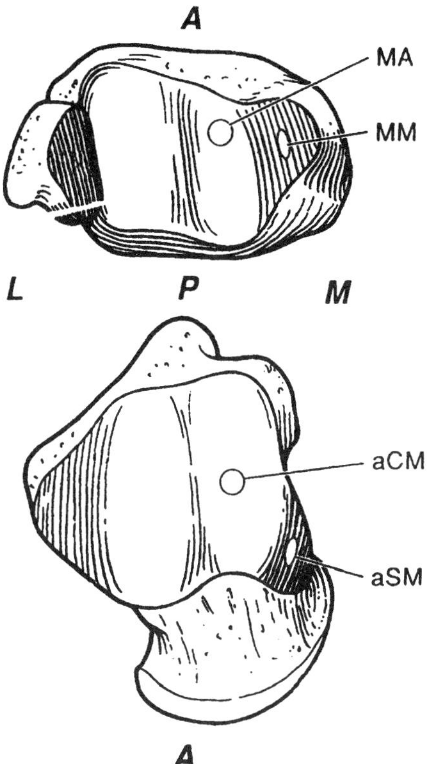

FIGURE 1.—A schematic diagram of the articulating surfaces of the tibiotalar joint. The biomechanical properties of articular cartilage were obtained at the following test sites: anterior medial porton of the tibia (*MA*), medial malleolus of the tibia (*MM*), central medial portion of the talus (*aCM*), and side medial portion of the talus (*aSM*). *A*, anterior; *M*, medial; *P*, posterior; *L*, lateral. (Courtesy of Anthanasiou KA, Fleischli JG, Bosma J, et al: Effects of diabetes mellitus on the biomechanical properties of human ankle cartilage. *Clin Orthop* 368:182-189, 1999.)

▶ Diabetes affects both injury rate and healing rate; persons with diabetes experience more musculoskeletal injuries and prolonged healing compared with those without diabetes. Diabetes is known to produce glycosylation of articular cartilage, which is associated with limited joint motion; as well, protein and collagen metabolism are decreased significantly. Comparison of cadaver ankle cartilage from patients with diabetes and normal patients revealed that cartilage from those with diabetes had inferior biomechanical properties, including lower indices of stiffness and larger permeability. These changes are likely caused by the altered tissue metabolism associated with diabetes. This study provides a clear biomechanical explanation of increased osteoarthritic changes in patients with diabetes.

M. J. L. Alexander, PhD

Quadriceps Strength in Women With Radiographically Progressive Osteoarthritis of the Knee and Those With Stable Radiographic Changes

Brandt KD, Heilman DK, Slemenda C, et al (Indiana Univ, Indianapolis)
J Rheumatol 26:2431-2437, 1999   4–29

Background.—In a recent cross-sectional analysis of a community-based cohort of elderly persons, quadriceps weakness was found in women with radiographic evidence of knee osteoarthritis (OA) who had no history of knee pain. The relationship between lower extremity weakness and the progression of established radiographic changes of knee OA was further investigated.

Methods.—Three hundred forty-two elderly persons were recruited. Seventy-nine had definite radiographic changes of unilateral or bilateral knee OA at baseline and also had available baseline data on lower extremity muscle strength and lean tissue mass and baseline and follow-up assessments of knee pain. Radiographs were graded for OA severity, and knee pain was assessed at baseline and again about 2.5 years later. Knee flexor and extensor strength was determined bilaterally at baseline by isokinetic dynamometry, and lower extremity muscle mass by dual-energy x-ray absorptiometry.

Findings.—Mean peak knee extensor strength in women with progressive OA before and after adjusting for lower extremity muscle mass was about 9% lower than in women with stable radiographic changes. However, this difference was not significant statistically. The 2 groups did not appear to differ in knee flexor strength. Compared with women with stable OA, the decline in quadriceps strength among women with progressive OA did not seem to be attributable to knee pain. In addition, knee extensor strength at baseline was apparently unrelated to the development or progression of knee pain among those with OA.

Conclusions.—Previous research has suggested that quadriceps weakness may be etiologically important in the development of knee OA. In the current study, the absence of a significant difference in quadriceps strength between persons with radiographically stable OA and those with joint damage progression suggests that factors other than quadriceps weakness are more important determinants of OA progression.

▶ It has been previously reported that weakness of the quadriceps muscle is common in patients with knee OA, likely caused by muscle atrophy related to disuse. Knee strength and radiographic changes were evaluated at baseline and again 2.5 years later, and the group with measured radiographic changes was also weaker. However, the strength changes were not statistically significant, likely because of the greater body weight of those with the increased joint damage. The greater body weight required more muscle mass to support the weight, so even though joint damage had progressed, strength was maintained. It is likely that other risk factors, such as obesity or inactivity, are more important determinants of joint damage than quadriceps strength.

M. J. L. Alexander, PhD

Effect of Seeding Duration on the Strength of Chondrocyte Adhesion to Articular Cartilage
Schinagl RM, Kurtis MS, Ellis KD, et al (Univ of California, San Diego, La Jolla)
J Orthop Res 17:121-129, 1999   4–30

Introduction.—Several strategies to enhance healing of articular cartilage have been based on the production of new extracellular matrix and integration of new host tissue. For such strategies to succeed, the transplanted chondrocytes must remain in a position from which their biosynthetic products can influence the repair. However, the articular cartilage may not provide a good surface for cell attachment. In vitro cell-adhesion studies were performed to determine the effects of seeding time on chondrocyte adhesion to cartilage.

Methods.—Cultured bovine articular chondrocytes were infused into a parallel-plate shear-flow chamber, where they settled onto sections of bovine articular cartilage. The chondrocytes (approximate density, 20,000

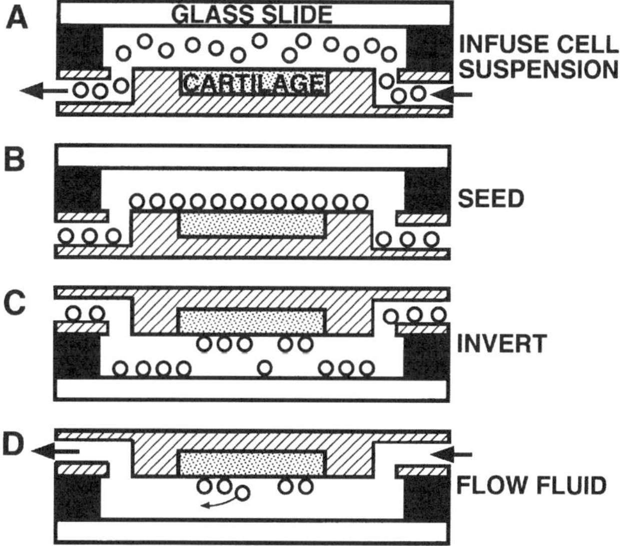

FIGURE 2.—Schematic illustration of the cell-detachment assay. **A,** Chondrocyte suspension was infused into parallel-plate shear-flow chambers holding cartilage sections. **B,** Cells settled to the cartilage surface by gravity. **C,** The chamber was inverted onto a microscope stage, and weakly adherent cells detached. **D,** Fluid flow-induced shear stress was applied to cause cell detachment. (Courtesy of Schinagl RM, Kurtis MS, Ellis KD, et al: Effect of seeding duration on the strength of chondrocyte adhesion to articular cartilage. *J Orthop Res* 17:121-129, 1999.)

cells/cm²) seeded and were allowed to attach to the cartilage for periods of 5 to 40 minutes. They were then exposed to flow-induced shear stress of 6 to 90 Pa, and the percentage of cells detached at each level of shear stress was calculated (Fig 2).

Results.—Shear stress durations of 1 minute were needed to induce steady-state cell detachment. The longer the duration of chondrocyte seeding, the firmer their attachment to cartilage. With a 9-minute seeding time, 50% of the cells were detached by force of gravity alone. However, with a 40-minute seeding time, 26 Pa of shear stress was needed to achieve the same level of detachment.

Conclusions.—Increased chondrocyte-seeding times are associated with increased resistance to shear stress–induced cell detachment from articular cartilage. These in vitro results suggest that, in a fresh cartilage section, 50% cell detachment would be induced by gravity after a 25-minute seeding time and by 2.3 Pa of shear stress after a 40-minute seeding period. Thus, when cartilage transplantation is performed for cartilage repair, chondrocytes should be allowed to stabilize for some time without any applied load.

▶ Articular cartilage does not heal well after injury because of the poor blood supply and the low density of chondrocytes in the tissue. One technique used in medicine to facilitate healing of cartilage is to transplant isolated chondrocytes into the site of the defect. However, articular cartilage provides a relatively antiadhesive surface for cell attachment, and shear stress because of joint movement can cause detachment of the cells. In this study, cell detachment was examined at several time intervals after seeding, and it was concluded that chondrocytes are more resistant to detachment with increasingly long seeding times. Patients who receive transplanted chondrocytes to repair injured cartilage should avoid loading the tissue for as long as possible after the procedure to ensure adhesion of the cells to the surrounding tissue.

M. J. L. Alexander, PhD

Level of Physical Activity and the Risk of Radiographic and Symptomatic Knee Osteoarthritis in the Elderly: The Framingham Study
McAlindon TE, Wilson PWF, Aliabadi P, et al (Boston Univ; Natl Heart, Lung and Blood Inst, Framingham, Mass; Brigham and Women's Hosp, Boston)
Am J Med 106:151-157, 1999   4–31

Objective.—The association between physical activity and osteoarthritis is controversial. The association between reported level of physical activity and incidence of radiographic and symptomatic knee osteoarthritis and the possibility that high body mass index (BMI) might exacerbate the effects of physical activity on knee arthritis were evaluated.

Methods.—Knee radiographs were obtained in 473 Framingham Heart Study participants (178 men), aged 63 to 91 years, at examinations 18

TABLE 2.—Incidence of Radiographic Knee Osteoarthritis by Level of Habitual Physical Activity

Type of Physical Activity (Hours Per Day)	Knees With Incident Osteoarthritis (%)	Odds Ratio (95% Confidence Interval)	Adjusted Odds Ratio (95% Confidence Interval)*	P for Trend
Heavy				
0	33 (6)	1.0	1.0	
1	25 (12)	2.2 (1.2-4.0)	2.2 (1.2-4.2)	
2	10 (8)	1.4 (0.6-3.4)	1.7 (0.7-4.1)	
3	7 (15)	2.9 (1.1-7.4)	2.9 (1.2-6.9)	
≥4	8 (24)	4.9 (1.6-15)	7.2 (2.5-21)	0.00009
Moderate				
0	19 (8)	1.0	1.0	
1	26 (9)	1.1 (0.6-2.)	1.3 (0.6-2.7)	
2	10 (7)	0.9 (0.4-2.1)	1.1 (0.5-2.7)	
3	14 (10)	1.2 (0.5-2.8)	1.5 (0.6-3.5)	
≥4	14 (11)	0.7 (0.3-1.7)	1.6 (0.6-4.1)	0.5
Light				
0	8 (6)	1.0	1.0	
1	38 (9)	1.7 (0.6-4.3)	1.7 (0.7-4.5)	
2	22 (10)	2.0 (0.7-5.3)	2.0 (0.7-5.4)	
3	10 (8)	1.7 (0.6-5.1)	1.9 (0.7-5.6)	
≥4	5 (8)	1.4 (0.4-5.5)	1.5 (0.4-5.6)	1.0

*Adjusted for age, sex, body mass index, weight loss, knee injury, health status, current smoking, and total caloric intake.
(Courtesy of McAlindon TE, Wilson PWF, Aliabadi P, et al: Level of physical activity and the risk of radiographic and symptomatic knee osteoarthritis in the elderly: The Framingham Study. *Am J Med* 106:151-157, copyright 1999, with permission from Excerpta Medica Inc.)

(1983-1985) and 22 (1992-1993) and were scored on a modified Kellgren and Lawrence scale from 0 to 4. Physical activity assessments were made from responses of participants to the Framingham Physical Activity Index at examination 20. BMI was calculated. The outcome measure was development of radiographic or symptomatic knee osteoarthritis. Risk for development of knee osteoarthritis was compared with hours spent in physical activity, number of flights of stairs climbed, and number of city blocks walked daily.

Results.—Radiographic osteoarthritis developed in 83 of 940 evaluable knees, and symptomatic osteoarthritis developed in 20 knees. Sixteen participants had bilateral osteoarthritis. Correlation (*r*) between BMI and hours per day of physical activity were −0.08 for light, −0.12 for moderate, and −0.02 for heavy exercise. The risk for osteoarthritis was significantly associated with the number of hours per day spent in heavy exercise for both men (6.4) and women (5.1) (Table 2). Age, sex, BMI, weight loss, knee injury, health status, total energy intake, and current smoking increased the risk for knee osteoarthritis with heavy exercise (odds ratio [OR], 7.0 for ≥4 h/d). There was no correlation for those who exercised lightly or moderately. Obesity increased the risk for knee osteoarthritis in those who engaged in heavy exercise (OR, 13 for ≥3 h/d). Results were similar for symptomatic osteoarthritis.

Conclusion.—Heavy physical activity increases the risk for knee osteoarthritis in older individuals, particularly if they are obese. There does not appear to be an increased risk for individuals who engage in moderate or light physical activity.

▶ Previous studies of long-distance runners have led to the optimistic conclusion that, despite the substantial loads imposed on the knees by such activity, the incidence of osteoarthritis was not increased.[1,2] However, the article by McAlindon et al draws what at first inspection seems the disturbing conclusion that prolonged heavy exercise can cause a 7-fold increase in risk. They suggest that 1 reason why their findings seem to differ from earlier reports is that their sample was older (an average age of 70 years). The sample was quite large (473 participants in the Framingham Study), but the 7-fold increase in risk was based on only 8 subjects. Further, unlike runners (where the type of exercise is well established), information on physical activity patterns was drawn from a limited (five-question) self-report. The physical activity that caused problems was *very* prolonged (averaging >4 h/d), and the 8 individuals who fell into this category may have included people working in heavy occupations as well as those who engaged in sports likely to cause knee injuries. It would thus seem that further research is needed before we accept without question the authors' claim that "heavy physical activity is an important risk factor for the development of knee osteoarthritis in the elderly."

R. J. Shephard, MD, PhD, DPE

References

1. Lane NE, Michel B, Bjorkengren A, et al: The risk of osteoarthritis with running and aging: A 5-year longitudinal study. *J Rheum* 20:461-468, 1993.
2. Panush RS, Schmidt C, Caldwell JR, et al: Is running associated with degenerative joint disease? *JAMA* 255:1152-1154, 1986.

Risk of Degenerative Ankle Joint Disease in Volleyball Players: Study of Former Elite Athletes
Gross P, Marti B (Swiss Sports School, Magglingen, Switzerland)
Int J Sports Med 20:58-63, 1999   4–32

Background.—Osteoarthritis is more common in the hands, spine, knee, and hips than in the ankle. However, it is known to occur after trauma involving intra-articular fractures. The most common sports and recreational injuries are injuries to the ankle, and it is possible that long-term instability of the ankle could be a significant risk factor for the premature development of osteoarthritis. The effects of long-term, high-intensity participation in volleyball on the risk for premature osteoarthritis were studied.

Methods.—A group of 22 former elite volleyball players, aged 34 ± 6 years, and 19 healthy, untrained control subjects, aged 35 ± 6 years, participated in this Swiss study. The volleyball athletes had played for at least 3 years in the most elite league in Switzerland and averaged 5.5 hours

(± 2 hours) of play per week. The volleyball athletes completed a questionnaire regarding their exercise habits, history of sports-related injury, and medical history. They underwent an orthopedic examination, including range-of-motion assessment and stability tests in the upper ankle joint. The anterior drawer and talar tilt test were used to test mechanical stability. Functional instability was assessed with a modified Freeman's test. Both the athlete and control groups underwent radiographic examinations.

Results.—Among the athlete group, 20 of the 22 players had experienced at least 1 ankle sprain. Ten athletes had ruptured the lateral ligaments, with 8 undergoing surgical repair. Significant mechanical instability was seen in 4 of the athletes, and 5 of them had a varus tilt of more than 8 degrees according to the stress radiograph. There was a greater prevalence of subchondral sclerosis and osteophytes among athletes than among control subjects. However, the differences between the 2 groups in joint space were not significant. A radiologic score indicating degenerative ankle disease was higher in 19 of the 22 volleyball players but in only 2 of the 19 control subjects. Multiple regression analysis of the data gathered from the questionnaires and physical examinations indicated that the only significant, independent predictors of increased radiologic index were the anterior drawer sign and a sense of instability.

Conclusion.—There were significantly more radiologic findings among the athletes than among the control subjects. However, high-intensity participation in volleyball could not be confirmed as an independent risk factor for osteoarthritis of the ankle joint. It is possible that the risk of osteoarthritis of the ankle is marginally greater with a combination of high-intensity volleyball competition and chronic lateral instability in the ankle.

▶ The clear inference is that chronic lateral ankle instability, and not intensive volleyball playing, increases the risk of ankle osteoarthritis. It seems that this observation would be true regardless of the activity.

J. S. Torg, MD

Physical Exercise in Outpatients With Epilepsy
Nakken KO (Natl Ctr for Epilepsy, Sandvika, Norway)
Epilepsia 40:643-651, 1999   4–33

Objective.—Many epileptic patients are hypoactive and rarely participate in organized physical activities, even though there is evidence that exercise rarely triggers seizures. The exercise habits of a selected group of adult outpatients with epilepsy were compared with those of age- and sex-matched healthy controls to determine if fear of exercise-induced seizures and the risk of seizure-related injuries as a result of exercise may be overestimated in patients with epilepsy.

TABLE 5.—Patients' Reports of Activities Most Often Associated With
Seizures (n = 96)

Activity	Number of Patients
Ball games	36 (37%)
Jogging	29 (30%)
Hiking	27 (28%)
Aerobics	21 (22%)
Bicycling	21 (22%)
Dancing	12 (12%)
Swimming	11 (11%)
Cross-country skiing	8 (8%)
Alpine sports	4 (4%)
Weight lifting	4 (4%)
Gardening	3 (3%)
Sexual intercourse	3 (3%)

(Courtesy of Nakken KO: Physical exercise in outpatients with epilepsy. *Epilepsia* 40:643-651, 1999, copyright International League Against Epilepsy.)

Methods.—Two questionnaires regarding seizures and exercise were completed by 90% of 233 adult patients with epilepsy; 204 (101 female), aged 16 to 66, supplied sufficient data to be included in the study. Exercise-induced seizures were defined as those occurring in more than 50% of the training sessions.

Results.—The proportion who never exercised was significantly higher in the patient group than in the average Norwegian. Patients preferred nonaerobic activities, whereas the controls preferred aerobic activities. Patients exercised significantly more often with friends and in fitness centers, whereas controls preferred athletic clubs. There were 109 patients (53%) who had never had a seizure while exercising, 23 (11%) who claimed to have had a seizure in more than 10% of training sessions, and 4 (2%) who had exercise-induced seizures in more than 50% of training sessions. There were 128 patients who never had a seizure after exercise, 17 (8%) who had frequent seizures immediately after exercise, and 4 (2%) who had seizures after > 50% of training sessions. Many patients with exercise-induced seizures had symptomatic localization-related epilepsy. About 80% of patients with exercise-induced seizures experienced them after strenuous exercise (Table 5). Seventy-eight (38%) patients said they had experience with how exercise affected their seizure frequency, with 41 (53%) stating that exercise had no influence, 20 (36%) claiming they had better control of their seizures because of regular exercise, and 9 (11%) saying exercise had a negative influence on seizure frequency. These 9 patients were the same individuals who claimed to have had seizures in more than 10% of training sessions. Twenty patients had been injured as a result of seizures during exercise.

Conclusion.—Patients with epilepsy are more physically active than previously thought. Only about 10% experience exercise-induced seizures. Most had no deleterious effects from exercise, and 36% claimed exercise, improved seizure control.

▶ Patients with epilepsy continue to be overprotected, and many remain relatively inactive, in part because several anecdotal reports have linked exercise with the precipitation of seizures.[1-3] The present report, based on a substantial series of 204 patients, puts such perceptions in perspective. More than half the patients claimed they never had epilepsy attacks during or after exercise. About one third of such individuals thought that exercise had a favorable impact on the frequency of seizures. Nevertheless, in 10% of cases (mostly those with an underlying structural brain lesion), exercise was a precipitant of attacks, and in 2%, it frequently caused seizures. Negative features of exercise included a high intensity of effort and exercise at high altitude.

R. J. Shephard, MD, PhD, DPE

References

1. Bennett DR: Epilepsy and the athlete, in Jordan BD, Tsairis P, Warren RF (eds): *Sports Neurology*. Rockville, MD, Aspen Publishers, 1989, pp 116-126.
2. Ogyniemi AO, Gomez AR, Klass DK: Seizures induced by exercise. *Neurology* 38:633-634, 1988.
3. Schmitt B, Thun-Hohenstein L, Vontobel H, et al: Seizures induced by physical exercise: Report of two cases. *Neuropediatrics* 25:51-53, 1994.

Cardiorespiratory Responses to Arm Cranking and Electrical Stimulation Leg Cycling in People With Paraplegia
Raymond J, Davis GM, Climstein M, et al (Univ of Sydney, Australia)
Med Sci Sports Exerc 31:822-828, 1999   4-34

Background.—In patients with paralysis of the lower limbs, arm exercise induces an altered circulatory response, counterbalanced by an increased heart rate, but accompanied by reduced ventricular stroke volumes and early fatigability. Electrical stimulation (ES)–induced muscle contractions are used to activate the venous "muscle pump," thus improving central and peripheral circulation. However, the resulting rise in oxygen uptake or cardiac output is lower than that seen with voluntary arm exercise. It has been suggested that adding lower-limb ES to arm-cranking exercise (ACE) may improve upper body exercise tolerance. Cardiorespiratory responses to ACE in the presence and absence of ES-induced leg cycling exercise (ES-LCE) were assessed in patients with paraplegia.

Methods.—The study included 10 men with T5 to T12 spinal cord injuries and paraplegia. On different days, the patients performed 4 different tests in randomized order: maximal and submaximal ACE, with and without ES-LCE. The metabolic and respiratory responses to each form of exercise were assessed.

Results.—Submaximal, steady-state ACE plus ES-LCE was associated with a 0.25-L/min increase in $\dot{V}O_2$, a 13-mL increase in stroke volume, and a 9.4-L/min increase in expired ventilation compared with submaximal ACE alone. The 2 submaximal exercise sessions were not associated with any difference in heart rate, cardiac output, or power output. Maximal ACE plus ES-LCE was associated with a 0.23-L/min increase in $\dot{V}O_2$ compared with maximal ACE alone. Otherwise, the 2 maximal exercise sessions were similar in terms of power output, heart rate, and expired ventilation.

Conclusions.—In paraplegic patients, adding ES-LCE to submaximal or maximal ACE significantly increases metabolic stress. Submaximal ACE plus ES-LCE is associated with a significantly increased stroke volume and no rise in heart rate. This is consistent with reduced venous blood pooling in the lower limbs and greater cardiac volume loading. Aerobic fitness of patients with paraplegia may be increased by adding ES-LCE to the ACE training program.

▶ When individuals with paraplegia undertake a training regimen, the cardiovascular response tends to be limited, in part, because a small muscle mass is activated and, in part, because blood pools in the veins of the paralyzed lower limbs.[1,2] It is thus logical to suggest that the training response might be enhanced by the addition of functional ES to the plan of treatment. This increases the active muscle mass and reduces the tendency for venous pooling. The observed augmentation of stroke volume might suggest that the training stimulus is indeed greater, but there is a pressing need to demonstrate the impact on training by more than a single comparison of the 2 patterns of exercise!

R. J. Shephard, MD, PhD, DPE

References

1. Shephard RJ: *Fitness in Special Populations.* Champaign, Ill, Human Kinetics, 1991.
2. Glaser RM, Janssen TWJ, Shuster DB: Exercise and cardiopulmonary fitness in individuals with spinal cord injury, in Shephard RJ, Miller HS (eds): *Exercise and the Heart in Health and Disease.* New York, Marcel Dekker, 1999, pp 505-540.

Effect of a Single Bout of Acute Exercise on Plasma Human Immunodeficiency Virus RNA Levels
Roubenoff R, Skolnik PR, Shevitz A, et al (Tufts Univ, Boston)
J Appl Physiol 86:1197-1201, 1999   4–35

Objective.—HIV causes a catabolic disease that reduces exercise capacity. Exercise, particularly high-intensity exercise which is known to activate the immune system in healthy adults, could improve the immune system in HIV-infected patients or increase replication of the virus. The effect of a single bout of strenuous exercise on plasma HIV RNA was tested in 25 adults with HIV infection.

Methods.—Blood samples were drawn for RNA testing from 25 HIV-infected patients (4 women), with an average age of 38 years, before and

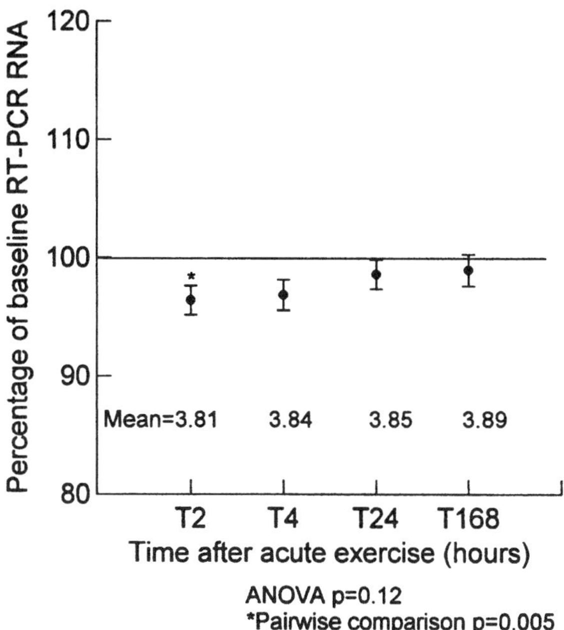

FIGURE 3.—Serum HIV RNA measured by reverse transcriptase-polymerase chain reaction at baseline and 2, 6, 24, and 168 hours (1 week) after 15 minutes of acute exercise, expressed as a percentage of baseline value for each subject. Mean log concentration for each follow-up time is also shown (**Bottom**). *Error bars*, indicate SE. There was no significant change in RNA after exercise ($P = .12$, repeated-measures analysis of variance [ANOVA]), although a statistically significant, but biologically unimportant, decline in RNA was seen 2 hours after exercise compared with baseline ($P < .01$), post hoc pairwise analysis. (Courtesy of Roubenoff R, Skolnik PR, Shevitz A, et al: Effect of a single bout of acute exercise on plasma human immunodeficiency virus RNA levels. *J Appl Physiol* 86:1197-1201, 1999.)

at 2, 6, 24, and 168 hours after 15 minutes of a 60-cm step aerobic exercise protocol.

Results.—Circulating neutrophil counts, creatine phosphokinase, and 3-methylhistidine increased after acute exercise, but viral loads did not (Fig 3). Although these results should not be generalized to long-duration or very high intensity exercise programs, a moderate level of exercise should not increase viral load in HIV-infected patients. It is possible that the high viral load present initially in patients resulted in a "ceiling effect" that made it difficult to see increases in HIV RNA.

Conclusion.—HIV-infected patients appear to benefit from regular exercise programs aimed at increasing muscle mass, reducing fat mass, and improving strength and functional status without activating HIV replication.

▶ During the 1980s and 1990s, there was some hope among exercise immunologists that exercise training could be used as a method to delay the progression from HIV infection to AIDS. Unfortunately, none of the studies conducted thus far have provided good evidence that HIV subjects randomized to exercise training regimens have improved in immune function relative to controls.[1] One conclusion, however, that has been made from these studies is that appropriately supervised exercise training does not appear to adversely affect HIV-infected individuals. Several potential benefits of both aerobic and strength training by HIV-infected individuals, especially when initiated early in the disease state, include improvement in psychological coping, and maintenance of health and physical function for a longer period.

Does one 15-minute exercise bout have an effect on plasma HIV RNA levels? Roubenoff et al provide important data indicating that a moderately intensive bout of exercise (in this study, 15 minutes of bench stepping) is not associated with an increase in HIV load. It should be emphasized, however, that 15 minutes of bench stepping has a very small influence on the immune system. Some HIV patients exercise intensively for long periods of time and engage in marathon race competitions. Such exercise causes large elevations in stress hormones and plasma cytokine levels and numerous changes in immune function that have been interpreted as negative. Further research is needed to study the effect of prolonged and intensive exertion on plasma HIV RNA levels.

D. C. Nieman, DPH

Reference

1. Shephard RJ: Exercise, immune function and HIV infection. *J Sports Med Phys Fitness* 38:101-110, 1998.

Moderate and High Intensity Exercise Training in HIV-1 Seropositive Individuals: A Randomized Trial
Terry L, Sprinz E, Ribeiro JP (Hosp de Clinicas de Porto Alegre, Brazil; Federal Univ of Rio Grande do Sul, Porto Alegre, RS, Brazil)
Int J Sports Med 20:142-146, 1999   4–36

Objective.—Results of studies of the effect of exercise on immunologic parameters of HIV-infected individuals are controversial. A trial of HIV-1–seropositive individuals randomly allocated to a moderate or high-intensity exercise program measured exercise capacity, immunologic markers, anthropomorphic variables, and depression scores.

Methods.—The effects of a 12-week moderate or high-intensity exercise program (1 hour 3 times weekly) were assessed in 21 volunteers (14 women), average age, 31 years, with inactive HIV-1 infection. Immunologic markers were measured at baseline, at 6 weeks, and at the end of the program. Height, body mass, and skinfold thickness were measured at baseline and after the program. Maximum exercise capacity was determined and a psychologic evaluation was performed before and after the program.

Results.—Eleven volunteers (3 women) in the high-intensity group and 10 (4 women) in the moderate-intensity group completed the study. Heart rate increased significantly more in the high-intensity group than in the moderate-intensity group (84% vs 60%). Exercise capacity as measured

TABLE 2.—Immunologic Variables (Mean ± SD) Measured at Baseline, in the Middle, and at the End of the Exercise Program

	Baseline	6 Weeks	12 Weeks
Leukocytes (cells·mm^{-3})			
Moderate Intensity	6344 ± 1315	6400 ±1403	6930 ± 1972
High intensity	6225 ± 1028	6282 ± 1717	6473 ± 2501
Lymphocytes (cells·mm^{-3})			
Moderate Intensity	2148 ± 560	2627 ± 761	2638 ± 682
High intensity	2475 ± 821	2585 ± 824	2511 ± 837
CD4 (cells·mm^{-3})			
Moderate Intensity	592 ± 245	614 ± 217	683 ± 291
High intensity	590 ± 242	651 ± 297	586 ± 316
CD4 (%)			
Moderate Intensity	28 ± 7	24 ± 7	26 ± 7
High intensity	25 ± 8	25 ± 7	23 ± 8
CD8 (cells·mm^{-3})			
Moderate Intensity	1030 ± 252	1242 ± 374	1252 ± 338
High intensity	1353 ± 492	1389 ± 470	1413 ± 500
CD8 (%)			
Moderate Intensity	49 ± 10	48 ± 9	48 ± 10
High intensity	55 ± 9	53 ± 6	57 ± 9
CD4:CD8 ratio			
Moderate Intensity	0.59 ± 0.26	0.51 ± 0.22	0.56 ± 0.26
High intensity	0.47 ± 0.19	0.48 ± 0.16	0.43 ± 0.18

(Courtesy of Terry L, Sprinz E, Ribeiro JP: Moderate and high intensity exercise training in HIV-1 seropositive individuals: A randomized trial. *Int J Sports Med* 20:142-146, 1999; Georg Thieme Verlag.)

with the treadmill test increased significantly, from 680 to 750 seconds in the moderate-intensity group and from 651 to 841 seconds in the high-intensity group. The increase in exercise capacity was significantly larger in the high-intensity group compared with the moderate-intensity group. Peak systolic blood pressure increased significantly in the high-intensity group only. Peak heart rate, blood tests, body mass, estimated body density, percentage of body fat, and immunologic parameters did not change significantly for either group (Table 2).

Conclusion.—Exercise capacity increases in HIV-seropositive patients who undertake moderate and high-intensity exercise. Immunologic parameters are not affected.

▶ There have been relatively few trials of exercise responses in HIV-positive individuals.[1,2] Despite fears that the disease-induced loss of immunocompetence would be made worse by an exercise training program, experience to date has been positive, at least in the early stages of the disease; resting immune function has not been further suppressed, and exercise has helped to avert the normal disease-linked loss of lean tissue and deterioration in mood state. The report of Sprinz and associates concerns patients in the very early stages of the disease, with little or no apparent decrease in CD4$^+$ cell count, although the CD4$^+$/CD8$^+$ ratio is lower than in most healthy patients. Although the trial is randomized, it is important to note that there is no control group, and the measure of training response (the increase in treadmill endurance time) is a relatively weak one. Nevertheless, the findings support the view that patients can tolerate quite vigorous exercise in the early stages of HIV infection.

R. J. Shephard, MD, PhD, DPE

References

1. Shephard RJ, Shek PN: Exercise and CD4+/CD8+ cell counts: Influence of various contributing factors in health and HIV infection. *Exp Immunol Rev* 2:65-83, 1996.
2. Birk TJ: HIV and exercise. *Exp Immunol Rev* 2:84-95, 1996.

Sports-related Cutaneous Reactions: Part II. Allergic Contact Dermatitis to Sports Equipment
Fisher AA
Cutis 63:202-204, 1999   4–37

Introduction.—Diving and swimming equipment can produce allergic contact dermatitis.

Allergic Contact Dermatitis Associated With Swimming and Diving.— Masks and mouthpieces can cause severe, painful, and at times disabling "mask burn." The oral mucosa, gingiva, and tongue may be affected. Facial dermatitis is most often caused by N-isopropyl-N-phenyl-paraphenylenediamine, an antioxidant. Patch tests produce a reaction within 48 to 96 hours (Table 1). Nose clips, ear plugs, fins, and fin straps can also cause contact dermatitis. Hypoallergenic masks and mouthpieces are available

---

TABLE 1.—Routine Patch Test Series

Mercapto Mix (contains 0.33% each)
  N-Cyclohexyl-2-benzothiazolesulfenamide
  2,2'-Benzothiazyl disulfide
  4-Morpholinyl-2-benzothiazyl disulfide
Thiuram Mix (contains 0.25% each)
  Dipentamethylenethiuram disulfide
  Tetramethylthiuram disulfide
  Tetramethylthiuram monosulfide
  Tetraethylthiuram disulfide
PPD (Black Rubber) Mix
  (contains 0.1% IPPD, 0.25% CPPD, and 0.25% DPPD)
  N-Phenyl-N-cyclohexyl-*p*-phenylenediamine
  N-Isopropyl-N-phenyl-*p*-phenylenediamine
  N,N'-Diphenyl-*p*-phenylenediamine
Carba Mix (contains 1% each)
  1,3-Diphenylguanidine
  Zinc diethyldithiocarbamate
  Zinc dibutyldithiocarbamate
Dibetanaphthyl-*p*-phenylenediamine 1%
Mercaptobenzothiazole 1%

---

from selected manufacturers. Other sports equipment, including billiard cues and kneeguards, can also cause contact dermatitis.

Comments.—The rash disappears when the allergen no longer touches the skin. After treating the dermatitis, allergy-free alternative equipment should be recommended.

Rubber Compounds.—Sensitizers include ethylbutylthiourea, *N,N*-diethylurea, and ethylene thiourea, which can cross react. Other sensitizers that do not cross react include mercaptobenzothiazole and thiuram. Ethylbutylthiourea, a component of some insoles and diving suits, can cause contact dermatitis. Alternative insoles are available.

▶ In another life, I worked with an organization that manufactured respirators, and I still recall the many problems that were encountered with the various types of rubber available to us. A variety of additives seemed capable of provoking serious skin reactions in users. It is useful to be reminded that a number of types of sports equipment can also cause painful and even disabling allergic dermatitis.

R. J. Shephard, MD, PhD, DPE

Prevention of Tinea Corporis in Collegiate Wrestlers
Hand HW, Wroble RR (Ohio Univ, Athens; Sportsmedicine Grant, Columbus, Ohio)
J Athletic Train 34:350-352, 1999   4–38

Objective.—Ringworm disqualifies wrestlers from athletic competition until they are no longer contagious. A comprehensive skin disease prevention protocol in combination with a barrier cream was developed and tested during the collegiate wrestling season (Table 1).

Methods.—During a 16-week period, 22 male collegiate division I wrestlers, aged 18.1 to 23.2 years, were studied. During the first 8 weeks, no special precautions were taken. During the second 8 weeks, wrestlers followed the protocol with half using a barrier cream and half using a

---

TABLE 1.—Prevention Protocol for Skin Infections

Clean and dry mats at least once daily. We use Kenmat (Kennedy Industries, Maple Glen, PA) mat
    disinfectant made especially for this purpose. The wrestling room is well ventilated and help
    dry the mat and reduce the humidity.
Wash and dry workout gear *every* day, after *every* workout.
Shower after *every* workout and after *every* event with an antibacterial soap.
Do not leave wet towels or gear in lockers overnight.
Athletic trainers should examine wrestlers for skin lesions.
All athletes with skin infections or lesions are referred to a physician for diagnosis and treatment.
Infected wrestlers are excluded from practice until lesions are no longer infectious.
Ringworm is considered noninfectious and can be covered by a nonpermeable dressing after 48 to 72
    hours of treatment if lesion is "dry" or no longer scaly.

(Courtesy of Hand HW, Wroble RR: Prevention of tinea corporis in collegiate wrestlers. *J Athletic Train* 34:350-352, 1999.)

---

placebo. Skin was checked daily, and lesions were diagnosed by the same physician.

Results.—There were 10 cases of ringworm before and 1 after the protocol was instituted. The single case after institution of the protocol occurred in a placebo group wrestler. All wrestlers were treated successfully with Kenshield (Kennedy Industries, Maple Glen, Pa), and no wrestler had a recurrence. There were no adverse reactions to the cream.

Conclusion.—The prevention protocol significantly reduced the incidence of tinea corporis in wrestlers.

▶ Infectious skin disease lesions usually found in wrestlers can be decreased if a prevention protocol is followed. This protocol includes proper cleaning of the mats, using clean gear, showering with antibacterial soap, and having a skin check by a certified athletic trainer. All infectious lesions are referred to a physician and the athlete is not allowed to wrestle until the lesions are not infectious.

F. J. George, ATC, PT

5 Physical Activity, Exercise, and Training: Physiology, Biochemistry, and Immune Function

Accumulation of Physical Activity for Health Gains: What Is the Evidence?
Hardman AE (Loughborough Univ, Leicestershire, UK)
Br J Sports Med 33:87-92, 1999   5–1

Objective.—The intensity level and duration of exercise necessary for a healthy lifestyle is controversial. Results of a study of the effectiveness of several short sessions of physical activity a day are presented.

Methods.—A search of MEDLINE found only 5 articles describing studies comparing the effects of several short sessions versus 1 long session daily of physical activity. Observational studies showed more favorable health outcomes with exercises performed at least partly on an intermittent basis. Results of epidemiologic studies suggest that exercises need not be performed in single longer sessions to be beneficial. Several studies have documented similar weight loss in sedentary or obese individuals who exercised for a long period (>20 minutes) once daily and those who exercised for 10 minutes several times a day.

Results.—Increasing energy expenditure reduces the risk for cardiovascular and metabolic disease by decreasing harmful lipid levels and the amount of abdominal visceral fat. Skeletal health is improved by infrequent loading events. Long periods of repetitive activity are not necessary to increase bone mineral density. Walking and cycling to work, on average 3 and 10 km, respectively, confer significant health benefits by increasing maximal oxygen intake and high-density lipoprotein cholesterol.

Conclusion.—The benefit from short bouts of exercise is assumed to be the result of an increase in total energy expenditure. As yet there is no definitive connection between the contribution of multiple sessions of exercise and total energy expenditure. Although longer sessions are necessary to improve cardiovascular conditioning, shorter multiple sessions avert the risks of vigorous exercise, particularly in sedentary individuals, and may be effective in correcting obesity and enhancing bone mineral density.

▶ Controversy regarding an optimal dose of physical activity has been resuscitated by recent changes in recommendations by the US Surgeon General and other authoritative groups.[1-3] The problem is that the establishment of a clear dose-response relationship for each and every disease in many different categories of patients is a monumental task, and despite the prognostications of "experts," such research has yet to be carried out. Cynics have suggested that the reason for lowering the recommended dose of exercise was not the access of new knowledge; rather, US Public Health authorities were afraid that the targets they had set themselves for increasing the physical activity of the population were unlikely to be met. Certainly, the assessment of any new knowledge has to date been somewhat incestuous, and better judgments may emerge from a Toronto conference held in October 2000, where evidence will be weighed by an outside panel with experience in evidence-based medicine. As reviewed here by Professor Hardman, one particularly controversial "new concept" has been the idea that one can "accumulate" the required 30 minutes of exercise on most days by undertaking several very brief periods of physical activity. As Professor Hardman points out, this concept stems from 2 relatively small-scale experiments.[4,5] Much depends on the type of benefit that is being sought. A response that is related to cumulative energy expenditure can build up over several sessions, and may even be enhanced if there are several periods of enhanced energy expenditure postexercise. However, responses that require cardiovascular conditioning intuitively seem likely to be favored by a continuous period of activity.

R. J. Shephard, MD, PhD, DPE

References

1. Pate RR, Pratt M, Blair SN, et al: Physical activity and public health: a recommendation from the Centers for Disease Control and Prevention and the American College of Sports Medicine. *JAMA* 273:402-407, 1995.
2. US Surgeon General: *Physical Activity and Health: A Report of the U.S. Surgeon General.* Atlanta, Ga: US Department of Health and Human Services, Centers for Disease Control and Prevention, 1996.
3. National Institutes for Health Consensus Development Panel. Physical activity and cardiovascular health. *JAMA* 276:241-246, 1996.
4. DeBusk RF, Stenestrand U, Sheehan M, et al: Training effects of long versus short bouts of exercise in healthy subjects. *Am J Cardiol* 65:1010-1013, 1990.
5. Ebisu T: Splitting the distance of endurance running: on cardiovascular endurance and blood lipids. *Jap J Phys Exerc* 30:37-43, 1985.

The Newcastle Exercise Project: A Randomised Controlled Trial of Methods to Promote Physical Activity in Primary Care

Harland J, White M, Drinkwater C, et al (Univ of Newcastle upon Tyne, England)

BMJ 319:828-832, 1999

5–2

Objective.—Regular exercise protects against a variety of physical and mental diseases and conditions. Although many "exercise on prescription" programs are available in England, few have been thoroughly evaluated. The effectiveness of promoting physical activity in primary care was analyzed in a randomized controlled study.

Methods.—Between March 1995 and March 1996, 523 patients (217 men), aged 40 to 64 years, in 1 urban general practice who met study criteria and were able to complete the submaximal exercise test, were randomly allocated to 1 of 4 intervention groups or a control group. Thirty participants were offered vouchers for free access to leisure facilities. Data were collected at baseline, at 12 weeks after baseline, and at 1 year after baseline. Patients underwent 1 brief interview or 6 intensive interviews over 12 weeks. Self-reported physical activity was assessed using the National Fitness Survey.

Results.—Response rates were 81% at 12 weeks and 86% at 1 year. Significantly more individuals in the intervention groups than in the control group had improved their physical activity scores at 12 weeks (38% vs 16%). Although neither the vouchers nor increased number of interviews alone had a significant effect on the results, both together increased the physical activity scores of 55% of those who were offered both, 39% more than in the control group. In the combined intervention groups, 29% of participants improved their physical activity compared with 11% in the control group, although there were no significant differences between intervention groups. Increases in physical activity reported by intervention groups at 12 weeks was not maintained at 1 year.

Conclusion.—Intensive physical activity intervention is the most effective, although gains at 12 weeks were not maintained at 1-year follow-up.

▶ The doctor's surgery remains an underexploited resource in health promotion. This report seems somewhat discouraging, in that even the most intensive of the interventions that were tried did not have a long-term impact on the behavior of patients attending routine surgeries. One possible factor in this disappointing result was that the motivation seems to have been external to the medical practitioner, with recruitment by a university research associate, and motivational intervention by a health visitor. Patients would probably have reacted more positively if the advice had been given directly by their family practitioner.

R. J. Shephard, MD, PhD, DPE

Assessment of Physical Activity in Older Individuals: A Doubly Labeled Water Study

Starling RD, Matthews DE, Ades PA, et al (Univ of Vermont, Burlington)
J Appl Physiol 86:2090-2096, 1999 5–3

Objective.—Although physical activity is important in maintaining overall health in older individuals, few methods have been developed to measure daily physical activity energy expenditure. The newly developed doubly labeled water (DLW) technique, the Minnesota Leisure Time Physical Activity Survey (LTA), Caltrac uniaxial accelerometer, and the Yale Physical Activity Survey (YPAS) were used to assess the physical activity in older women and men.

Methods.—Over a 10-day period, the DLW technique and resting metabolic rate were used to measure total daily energy expenditure in 35 Caucasian women and 32 Caucasian men volunteers, aged 45 to 84. Volunteers completed the YPAS and LTA.

Results.—Physical activity expenditure for women as measured by LTA (1621 kJ/d) and Caltrac (1592 kJ/d) was significantly lower than that measured by DLW (3666 kJ/d) and YPAS (3625 kJ/d). The corresponding physical activity expenditure measures for men were 1928, 2327, 5086, and 4649 kJ/d). The agreement between DLW and YPAS was poor (Fig 3).

Conclusion.—Although the LTA and Caltrac measures may significantly underestimate physical activity expenditure in older women and men, YPAS and DLW compare well and more accurately represent actual activity expenditure despite wide limits.

▶ Many epidemiologists in the United States have used lengthy and complex questionnaires in attempts to obtain an accurate assessment of habitual physical activity. However, our laboratory has long maintained that an almost equal amount of information can be obtained by asking 1 or 2 well-designed questions.[1] Until recently, there has been little in the way of a gold standard to evaluate questionnaires but, given a substantial budget, the analysis of DLW provides a very reliable and valid estimate of accumulated activity over a 2-week period. The present report demonstrates that the results obtained from some of the commonly used questionnaires deviate alarmingly from this "gold standard," at least in older individuals. For example, YPAS scores deviate from the criterion value by -5.48 kJ to + 6.35 kJ per day, a range that corresponds to more than the average dietary intake of a senior citizen! Estimates of habitual activity obtained for individual subjects thus have little meaning. As there is no systemic error with this methodology, the Yale questionnaire may still allow some conclusions to be drawn on the behavior of a large population sample. However, 2 other very popular approaches (the Minnesota LTA and the Caltrac accelerometer) are also marred by substantial systematic errors relative to the gold standard.

R. J. Shephard, MD, PhD, DPE

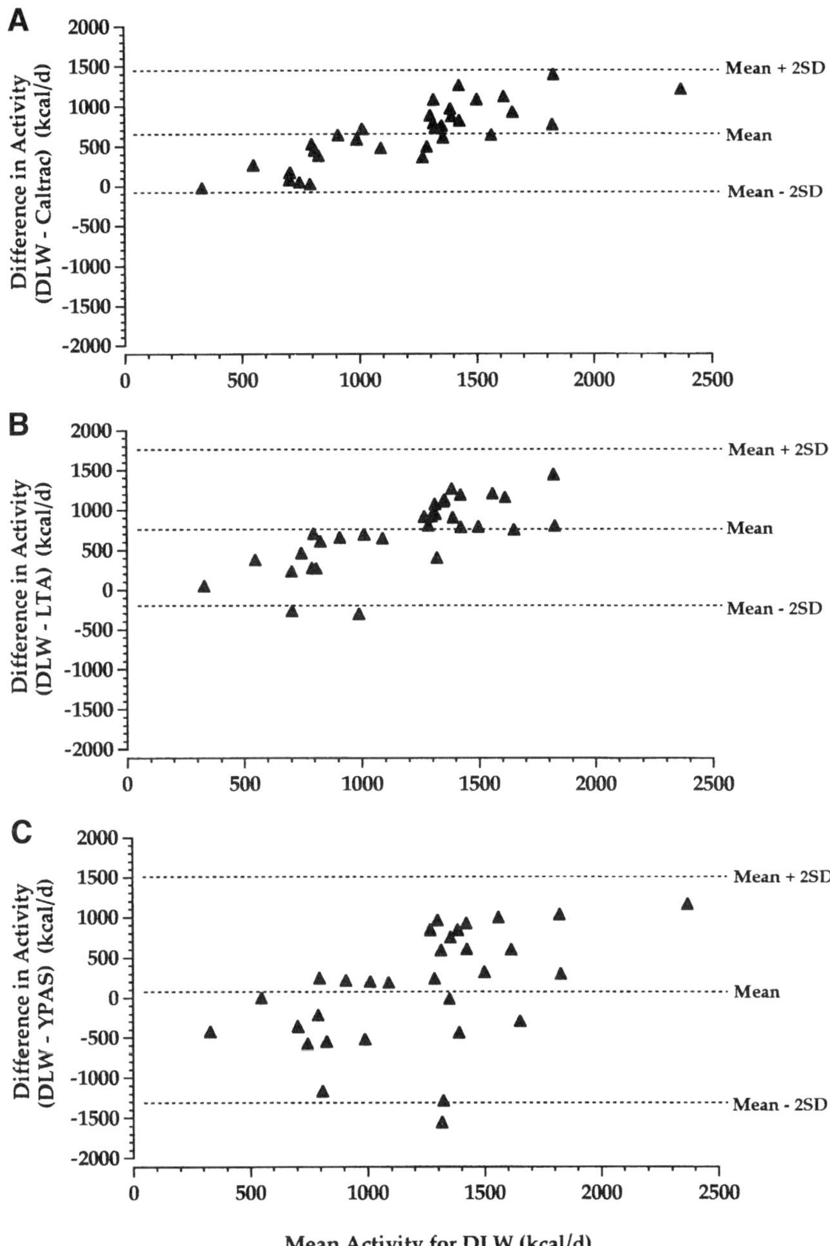

FIGURE 3.—Bland and Altman plots between doubly labeled water and Caltrac (**A**), Minnesota Leisure Time Physical Activity Survey (**B**), and Yale Physical Activity Survey (**C**) for 32 older men. Mean difference between doubly labeled water and the alternative method ± 2 SD are shown. (Courtesy of Starling RD, Matthews DE, Ades PA, et al: Assessment of physical activity in older individuals: a doubly labeled water study. *J Appl Physiol* 86:2090-2096, 1999.)

Reference

1. Godin G, Shephard RJ: A simple method to assess exercise behavior in the community. *Can J Appl Sport Sci* 10: 141-146, 1985.

Familial Aggregation of $\dot{V}O_{2max}$ Response to Exercise Training: Results From the HERITAGE Family Study

Bouchard C, An P, Rice T, et al (Laval Univ, Ste-Foy, Quebec; Washington Univ, St Louis; Indiana Univ, Bloomington; et al)
J Appl Physiol 87:1003-1008, 1999   5–4

Objective.—Maximal oxygen intake (VO_{2max}) appears to have a familial component. The VO_{2max} response to a standardized training regimen would be expected to exhibit familial aggregation, with some families having a high trainability pattern and others a low responsiveness. HERITAGE Family Study data on sedentary white individuals and individuals after 20 weeks of standardized endurance training were used to test this hypothesis.

Methods.—With a cycle ergometer, the average increase in VO_{2max} was measured in 481 sedentary adults from 98 2-generation families twice before and twice after 20 weeks of exercise training. Patients were stratified by age and sex.

Results.—The average training-induced increase in VO_{2max} differed significantly with age and sex, with VO_{2max} responses varying from an average 293 mL/min in mothers to 486 mL/min in sons (Fig 1). VO_{2max}

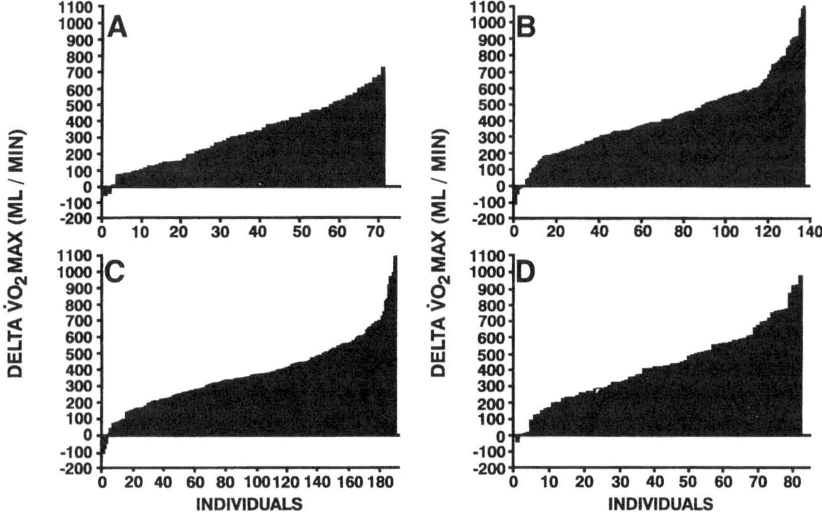

FIGURE 1.—Individual differences (delta) in increase in maximal oxygen uptake (VO_{2max}) with training for 481 individuals of the study distributed across the 4 clinical centers: Indiana (*A*), Minnesota (*B*), Quebec (*C*), and Texas (*D*). (Courtesy of Bouchard C, An P, Rice T, et al: Familial aggregation of VO_{2max} response to exercise training: results from the HERITAGE Family Study. *J Appl Physiol* 87:1003-1008, 1999.)

response was 2.5 times greater between families than within families (analysis of variance). Family membership was responsible for 39% of the variance. VO_{2max} response phenotype was not affected by age. The maximal heritability of VO_{2max} after adjusting for age and sex was 47%. The maximal maternal heritability was 28%.

Conclusion.—VO_{2max} is a highly familial trainable phenotype.

▶ The extent to which training response depends on an athlete's genes continues to attract controversy. Bouchard and associates have shown Fig 1 at many international meetings; the authors infer that some sedentary people show gains in aerobic power of 1 L or more as a result of training, while others, also supposedly sedentary, show almost no response. However, this argument neglects both interindividual differences in the degree of sedentariness and also the substantial error of test-retest measurements. The confidence limits for cycle ergometer measurements is about ± 450 mL/min, and given a mean training-related increase of 400 mL/min, the expected range of observed response would extend from −50 mL/min to 850 mL/min, in the absence of any inherited difference in response, almost exactly what we see in the figure! I am more convinced by other work from the same laboratory[1] showing greater similarities in training response in homozygous twins than in heterozygous twins. However, much more work is needed before we can be sure how important an influence genes have on training responses.

R. J. Shephard, MD, PhD, DPE

Reference

1. Bouchard C: Genetic determinants of endurance performance, in: Shephard RV, Åstrand PO, (eds): *Endurance in Sport.* Oxford, England, Blackwell Scientific, 1992, pp 149-159.

Elite Athletes and the Gene for Angiotensin-converting Enzyme
Taylor RR, Mamotte CDS, Fallon K, et al (Univ of Western Australia, Perth; Royal Perth Hosp, Western Australia; Australian Inst of Sport, Belconnen, Australian Capitol Territory; et al)
J Appl Physiol 87:1035-1037, 1999   5–5

Objective.—Because the deletion (D) allele of the angiotensin-converting enzyme (ACE) is involved in tissue repair and may be involved in several cardiovascular conditions, inheritance of the D allele may lead to enhanced athletic performance. ACE genotypes were analyzed in elite, aerobically fit, Australian athletes and compared with those of a community control group.

Methods.—ACE genotypic distribution was determined between 1994 and 1999 in 120 elite white athletes (81 men, 39 women; mean age, 30 years) and compared with ACE genotypic distribution in a community control group of healthy individuals (mean age, 40 years).

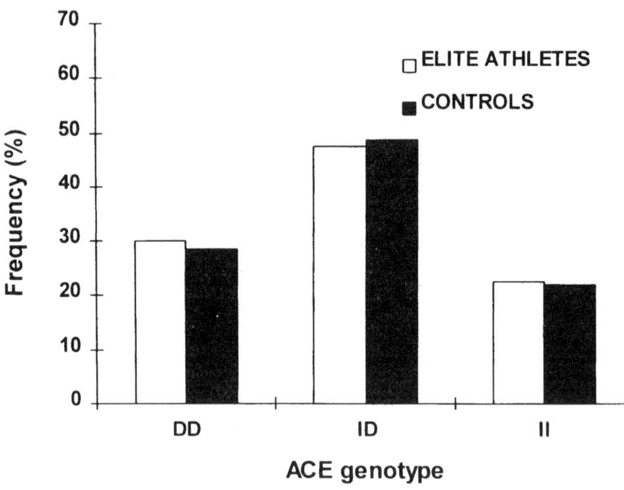

FIGURE 1.—Angiotensin-converting enzyme (*ACE*) genotype distribution in elite athletes and control subjects, showing close concordance between 2 groups. *Abbreviations*: *D*, Deletion allele; *I*, insertion allele. (Courtesy of Taylor RR, Mamotte CDS, Fallon K, et al: Elite athletes and the gene for angiotensin-converting enzyme. *J Appl Physiol* 87:1035-1037, 1999.)

Results.—There were no differences between the genotypic distributions of both groups (Fig 1).

Conclusion.—No difference in ACE genotypic distribution was found in a group of elite athletes compared with a community control group.

▶ The extent to which fitness is inherited remains a hot topic. Reports of linkages between changes of fat and nonfat mass during basic military training,[1] ability to climb to 7000 m without oxygen,[2] and ACE genotype were based on small populations. The findings encouraged some supporters of a strong constitutional impact. However, many factors other than aerobic fitness influence climbing ability, and the present comparison of a large sample of both national athletes and slightly older control subjects provides fairly convincing evidence that this particular gene is *not* a determinant of elite athletic performance. There remains scope for further investigation because the types of aerobic competitors examined were somewhat heterogeneous, and a larger sample would be needed to rule out all influence of ACE genotype on endurance performance.

R. J. Shephard, MD, PhD, DPE

References

1. Montgomery H, Clarkson P, Barnard M, et al: Angiotensin-converting enzyme gene insertion/deletion polymorphism and response to physical training. *Lancet* 353:541-545, 1999.
2. Montgomery HE, Marshall R, Hemingway H, et al: Human gene for physical performance. *Nature* 393:221-222, 1998.

Gastrointestinal Symptoms During Long-Distance Walking

Peters HPF, Zweers M, Backx FJG, et al (Utrecht Univ, The Netherlands; Netherlands Olympic Committee-Netherlands Sports Found, Arnhem; Ministry of Defense, Utrecht)
Med Sci Sports Exerc 31:767-773, 1999   5–6

Background.—Long-distance runners and triathletes commonly experience gastrointestinal (GI) symptoms during these grueling endurance events. Other studies have found incidence ranging from 10% to 81%. However, less attention has been paid to the frequency of GI symptoms during exercise of low intensity. The frequency and intensity of GI symptoms during a prolonged low-intensity exercise such as long-distance walking was examined.

Methods.—The study group consisted of 165 participants (79 men) in a 4-day walking event outside Nijmeegen, The Netherlands, in 1994. Questionnaires were sent to a random sample of 30- to 49-year-old registrants for the event. Data requested from the participants related to their dietary intake, the incidence and severity of symptoms, and their daily activities. The 165 participants were those subjects who completed both the questionnaire and a diary before and during the event. The men walked a total distance of 203 kilometers (averaging 51 km/day) during the 4-day event, while the women covered a total of 164 kilometers, averaging 41 km/day. Specific GI symptoms studied included nausea, flatulence, diarrhea, cramps, bloating, and stomach ache. Other related symptoms included headache, exhaustion, side ache, and muscle cramps. Gender differences, weight loss, exercise experience, and dietary intake before and during the walks were studied as they related to GI symptoms.

Results.—In the 3 days before the event, the incidence of GI symptoms was 1% or less and did not affect any of the participants' activities. During the event, an average of 24% of the participants experienced some GI symptoms. Only 4 to 5 walkers per day experienced symptoms severe enough to delay their walks. Of the 9 subjects who could not complete the walks, only 2 reported 1 GI symptom or more. The most common symptoms were nausea, flatulence, and headache, all of which occurred in 5% or more of the participants. Flatulence was the most significant of these symptoms reported, and lasted much longer for men than for women. Logistic regression analysis of the data indicated that the probability of finishing was much lower for subjects who experienced 1 GI symptom or more. Data from the participants also demonstrated that those whose diets included high amounts of fat and protein had a higher incidence of GI symptoms. In addition, participants who consumed alcohol the night before walking experienced a higher incidence of flatulence and stomach cramps. There was also a significant correlation between weight loss during the exercise and the occurrence of GI symptoms. However, body weight loss among the walkers in the study was less (2.5%) than that found among marathon runners (3.5%) in 1 study.

Conclusions.—As expected, GI symptoms were less frequent and less intense among these distance walkers (24%) than is typical for distance runners (20% to 50% in 1 study). Water consumption to prevent weight loss of more than 2.5% and avoidance of alcohol and high amounts of fats and proteins can help long-distance walkers avoid GI symptoms.

▶ Gastrointestinal complaints are common among endurance athletes but vary depending on the sport.[1] Several hypotheses have been developed including mechanical effects, reduction of splanchnic blood flow, GI hormones, stress, diet, dehydration, and alterations in intestinal absorption, but the etiology and pathophysiology are far from clear.[2]

In this study, as hypothesized, GI symptoms in long-distance walkers occurred at a lower frequency and intensity than reported in runners and cyclers. The few GI symptoms that did occur appeared to be related to dietary intake of fat, protein, and alcohol, and inadequate fluid consumption.

D. C. Nieman, PhD

References

1. Peters HP, Bos M, Seebregts L, et al: Gastrointestinal symptoms in long-distance runners, cyclists, and triathletes: Prevalence, medication, and etiology. *Am J Gastroenterol* 94:1570-1581, 1999.
2. Gil SM, Yazaki E, Evans DF: Aetiology of running-related gastrointestinal dysfunction. How far is the finishing line? *Sports Med* 26:365-378, 1998.

Effects of Acute Graded Exercise on Human Colonic Motility
Rao SSC, Beaty J, Chamberlain M, et al (Univ of Iowa, Iowa City)
Am J Physiol 276:G1221-G1226, 1999   5–7

Background.—Although observations suggest that exercise stimulates colonic motility, this has not been established. The immediate effects of graded exercise on colonic motility were investigated.

Methods.—Eleven healthy volunteers participated in the study. Colonic motility was determined at 6 sites by placing a solid-state probe colonoscopically. The volunteers were allowed to ambulate. The day after probe placement, the subjects exercised on bicycles at 25%, 50%, and 75% of peak oxygen intake for 15 minutes. Each session was followed by a 15-minute rest. Assessment included motor patterns, motility indexes, and regional variations before exercise, during exercise, during rest, and after exercise.

Findings.—An intensity-dependent reduction in the number and area under the curve of pressure waves was noted during exercise. In addition, the incidence of propagated or simultaneous pressure waves and cyclical events was reduced. The pressure activity reverted to baseline after exercise. However, the number and amplitude of propagated waves increased, and the simultaneous waves and cyclical events remained lower (Table 3).

TABLE 3.—Effects of Graded Exercise on Colonic Motor Patterns

	Control	25% $\dot{V}o_2$	Rest	50% $\dot{V}o_2$	Rest	75% $\dot{V}o_2$	Rest	Recovery 1	Recovery 2
No. of propagating waves	2.5 (2-4)	1.0 (0-1)*†	1.5 (1-4)	0 (0-0)*†	2.0 (1-2)	0 (0-1)†	1.0 (0-3)	3 (0-3)	3 (2-6)
Amplitude of propagating waves, mmHg	72 (56-91)	71 (55-92)	85 (71-97)	58 (0-63)*	88 (79-109)	0 (0-64)	81 (0-93)	77 (38-99)	107 (94-116)‡
No. of simultaneous waves	2 (0-3)	1 (0-3)	1 (0-2)	1 (0-1)	1 (0-2)	0 (0-0)†	0 (0-1)	0.5 (0-1)‡	1 (0-2)
No. of isolated waves	0.5 (0-3)	3 (1-4)	1 (0-2)	0.5 (0-2)	1 (0-3)	0 (0-1)†	1 (0-2)	0 (0-2)	1 (0-4)‡
No. of cyclical events	1 (0-2)	1 (1-3)	1 (1-2)	0.5 (0-2)	1 (0-2)	0 (0-0)†	0 (0-1)	1 (0-2)	0.5 (0-1)
Duration of cyclical events, min	8 (4-14)	5 (2-10)	6 (3-6)	1 (0-6)†	2 (0-9)	0 (0-0)†	0 (0-2)	5 (3-11)	7 (4-19)

Note: Values are medians with 25th-75th percentiles in parentheses.
*$P<.05$, exercise versus rest.
†$P<.05$, exercise versus control.
‡$P<.05$, control versus recovery.
(Courtesy of Rao SSC, Beaty J, Chamberlain M, et al: Effects of acute graded exercise on human colonic motility. *Am J Physiol* 276:G1221-G1226, 1999. Copyright the American Physiological Society.)

Conclusions.—These data show that acute graded exercise reduces colonic phasic activity, which may offer less resistance to colonic flow. The postexercise increase in propagated activity may increase colonic propulsion.

▶ The issue of the effect of exercise on colonic motility is important from 2 points of view. In the short term, there are the athletes who suffer from abdominal cramps and diarrhea,[1,2] and in the longer term, an increase in colonic motility has been suggested as the reason why regular physical activity protects against cancer of the descending colon. In the present study, the colonic motion during activity was actually decreased, although there was an increase post exercise. The authors note that earlier findings were for well-trained athletes, and sometimes restricted to those who suffered from exercise-induced diarrhea.[3] There is also some uncertainty as to the types of colonic movement that propagate the stool and decrease contact between the mucosa and potential toxins. Finally, prostaglandins may be implicated, and, if so, a stimulatory effect might require a longer period of activity than that tested by Rao and associates.

R. J. Shephard, MD, PhD, DPE

References

1. Moses FM: The effect of exercise on the gastrointestinal tract. *Sports Med* 9:159-172, 1990.
2. Riddoch C, Trinick T: Prevalence of running-induced gastrointestinal (GI) disturbances in marathon runners. *Br J Sports Med* 22:71-74, 1998.
3. Cheskin LJ, Crowell MD, Kamal N, et al: The effects of acute exercise on colonic motility. *J Gastrointest Motil* 4:173-177, 1992.

Gastrointestinal Symptoms in Long-Distance Runners, Cyclists, and Triathletes: Prevalence, Medication, and Etiology
Peters HPF, Seebregts L, Akkermans LMA, et al (Utrecht Univ, The Netherlands)
Am J Gastroenterol 94:1570-1581, 1999   5–8

Objective.—Gastrointestinal (GI) symptoms are common in endurance athletes. The prevalence of exercise-related symptoms and medication use in long-distance runners, cyclists, and triathletes were investigated.

Methods.—A questionnaire soliciting information about training, medication, GI symptoms, and diet during the previous 12 months was mailed to 606 endurance athletes: 114 male and 85 female long-distance runners, 98 male and 99 female cyclists, and 110 male and 100 female triathletes. Females were also asked about the use of oral contraceptives, regularity, and symptoms of the menstrual cycle. The relationship between, and importance of, these variables and GI symptoms was assessed using univariate and multivariate analysis.

TABLE 3.—Variables (**Left Column**) Significantly Related (*P*<.05) to **Upper** or **Lower** Gastrointestinal Symptoms During Competition in Runners, Triathletes, and Cyclists

Upper GI Symptoms		
Lower GI symptoms during competition	runners:	10.3 (3.5-30.7)
	triathletes:	6.0 (2.9-12.5)
	cyclists:	8.8 (4.3-18.3)
Upper GI symptoms during resting	runners:	6.6 (3.2-13.6)
	triathletes:	2.9 (1.5-5-9)
	cyclists:	6.1 (3.0-12.4)
Water intake before competition	runners:	3.3 (1.1-10.3)
Energy drink during the running part of a triathlon	triathletes:	2.3 (1.2-4.5)
Thirst quencher during the running part of a triathlon	triathletes:	2.1 (1.1-4.2)
Homemade product 2 h before competition	triathletes:	2.2 (1.1-4.5)
Solid food during cycling part of a triathlon	triathletes:	2.1 (1.1-4.1)
Lower age	cyclists:	27.8 ± 6.6 (n = 56) *vs* 25.3 ± 4.4 (n =(114) yr*
Lower GI Symptoms		
Lower symptoms during resting	runners:	4.0 (1.9-8.4)
	triathletes:	4.8 (1.6-15.1)
	cyclists:	3.2 (1.5-6.6)
Less running experience	runners:	13.4 ± 5.6 (n = 46) *vs* 11.5 ± 5.3 (n = 112) yr*
Energy drink during the running part of a triathlon	triathletes:	3.1 (1.5-6.2)
Thirst quencher during the running part of a triathlon	triathletes:	2.8 (1.4-5.6)
Solid food during the running part of a triathlon	triathletes:	3.2 (1.3-7.9)
Thirst quencher 2 h before competition	triathletes:	2.6 (1.3-5.3)

Notes: Variables are compared between subjects with and without upper or lower gastrointestinal symptoms using Fisher's Exact Test. Relative risks and 95% CI are indicated for each variable (**Right Column**).

*Students *t* test applied.

(Reprinted by permission of the publisher from Peters HPF, Seebregts L, Akkermans LMA, et al: Gastrointestinal symptoms in long-distance runners, cyclists, and triathletes: prevalence, medication, and etiology. *Am J Gastrointerol* 94:1570-1581, copyright 1999 by Elsevier Science, Inc.)

Results.—The response rate was 96% and 84% of male and female distance runners, 88% and 89% of cyclists, and 68% and 79% of triathletes. In these groups, 22, 6, and 9 questionnaires, respectively, could not be used. The prevalence of lower GI symptoms was higher than upper GI symptoms at rest and in all modes of activity except for female cyclists during competition and for male cyclists after competition (Table 3). Bloating, diarrhea, and flatulence occurred more at rest in endurance athletes. Younger cyclists had more GI symptoms than older cyclists, and women had more GI problems than men. Eating within 30 minutes before exercise and ingesting orange juice, coffee, a high-fat and high-protein diet, solid foods, hypertonic beverages, or fiber-rich foods during exercise increased the risk of GI symptoms. The percentage of athletes taking medication at rest and during exercise was 39% in distance runners, 50% in cyclists, and 35% in triathletes.

Conclusion.—Long-distance runners experience lower GI symptoms and cyclists and triathletes experience lower and upper GI symptoms. The percentage of athletes taking medication for GI symptoms is relatively high.

▶ The occurrence of GI symptoms during long-distance events is a well-recognized factor with potential to impair competitive performance.[1] However, in many studies, the prevalence of the problem may have been biased by the fact that questionnaires submitted immediately after a race were completed mainly by those with GI complaints. This report was based on a substantial sample (606 endurance athletes), was submitted outside the context of a race, was completed with a satisfactorily high response rate, and made allowance for GI problems when not engaged in heavy exercise. As in an earlier study,[2] bloating, diarrhea, and flatulence were reported more at rest than during competition, although retching, stitches, and fecal incontinence were associated with endurance exercise. Lower abdominal symptoms are more frequent in running than in cycling, presumably because of the biomechanical vibration induced by running.[3] Precipitating factors are hard to identify. Repeated drinking apparently reduces complaints,[1] and it is possible that the intake of water **after** dehydration has developed aggravates intestinal ischemia.[4]

R. J. Shephard, MD, PhD, DPE

References

1. Rehrer NJ, Janssen GM, Brouns F, et al: Fluid intake and gastrointestinal problems in runners competing in a 25-km race and a marathon. *Int J Sports Med* 10 (Suppl 1): S22-S25, 1989.
2. Sullivan SN, Wong C, Heidenheim P: Does running cause gastrointestinal symptoms? a survey of 93 randomly selected runners compared with controls. *N Z Med J* 107:328-331, 1994.
3. Dupuis HJ, Draeger J, Hartung E: Vibrations transmission to different parts of the body by various locomotions, in: Komi PV (ed): Biomechanics VA. Baltimore: University Park Press, 537-543, 1976.
4. Halvorsen FA, Ritland S: Gastrointestinal problems related to endurance event training. *Sports Med* 14:157-163, 1992.

Short-term Effects of Marathon Running: No Evidence of Cardiac Dysfunction

Lucía A, Serratosa L, Saborido A, et al (Universidad Europea de Madrid; Universidad Complutense de Madrid; Centro Nacional de Medicina del Deporte del Consejo Superior de Deportes, Madrid; et al)

Med Sci Sports Exerc 31:1414-1421, 1999   5–9

Background.—The physical fitness levels of participants in marathon running can vary widely. Because the cardiac effects of running a marathon

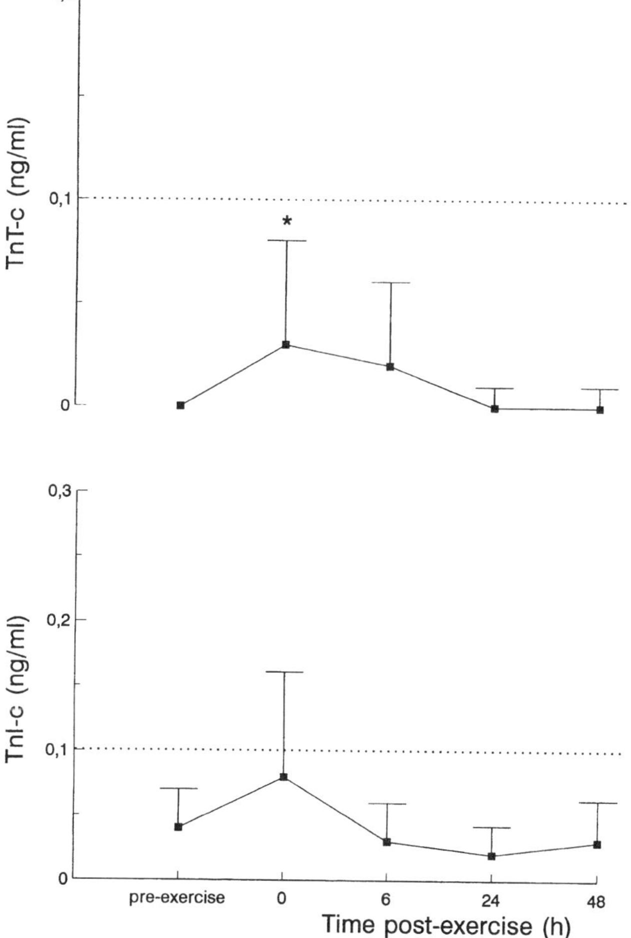

FIGURE 3.—Markers of myocardial damage: cardiac TnT-c and TnI-c. Values are mean ± SD, and dotted lines represent normal upper limits. * 0 hours postexercise versus preexercise, and 24 and 48 hours postexercise, respectively. *P* < .05. No significant differences existed for TnI-c levels. (Courtesy of Lucía A, Serratosa L, Saborido A, et al: Short-term effects of marathon running: No evidence of cardiac dysfunction. *Med Sci Sports Exerc* 31:1414-1421, 1999.)

were unknown, this study proposed to measure whether cardiac damage, evidenced by certain biochemical markers, resulted.

Methods.—Twenty-two runners (17 men, 5 women) qualified for the study. Five blood samples were collected from each runner: 48 hours before the race began, immediately after the race, and 6, 24, and 48 hours later. Blood levels of total creatine kinase activity (total CK), mass concentration of creatine kinase isoenzyme MB (CK-MB mass), myoglobin, and cardiac troponin T (TnT-c) or I (TnI-c) were measured. In addition, each runner underwent a baseline echocardiographic study 2 to 5 days before the race, within 30 minutes of completing the race, and 24 to 36 hours later. The focus was on left ventricular systolic and diastolic function.

Results.—Levels of TnT-c and TnI-c were normal before and after the race in all subjects but 1 (Fig 3), and no changes were noted in overall left ventricular systolic function. Diastolic function was significantly affected after the race but returned to resting levels in 24 to 36 hours.

Conclusions.—The marathon experience did not appear to produce any deleterious effects on the hearts of runners, regardless of their degree of physical fitness.

▶ The issue of whether extreme endurance exercise has a negative effect on cardiac function remains controversial. Lucía and associates are a little dated in their suggestion that there have been no reports showing both the release of markers of myocardial damage and echocardiographic abnormalities.[1] Nevertheless, the event concerned, the Hawaii Ironman triathlon, is one of the most demanding of endurance competitions. In contrast, Lucía et al examined only moderate performers in a marathon race that was run under relatively cool conditions. These authors claim that earlier reports of cardiac muscle damage were due to use of TnT-c as a marker; this protein is suppressed in normal skeletal muscle, but may be reactivated by muscle injury.[2] However, Rifai and associates[1] also showed increments in the more specific TnI-c marker of injury after the Ironman event. So, there does seem to be some evidence that, if you exercise hard enough, it is possible to produce at least transient damage to heart muscle.

R. J. Shephard, MD, PhD, DPE

References

1. Rifai N, Douglas PS, O'Toole M, et al: Cardiac troponin T and I, electrocardiographic wall motion analyses and ejection fractions in athletes participating in the Hawaii Ironman triathlon. *Am J Cardiol* 83:1085-1089, 1999.
2. Adams JE, Bodor GS, Dávila-Román VG, et al: Cardiac troponin I: A marker with high specificity for cardiac injury. *Circulation* 88:101-106, 1993.

Cardiac Troponin T and I, Electrocardiographic Wall Motion Analyses, and Ejection Fractions in Athletes Participating in the Hawaii Ironman Triathlon

Rifai N, Douglas PS, O'Toole M, et al (Children's Hosp, Boston; Beth Israel Deaconess Med Ctr, Boston; Univ of Tennessee, Memphis; et al)

Am J Cardiol 83:1085-1089, 1999   5–10

Objective.—Cardiac troponin T (cTnT) and I (cTnI) are markers of myocardial muscle injury. These markers were used to ascertain whether myocardial muscle injury was sustained in competitive athletes during participation in the 1994 Hawaii Ironman World Championship Triathlon.

Methods.—Nonfasting blood samples were obtained from 23 well-trained amateur athletes (11 men, average age, 33 years; 12 women, average age, 43 years), 2 days before and within 15 minutes after completion of the 1994 triathlon. Myoglobin creatine kinase (CK), CK-MB, cTnT, and cTnI concentrations were measured. Two-dimensional echocardiograms were obtained 2 to 5 days before and within 30 minutes after completion of the triathlon.

Results.—Whereas prerace myoglobin, CK, and CK-MB values were within normal ranges, postrace values were significantly elevated in all athletes (Table 1). Prerace cTnT and cTnI levels were undetectable. Postrace level of cTnT was positive in 11 athletes (6 men). Those with detectable cTnT levels had significantly higher CK levels after the race than did those with no postrace detectable levels of cTnT (2444 IU/L vs 778 IU/L). cTnT was significantly correlated with myoglobin ($r=0.57$) and CK ($r=0.70$). Two athletes had increases in cTnT and cTnI of ≥ 0.1 µg/L and ≥ 2.00 µg/L, respectively. Four athletes had moderate increases in cTnT of 0.4 to 0.5 µg/L but no detectable levels of cTnI. Whereas all prerace

TABLE 1.—Biochemical Markers for Muscle Injury and Echocardiographic Changes Before and After Triathlon

	Men (n = 11)			Women (n = 12)		
	Before	After	p Value	Before	After	p Value
Myoglobin (µg/L)*	31 ± 6	1033 ± 748	0.005	29 ± 9	586 ± 420	0.004
CK (IU/L)*	193 ± 39	1798 ± 1686	0.02	1235 ± 5	1530 ± 1090	0.001
CK-MB (µg/L)*	2.1 ± 1.6	28 ± 24	0.007	1.3 ± 0.9	29 ± 20	0.001
cTnT (ELISA)†	0/11	6/11	0.0001	0/12	5/12	0.002
cTnT (Enzymun)†	0/11	4/11	0.03	0/12	2/12	NS
cTnI†	0/11	2/11	NS	0/12	0/12	NS
Echo regional wall motion abnormality present†	0/7	6/7	0.001	0/5	3/5	0.05
Ejection fraction (%)	58 ± 7	46 ± 5	0.005	52 ± 3	46 ± 8	NS

Statistical differences between prerace and postrace values were determined by paired *t* test.
Only 12 athletes had echos for wall motion and 11 for ejection fraction, prerace and postrace.
*Values presented as mean ± SD.
†Values presented as number of positive observations/total observations.
(Reprinted from Rifai N, Douglas PS, O'Toole M, et al: Cardiac troponin T and I, electrocardiographic wall motion analyses, and ejection fractions in athletes participating in the Hawaii Ironman Triathlon. *Am J Cardiol* 83:1085-1089, copyright 1999 with permission from Excerpta Medica Inc.)

echocardiograms were normal, 9 postrace echocardiograms showed hypokinesia in 1 to 10 segments. The average number of abnormal segments was 6.5 for athletes with large cTnT and cTnI elevations, 2.3 for athletes with a moderate elevation in cTnT, and 1.7 for 6 athletes with no changes. Ejection fraction decreased significantly by 24% after the race. These results were corroborated by findings in the 1995 triathlon.

Conclusion.—Echocardiographic results and biochemical markers in the blood of triathletes confirm myocardial damage. Whether the damage is temporary or permanent remains to be elucidated.

▶ There have previously been reports of both general and regional abnormalities of ventricular wall motion following the very strenuous activity of Hawaiian Ironman triathlon participation.[1,2] However, it has been unclear whether this should be considered as evidence of injury to cardiac muscle (for example, from ischemia or an excessive exposure to free radicals). One factor inhibiting investigation has been the overlap between traditional markers of skeletal and cardiac muscle damage; for example, the MB isozyme of creatine kinase can be released not only from cardiac muscle but to a lesser extent from skeletal muscle. Early claims for specificity of the initial cTnT assay kit proved unfounded; indeed, in the present study it was no better than CK-MB. However, a cross-reactivity of less than 0.005% is claimed for second-generation assays of cTnT and cTnI.[3] The present study showed an intriguing correlation between regional abnormalities of wall motion and increased plasma levels of cTnT. However, it is still unclear whether the event gives rise to significant clinical injury. By analogy with skeletal muscle, it may be necessary to stress the heart to the point where there is some leakage of intracellular contents in order for hypertrophy to occur.

R. J. Shephard, MD, PhD, DPE

References

1. Douglas PS, O'Toole ML, Hiller WDB, et al: Cardiac fatigue after prolonged exercise. *Circulation* 76:1206-1213, 1987.
2. Douglas PS, O'Toole ML, Woolard J: Regional wall motion abnormalities after prolonged exercise in the normal left ventricle. *Circulation* 82:2108-2104, 1990.
3. Muller-Bardorff M, Hallermeyer K, Schroder A, et al: Improved troponin T ELISA specific for the cardiac troponin T isoform, I: development, analytical and clinical validation of the assay. *Clin Chem* 43:458-466, 1997.

Long-term Exercise and Atherogenic Activity of Blood Mononuclear Cells in Persons at Risk of Developing Ischemic Heart Disease

Smith JK, Dykes R, Douglas JE, et al (East Tennessee State Univ, Johnson City)
JAMA 281:1722-1727, 1999

5–11

Background.—Research suggests that atherosclerosis is an immunologically mediated disease in which atherogenic and atheroprotective cytokine secretion of infiltrating blood mononuclear cells is important. Whether long-term exercise directly affects this atherogenic, atheroprotective activity is unknown. The effect of long-term exercise on the atherogenic activity of blood mononuclear cells in persons at risk of ischemic heart disease development was studied.

Methods.—Forty-three volunteers completed the 6-month trial. All had a myocardial infarction risk ratio of 1.7 or greater based on serum complement, or C-reactive protein levels, or both, as well as normal exercise treadmill test results. Additional risk factors for ischemic heart disease were hypercholesterolemia, present in 65.1%; a family history of coronary heart disease, in 62.8%; inactivity, in 60.5%; hypertension, in 32.6%; obesity, in 25.6%; smoking, in 11.6%; and diabetes mellitus, in 4.7%. The volunteers exercised a mean 2.5 hours per week.

Findings.—After the exercise program, mononuclear cell production of atherogenic cytokines declined by 58.3%. The production of atheroprotective cytokines increased by 35.9%. After the exercise program, changes in transforming growth factor β-1 and phytohemagglutinin-induced atherogenic cytokine production were proportionate to the time the subjects spent doing repetitive lower body motion exercises, indicating a dose-response relationship. A 35% reduction in C-reactive protein serum levels reflected cellular function changes after the exercise program.

Conclusions.—Long-term exercise appears to reduce the atherogenic activity of blood mononuclear cells in persons at risk for ischemic heart disease. Thus, physical activity may protect against ischemic heart disease.

▶ There has been increasing recognition in recent years that the immune system can contribute to the onset of atherosclerosis.[1] Although we often regard the body's immune response as a favorable development, excessive secretion of proinflammatory cytokines can have many negative consequences. In the person who is vulnerable to atherosclerotic lesions, an excessive immune response can increase endothelial cell procoagulant activity, LDL oxidation, and foam cell formation, thus accelerating the formation of atherosclerotic plaques. The proinflammatory response is normally counterbalanced and controlled by an increase in the output of anti-inflammatory cytokines. In the study reported by Smith and associates, a 6-month bout of moderate aerobic exercise (average 2.5 h/wk) shifted the balance of proinflammatory and anti-inflammatory cytokine activity so that the risk of atherosclerosis was decreased. It is unfortunate that the authors did not provide more details concerning the amount of exercise that was undertaken, because excessive training can have a proinflammatory effect. Although normal volumes of aerobic activity reduce the risk for atherosclerotic disease, it would be interesting to see whether an excessive training volume, pursued over a long period, accelerates the process of atherosclerosis; one might even speculate that such a mechanism could explain the occasional coronary death in fanatic exercisers.

R. J. Shephard, MD, PhD, DPE

Reference

1. Wick G, Schett G, Amberger A, et al: Is atherosclerosis an immunologically mediated disease? *Immunol Today* 16:27-33, 1995.

Adverse Events Associated With Eccentric Exercise Protocols: Six Case Studies
Sayers SP, Clarkson PM, Rouzier PA, et al (Univ of Massachusetts, Amherst)
Med Sci Sports Exerc 31:1697-1702, 1999   5–12

Background.—Eccentric exercise protocols are used to study mild muscle damage. Rhabdomyolysis, a degeneration of muscle cells, can occasionally result from eccentric exercise protocols. When damage is extensive, myoglobin levels increase in the blood and can discolor the urine. Coupled with dehydration, this can lead to kidney failure. Some study participants may react more strongly than others to an eccentric exercise protocol. This report described adverse events that occurred after participation in an eccentric exercise study.

Study Design.—Six case reports were presented from 2 eccentric exercise studies. All study participants were male. The exercise protocol involved maximal eccentric action of the elbow flexors. Each participant performed 2 sets of 25 maximal eccentric actions, separated by 5 minutes of rest. Soreness, range of motion, and blood creatine kinase values were assessed. The first study, including 27 volunteers, resulted in 2 adverse events. The second study included 204 volunteers and caused 6 adverse events. The major adverse events were swelling and prolonged loss (up to 47 days) of the ability to generate force.

> *Case Study.*—Male, 27, participated in an eccentric exercise protocol. The baseline maximal isometric force was low (37.3 kg) and, immediately after exercise, decreased by 79%. Perceived muscle soreness peaked on day 3, but on day 5 extreme swelling was observed and muscle force declined to 16% of baseline. This participant required 47 days to return to baseline levels of muscle force.

Conclusion.—A small percentage of volunteers who participate in eccentric exercise protocols experience adverse reactions—including swelling, prolonged loss of muscle force, and elevated serum creatine kinase levels—consistent with rhabdomyolysis. Investigators using eccentric exercise regimens are urged to use extreme caution and to be aware of the potential for adverse events.

▶ Rhabdomyolysis is a potentially fatal condition, and it is important to be aware that there is a potential for such a complication after a relatively brief laboratory eccentric exercise protocol. One wonders why the present study was allowed to continue when there were as many as 6 incidents in a sample of 204 subjects; the report emphasizes the need for investigators to discuss adverse outcomes with their institutional ethics committee!

R. J. Shephard, MD, PhD, DPE

Relation Between Aerobic Fitness Level and Stress Induced Alterations in Neuroendocrine and Immune Function
Moyna NM, Bodnar JD, Goldberg HR, et al (Univ of Pittsburgh, Pa)
Int J Sports Med 20:136-141, 1999   5–13

Background.—Reduced plasma concentrations of catecholamines and cortisol have been associated with exercise at the same absolute power output after a program of endurance training. A generalized adaptation of the stress response system may be produced by an exercise training program of sufficient intensity or duration, and this adaptation may cause the neuroendocrine response to be either habituated or sensitized to a nonexercise stressor. However, results of studies in this area are mixed, with some showing evidence of an attenuation of catecholamine response among aerobically trained individuals during acute stressors in laboratory situations and other studies failing to detect any differences between trained and untrained individuals in hypothalamic-pituitary-adrenal and sympathoadrenal responses to stress. It has been shown that acute psychological stress can alter the number and function of circulating immune cells, which can affect the responsiveness of the immune system. The neuroendocrine and cellular immune responses of sedentary, moderately active, and aerobically trained subjects were investigated during acute psychological stress.

Methods.—The study group comprised 45 healthy men divided into 3 groups: aerobically trained (15), moderately active (15), and sedentary (15). Subjects fasted overnight and also abstained from caffeine, alcohol, and exercise for 24 hours before testing. An indwelling catheter was placed and blood drawn before, during, and 30 minutes after the subjects delivered a 3-minute speech for which they had 2 minutes to prepare. After 30 minutes of rest, the subjects were given the Spielberger State Anxiety Inventory. They also reported on their anxiety before and immediately after the speech.

Results.—Both the number and function of immune cells and the self-reported anxiety scores changed significantly as a result of the acute stressor task. However, there were no significant differences among the groups. Plasma levels of norepinephrine also increased during the speech but were lower in the aerobically trained subjects as compared with the moderately active and sedentary groups. The responses of the neuroendocrine and immune systems were found to be independent of the aerobic fitness levels of the subjects.

Conclusions.—It is probable that the sympathetic nervous system was responsible for the quantitative and qualitative changes in the immune system, because plasma cortisol levels did not change either during or after the stressor. The absence of a significant difference in immune response among the sedentary, moderately active, and aerobically trained groups may be related to the nature of the stressor task in this study as well as the fact that all subjects in this study were healthy young men whose resting immune parameters were within normal range.

▶ Individuals subjected to stressful psychological conditions experience an increase in heart rate, blood pressure, plasma catecholamines, and other measures of sympathetic nervous system activation. Although not all researchers agree, exercise training is typically associated with a reduction in cardiovascular reactivity to mental stress.[1] Acute psychological stress can also alter some aspects of immune function including T and natural killer cell function. Although it was hypothesized that aerobically trained versus untrained individuals would respond to a mental stress with less perturbation of immunity, results in this study did not support that. One problem was that the mental stress (a 3-minute speech) was too mild, and immune changes were small. Further research is warranted with a more significant stressor.

D. C. Nieman, PhD

Reference

1. Claytor RP: Stress reactivity: Hemodynamic adjustments in trained and untrained humans. *Med Sci Sports Exerc* 23:873-881, 1991.

The Effects of Carbohydrate Supplementation on Immune Responses to a Soccer-Specific Exercise Protocol
Bishop NC, Blannin AK, Robson PJ, et al (Univ of Birmingham, England)
J Sports Sci 17:787-796, 1999   5–14

Background.—There is increasing evidence that athletes involved in heavy prolonged training and competition are more likely to experience upper respiratory infection than less-active individuals. Various components of the immune system are suppressed temporarily as a result of strenuous exercise, in part by the actions of glucocorticoids, catecholamines, and other stress hormones. However, in recent studies, these effects were lessened by carbohydrate ingestion at regular intervals during prolonged exercise. Whether these effects also are found with carbohydrate ingestion during intermittent exercise, such as in soccer, which is characterized by periods of highly intense activity interrupted by periods of rest or reduced activity, was investigated.

Methods.—Eight healthy men from a university soccer team were enrolled in the study. Their mean age was 21, mean height 183 cm, and mean body mass 78.1 kg. The players were randomized to receive either carbohydrate or placebo beverages for use before, during, and after 2 soccer-specific exercise sessions of 90 minutes each. The soccer exercise sessions were divided into 45-minute intervals and were designed to mimic a typical soccer match in terms of distances covered and activities performed, and were spaced 3 days apart to mimic the time between games in a typical regular season. Players in the carbohydrate group received 400 mL of a lemon-flavored glucose solution 10 minutes before the start of each 45-minute exercise period and 5 minutes after exercise, and consumed 150 mL of the same solution at 14- and 29.5-minute points during each exercise period. Subjects in the placebo group received a lemon-flavored placebo drink according to the same protocol as the carbohydrate group.

Results.—In both groups, the plasma lactate concentration increased to approximately 4 mmol $\cdot$ 1^{-1} at 45 minutes and 90 minutes of exercise. However, plasma glucose concentration after 90 minutes was much lower among the placebo group (4.57 $\pm$ 0.12 mmol $\cdot$ 1^{-1}) than among the carbohydrate group (5.49 $\pm$ 0.11 mmol $\cdot$ 1^{-1}). There were no differences between the 2 groups in the patterns of change for plasma cortisol levels, circulating lymphocyte counts, and saliva immunoglobulin A secretion. Although blood neutrophil counts 1 hour after the trial were 14% higher in the placebo group than in the carbohydrate group, there were no differences in the degranulation response of blood neutrophils stimulated by bacterial lipopolysaccharide.

Conclusions.—Although studies of prolonged exercise have demonstrated attenuation of immunosuppressive effects with carbohydrate ingestion, these results were not found with the intermittent exercise protocol in this study. Carbohydrate ingestion appears to have a minor influence on the immune system's response to exercise when the overall intensity of the exercise is moderate and there are relatively small changes to levels of plasma glucose and cortisol and immune variables.

▶ Many components of the immune system exhibit adverse change after prolonged heavy exertion. During this "open window" of impaired immunity (which may last from 3 to 72 hours, depending on the immune measure), viruses and bacteria may gain a foothold, increasing the risk of subclinical and clinical infection. Compared with placebo, carbohydrate beverage ingestion before, during, and after heavy exertion has been associated with higher plasma glucose levels, an attenuated cortisol and growth hormone response, fewer perturbations in blood immune cell counts, and a diminished proinflammatory and anti-inflammatory cytokine response. Overall, these data indicate that the physiologic stress to the immune system is reduced when endurance athletes use carbohydrates before, during, and after prolonged and intense exertion.

The immunomodulatory effects of carbohydrate ingestion do not occur, however, when the exercise is intermittent and changes in blood hormone and immune parameters are minimal, such as occurs during soccer or rowing drills.[1] In other words, the exercise bout must test the limits of body carbohydrate stores before exogenous carbohydrate can be expected to ameliorate hormonal and immune responses.

D. C. Nieman, PhD

Reference

1. Nieman DC, Nehlsen-Cannarella SL, Fagoaga OR, et al: Immune response to two hours of rowing in female elite rowers. *Int J Sports Med* 20:476-481, 1999.

Effects of Maximal Exercise on Natural Killer (NK) Cell Cytotoxicity and Responsiveness to Interferon-α in the Young and Old
Woods JA, Evans JK, Wolters BW, et al (Univ of Illinois at Urbana/Champaign)
J Gerontol 53A:B430-B437, 1998   5–15

Objective.—The elderly have higher rates of cancer, autoimmune disease, and infection, probably as a result of age-related dysregulation of the immune system. Even though the elderly have greater numbers of natural killer (NK) cells, the cytotoxic ability of NK cells to respond to interferon (IFN)-α, interleukin-2, and interleukin-12 appears to be impaired. Because exercise appears to stimulate basal and interleukin-2 stimulated NK cell

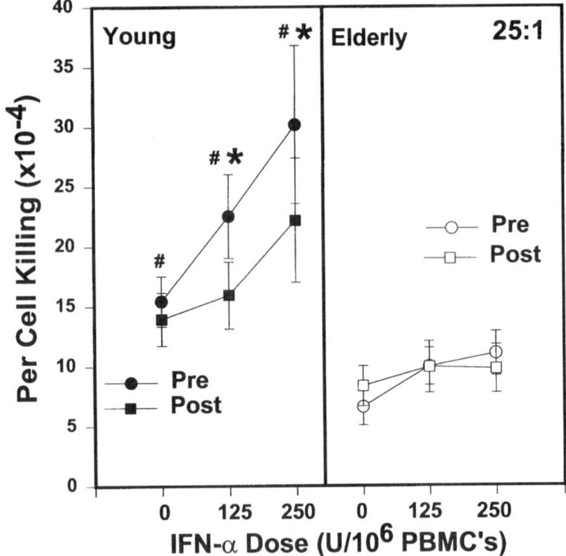

FIGURE 3.—Per natural killer cell killing of K562 target cells as a function of interferon (IFN)-α dose at an E:T ration of 25:1 (similar results seen at 50 and 12.5:1 ratios). Significant age and dose main effects were found at all E:T ratios. *Number sign* denotes a significant increase in young pre-exercise values when compared with old pre-exercise values at the same E:T ratio. *Asterisk* indicates a significantly greater value than that of the unstimulated culture in the pre-exercise sample within age group. In addition, significant dose × age interactions were found, indicating that the young and old do not respond in the same way to IFN-α stimulation and significant dose × time interactions, indicating that exercise affected IFN-α responsiveness. This was apparent in the young subjects. (Courtesy of Woods JA, Evans JK, Wolters BW, et al: Effects of maximal exercise on natural killer (NK) cell cytotoxicity and responsiveness to interferon-α in the young and old. *Journal of Gerontology* 53A(6)B430-B437, 1998. Copyright, The Gerontological Society of America, 1030 15th Street, NW, Suite 250, Washington, DC 20005. Reproduced by permission of the publisher via Copyright Clearance Center, Inc.)

cytotoxicity (NKCC), the effects of age and acute maximal exercise on the IFN-α stimulated generation of LAK cells to mediate killing of NK-insensitive Daudi target cells were examined.

Methods.—A total of 33 healthy individuals, aged 58 to 77 years, and 14 healthy controls, aged 18 to 27 years and not taking immunosuppressive medications, performed the modified Balke graded maximal exercise treadmill test to volitional fatigue. Peripheral mononuclear cells were analyzed in venous blood samples drawn before and immediately after exercise.

Results.—Although there was no dose X time or age X time interaction after exercise, exercise did decrease the per cell killing ability of IFN-α–stimulation in young controls compared with elderly participants (Fig 3). Age had no effect on unstimulated NKCC cytotoxicity regardless of cell type, even though elder participants had significantly higher levels of CD56+ cells in the peripheral blood mononuclear cell fraction. When unstimulated NK tumor killing was expressed on a per NK (CD56+) cell basis, there was a decrease in killing of K562 but not of Daudi cells in elderly participants. There was decreased IFN-α responsiveness in NK cells isolated from elderly participants.

Conclusion.—Although NK cells increase significantly in the elderly, their cytolytic ability is decreased as is their ability to respond to IFN-α stimulation. Exercise in the elderly increases the number of NK and NKCC cells and may improve immune response.

▶ Immunesenescence or age-associated immune deficiency (in particular, dysregulation of T-cell function) appears to be partly responsible for the afflictions of old age. A new and growing area of research is the study of the relationship between certain lifestyle factors (in particular, physical activity and diet) and immunesenescence.

Can regular physical activity attenuate alterations in immunity in old age? Very few human studies have been conducted in this area. The most interesting results come from cross-sectional studies of highly active elderly subjects and their sedentary peers. Mitogen-induced lymphocyte proliferation (a measure of T-cell function) and NK cell activity have been shown to be significantly higher in elderly athletes versus sedentary controls.[1]

In this study, Woods et al measured the response of NK cells (under varying conditions) to an acute maximal exercise bout in young and old subjects, extending the work of Fiatarone et al.[2] The most important finding was that maximal exercise increased NK cell activity and NK cell number to a similar extent in young and old subjects. Single NK cells from the old subjects, however, showed an intrinsic defect in their ability to kill target cancer cells and respond to IFN-α (an activator of NK cell activity), confirming the results of other studies.

D. C. Nieman, PhD

References

1. Nieman DC, Henson DA: Role of endurance exercise in immune senescence. *Med Sci Sports Exerc* 26:172-181, 1994.

2. Fiatarone MA, Morley JE, Bloom ET, et al: The effect of exercise on natural killer cell activity in young and old subjects. *J Gerontol Med Sci* 44:M37-M45, 1989.

The Effect of Physical Activity and Fitness on Specific Antibody Production in College Students

Schuler PB, Lloyd LK, Leblanc PA, et al (Univ of West Florida, Pensacola; Univ of Alabama, Tuscaloosa; Mississippi State Univ)
J Sports Med Phys Fitness 39:233-239, 1999   5–16

Background.—The best expression of the relationship between exercise and the immune system appears to be a bell-shaped curve, with the negative effects of exhaustive exercise and no exercise at the extreme ends and the enhanced benefits of moderate exercise at the top of the bell. In view of the lack of data regarding the effects of moderate exercise on the immune system, its effects on the immune response to a specific antigen—the H1 and H3 components of the 1995-1996 influenza virus vaccine—were investigated.

Methods.—The authors proceeded on the hypothesis that the amount of immunoglobulins produced in response to a specific antigen would accurately reflect the body's immune response, and that this response could be measured accurately in blood samples from the peripheral circulation. The study group comprised 67 college students (43 women) from 18 to 29 years old. Height, weight, skinfold thickness, blood pressure, resting heart rate, and percentage of body fat were assessed. Blood samples were drawn, and the researchers evaluated physical activity by means of the Stanford 7-Day Physical Activity Recall Questionnaire. A graded submaximal cycle ergometer test was used to assess the subjects' level of physical fitness. The students then were vaccinated with the 1996 influenza vaccine, and were asked to return to the laboratory at 1, 2, 4, and 6 weeks for more blood samples, which were then assayed for hemagglutinin inhibition response. Subjects were divided into less-fit, moderately fit, and highly fit groups for repeated ANOVA analysis of the effects of various levels of physical activity and fitness on antibody production.

Results.—Titers were significantly increased for both antigens after vaccination and were highest at week 4 for the H1 component and week 6 for the H3 component. However, there were no significant differences between groups for the 2 antigens, and no significant interaction. Because blood samples taken before vaccination had a large amount of antibodies to the H1 component, researchers believe the H1 titers represented a secondary antibody response and the H3 titers a primary response.

Conclusions.—Results of this study are similar to those of other studies, which have demonstrated that exercise does not affect the primary antibody response to a specific antigen. Among this population of college students, physical fitness and activity had no effect on the production of a specific antibody at any level of activity or fitness.

► Several studies have shown that, despite altered immunity after prolonged and intensive exercise, the ability of the immune system to mount an antibody response to vaccination over the 2- to 4-week postexercise period is not affected. In a study by Bruunsgaard et al, male triathletes, when compared with sedentary controls, had normal antibody production to pneumococcal, tetanus, and diphtheria vaccines after a half-Ironman triathlon despite a significantly reduced delayed-type hypersensitivity skin response.[1]

This cross-sectional study contributes to the exercise immunology literature by showing that varying levels of physical activity and fitness within a relatively homogenous group of college students is not related to antibody production after an influenza vaccination. Further research is warranted to determine whether moderate exercise training influences antibody production in populations that have reduced immunosurveillance such as the elderly or HIV-infected individuals.

D. C. Nieman, PhD

Reference

1. Bruunsgaard H, Hartkopp A, Mohr T, et al: In vivo cell-mediated immunity and vaccination response following prolonged, intense exercise. *Med Sci Sports Exerc* 29:1176-1181, 1997.

Effects of Sleep and Sleep Deprivation on Catecholamine and Interleukin-2 Levels in Humans: Clinical Implications
Irwin M, Thompson J, Miller C, et al (Univ of California, San Diego; San Diego Veterans Affairs Med Ctr, Calif)
J Clin Endocrinol Metab 84:1979-1985, 1999   5–17

Objective.—Sleep appears to regulate the immune system, to play a role in the homeostatic regulation of the sympathetic nervous system and possible cardiovascular disorders, and to induce a decrement in natural killer (NK) cell activity after a partial night of sleep deprivation. The correlation between changes in NK activity and changes in catecholamine and interleukin-2 levels after sleep loss was explored.

Methods.—Seventeen male volunteers participated in a 3-night sleep protocol. Volunteers adapted to the conditions on the first night, had sleep monitored and nocturnal blood samples drawn during the second night, and submitted to partial sleep deprivation–late night (PSD-L) between 3 and 6 AM on the third night during which time sleep was again monitored, nocturnal blood samples were drawn, behavior was observed, and electroencephalograms were obtained.

Results.—On the baseline night, volunteers slept an average of 6.7 hours, and on the PSD-L night, the total amount of sleep averaged 3.8 hours. On the baseline night, circulating levels of norepinephrine and epinephrine declined significantly until about 1 hour after sleep began; but on the PSD-L night, levels of both catecholamines increased sharply with awakening during the deprivation period (Fig 2A). During sleep stages 3

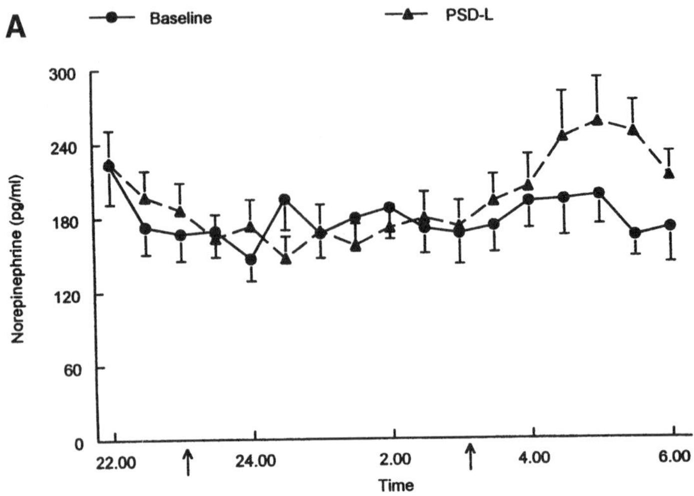

FIGURE 2.—A, Mean (±SEM) circulating levels of norepinephrine in subjects during the baseline and partial sleep deprivation (*PSD=L*) nights. The *arrow* at 2300 hours indicates the average time that the subjects were asleep on the baseline night; the *arrow* at 0300 hours indicates the time that the subjects were awakened on the PSD-L night. (Courtesy of Irwin M, Thompson J, Miller C, et al: Effects of sleep and sleep deprivation on catecholamine and interleukin-2 levels in humans: Clinical implications. *J Clin Endocrinol Metab* 84(6)1979-1985, 1999. Copyright, The Endocrine Society.)

and 4, norepinephrine levels were significantly lower compared with concentrations during the awake period, stages 1 and 2 sleep, and rapid eye movement sleep. Interleukin-2 levels were unchanged. Mean NK lytic activity was reduced 45% after the PSD-L night.

Conclusion.—Sleep deprivation appears to cause an elevation in circulating catecholamine levels that may contribute to the development of cardiovascular disease.

► Sleep disorders are common among humans worldwide. According to a report issued by the National Commission on Sleep Disorders Research, as many as 80 million Americans have serious, incapacitating sleep problems, 20% to 40% have insomnia, and nearly half of older adults say they cannot get a solid night's rest. Poor sleep can result in fatigue, increasing the opportunity for human error and accidents. Insomnia early in adult life is a risk factor for the development of clinical depression and psychiatric distress.

Now we have another reason to worry when sleep is disrupted. In this study, when subjects were awakened at 3 AM and kept awake until 6 AM (after sleeping a little under 4 hours), norepinephrine and epinephrine values increased above normal sleeping levels. This increase in sympathoadrenal activity could potentially link sleep loss, according to these researchers, with a decrease in NK cell activity (an important measure of immune function) and an increase in cardiovascular disorders.

D. C. Nieman, PhD

6 Metabolism, Nutrition, and Fluids

Collegiate Coaches' Knowledge of Eating Disorders
Turk JC, Prentice WE, Chappell S, et al (Univ of North Carolina at Chapel Hill)
J Athletic Train 34:19-24, 1999   6–1

Purpose.—Surveys suggest that eating disorders are a common problem among collegiate athletes. Coaches in many sports may encourage their athletes to diet and lose weight, which could trigger an eating disorder in a susceptible athlete. Collegiate coaches were surveyed regarding their knowledge of eating disorders.

Methods.—A questionnaire was developed and sent to 258 National Collegiate Athletic Association Division I-A coaches from 5 universities. The survey included questions assessing the coaches' knowledge of eating disorders, including cause, signs and symptoms, risk factors, prevention and education, and management and treatment. The role of the athletic department in educating coaches and athletes about eating disorders was assessed as well.

Results.—The final response rate was 53.5% Sixty-one percent of coaches said their team had not attended an educational program regarding eating disorders within the past year. Most respondents were unaware of educational resources regarding eating disorders available from their athletic department. The percentage of correct responses fell into a normal distribution: only 4% of respondents scored 90% correct or greater, whereas 32% scored between 70% and 80%. The coaches had the lowest percentage of correct responses in the education and prevention domain, which also had the highest mean confidence response.

Conclusion.—The findings underscore the need to improve collegiate coaches' knowledge about eating disorders. The researchers recommend annual education programs, preferably sponsored by the athletic department. More research is needed to validate the current findings, to assess the effectiveness of preventive measures, and to assess coaches' knowledge by sport coached and by coach and team sex.

▶ Coaches can have a tremendous influence on their athletes' behavior. It is imperative that coaches be well educated in eating disorders. Athletic departments should sponsor eating disorder programs for coaches as well as athletes.

F. J. George, ATC, PT

Economic Costs of Obesity and Inactivity
Colditz GA (Harvard Med School, Boston)
Med Sci Sports Exerc 31:S663-S667, 1999   6–2

Background.—Inactivity is a major factor in impaired glucose tolerance and several other causes of morbidity and mortality, notably cardiovascular disease, colon cancer, osteoporosis, hip fracture, and type II diabetes. The adverse effects of inactivity on these conditions are independent of body weight, so the costs of inactivity can be added to those that can be attributed to obesity. Studies have estimated the mortality from diet and inactivity at 14%, while sedentary lifestyle contributes to 23% of deaths from leading chronic diseases. The economic costs, direct and indirect, of obesity and inactivity represent part of the impact on public health of increasingly sedentary lifestyles of residents of developed countries. The economic costs of inactivity, including those costs attributable to obesity, were studied.

Methods.—The authors found studies in the MEDLINE database that reported on the economic costs of obesity or inactivity and the cost of illness. References relating to obesity or conditions attributable to obesity were then reviewed, as were references relating to chronic conditions involving inactivity, such as coronary heart disease, hypertension, type II diabetes, gallbladder disease, osteoarthritis, and cancer of the breast, colon, and endometrium. Population-attributable risk percent was then calculated to estimate the proportion of disease that could be prevented by eliminating inactivity or obesity. The prevalence-based cost of illness was calculated in 1995 dollars.

Results.—The lack of physical activity, which was defined as the absence of physical activity in leisure time, had a direct cost of $24 billion, 2.4% of health care expenditures in the United States (Table 1). The direct costs

TABLE 1.—Costs of Inactivity (Billion $), in the United States, 1995

Condition	Relative Risk	PAR%	Direct Costs
Type 2 diabetes	1.5	12%	6.4
CHD	2	22%	8.9
Hypertension	1.5	12%	2.3
Gall bladder disease	2	22%	1.9
Cancer			
Breast	1.2	5%	0.38
Colon	2	22%	2.0
Osteoporotic fractures	2	18%	2.4
Total			24.3 billion

(Courtesy of Colditz GA: Economic costs of obesity and inactivity. *Med Sci Sports Exer* 31:S663-S667, 1999.)

TABLE 2.—Costs ($ Billions) of Obesity (BMI > 30) in the United States, 1995

Condition	Relative Risk	PAR%	Direct Costs
Type 2 diabetes	11	69%	36.6
CHD	4	40%	16.2
Hypertension	4	40%	7.6
Gall bladder disease	5.5	50%	4.3
Cancer			
Breast	1.3	7%	.53
Endometrium	2.5	27%	.23
Colon	1.5	10%	0.89
Osteoarthritis	2.1	20%	3.6
Total		70 billion	

Using prevalence of obesity = 22.5% as reported in the National Health and Nutrition Examination Survey III and for breast and endometrial cancer using prevalence of 24.9% as reported by Flegal et al, 1998.

(Courtesy of Colditz GA: Economic costs of obesity and inactivity. *Med Sci Sports Exerc* 31:S663-S667, 1999.)

of obesity, which was defined as body mass index greater than 30, totaled $70 billion in 1995 dollars (Table 2). The sum of these inactivity (2.4%) and obesity (7%) costs was used to estimate the total direct cost of inactivity at 9.4% of health care expenditures in the United States.

Conclusions.—Estimates of the proportion of deaths attributable to inactivity and obesity range from 14% to 23% of total US mortality, which represents a significant public health burden not only for mortality but for chronic conditions as well. Inactivity has a wide range of negative health consequences and is a major avoidable factor in the cost of illness in the United States as well as in other developed countries where sedentary occupations and reliance on motorized transportation have increased while physical labor has declined.

▶ Inactivity and obesity are both associated with numerous comorbidities and early mortality. Estimates of the proportion of US deaths caused by these factors range from 14% to 23%. Inactivity and obesity also cause many chronic conditions that negatively impact quality of life and work productivity. In this article, lack of physical activity and obesity were related to 9.4% of the US national health care expenditures (about $94 billion). The costs of inactivity and obesity are similar to the total estimated impact of cigarette smoking in the United States.

D. C. Nieman, PhD

Comorbidities of Overweight and Obesity: Current Evidence and Research Issues

Pi-Sunyer FX (Columbia Univ, New York)
Med Sci Sports Exerc 31:S602-S608, 1999

6–3

Background and Method.—The relevant English-language literature was reviewed to determine the current state of knowledge regarding the association of overweight and obesity with other medical comorbidities, as well as the relationship of body fat distribution to comorbidities.

Results.—The review found associations with Type II diabetes mellitus, hypertension, dyslipidemia, coronary heart disease, gall bladder disease, respiratory disease, cancer, and osteoarthritis. Body fat distribution was found to be associated with hypertension, Type II diabetes mellitus, dyslipidemia, and cardiovascular disease. There also appear to be clearly established links between obesity and coronary artery disease, heart failure, cardiac arrhythmia, stroke, and menstrual irregularities. Issues that should have research priority include the need for more-definitive data regarding the relationship of central fat to comorbidities and the importance of visceral fat versus subcutaneous fat in comorbidities; the relationship of obesity to psychiatric disorders; genetic components of obesity and related comorbidities; and the associations of diet and sedentariness with the various comorbidities, as well as the effects of race, gender, intensity and duration of obesity on those associations.

Conclusions.—A great deal of evidence links obesity to a number of medical comorbidities; however, the strength of the associations varies depending on the specific disease. More research on causation is needed as well as into other factors that may have a role in the interaction between overweight and obesity and the medical comorbidities with which they are associated.

▶ Although it was long suspected that obesity is related to numerous health risks and early death, it was not until 1985 that the health hazards of obesity were first officially recognized by the National Institutes of Health.[1] Most experts now feel that obesity constitutes 1 of the more important medical and public health problems of our time. In this brief but thorough review, the current status of knowledge on obesity and comorbidities is outlined, with an emphasis on research priorities.

D. C. Nieman, PhD

Reference

1. National Institutes of Health. Consensus development conference statement: Health implications of obesity. *Ann Intern Med* 103:981-1077, 1985.

Physical Activity in the Treatment of the Adulthood Overweight and Obesity: Current Evidence and Research Issues
Wing RR (Brown Univ, Providence, RI)
Med Sci Sports Exerc 31:S547-S552, 1999   6–4

Background.—The literature was reviewed regarding the role of exercise in treating overweight and obesity in adults. The researchers asked 3 questions: (1) Does exercise alone produce weight loss? (2) Does exercise combined with diet produce greater weight loss than diet alone? (3) Does a combination of diet and exercise produce better maintenance of weight loss than diet alone?

Methods.—The Expert Panel on the Identification, Evaluation, and Treatment of Overweight and Obesity in Adults selected randomized, controlled trials of at least 4 months' duration for review. For the question of exercise versus no treatment, the panel chose 13 articles for review; for the question of exercise plus diet versus exercise alone, it chose 15 articles. Three meta-analyses were also used. For the review, the number of studies showing significant differences favoring exercise was used as the criterion for evaluation of the effect of exercise on weight loss.

Results.—There was significantly more weight loss in exercise alone versus no treatment in 6 of 10 randomized studies. The average weight loss in these studies was 1 to 2 kg. For diet plus exercise, just 2 of 13 studies found a significant difference in initial weight loss; however, results in all of the studies indicated a trend in this direction. In 6 studies with maintenance periods of a year or more, 2 demonstrated significant long-term differences in favor of a combination of diet plus exercise; however, every study considered in the review pointed in this direction. Correlations analyses consistently indicated that exercise has positive effects on weight loss, although in many cases, the effects are modest. Specific findings that would improve weight loss include a need for better assessment of physical activity, improvement in long-term adherence to exercise through multiple short bouts as opposed to single longer bouts, and the need for high-intensity exercise to maximize weight loss. One study found that those who best maintained their weight loss were in the top quartile of physical activity at the end of the study. Other data suggest that energy expenditure of about 10,465 kJ/wk^{-1} is needed to maintain weight loss. A recent study pointed to an average threshold of physical activity of 80 min/d^{-1} of moderate activity or 35 min/d^{-1} of vigorous activity. Whether resistance training or aerobic exercise is more beneficial to weight loss is still an open question.

Conclusions.—This review of relevant literature indicates that exercise has beneficial effects on weight loss, but they are often modest. Better methods of measuring exercise and promoting long-term adherence to exercise are necessary to identify the doses and kinds of exercise needed to best promote long-term weight loss.

▶ Is physical activity a powerful tool in the treatment of obesity? Although there is increasing support for the role of physical activity in preventing obesity, and in the ability to maintain weight loss over the long term after periods of energy restriction, most well-designed studies have failed to support the connection between physical activity and significant weight loss during obesity treatment programs.[1] Part of the problem is that obese individuals are often incapable of expending enough energy during exercise to have a meaningful impact on reduction in body fat stores. As this article reports, exercise expending at least 10,465 kJ/week (about 80 minutes per day of moderate activity) is necessary before meaningful weight loss occurs.

Few obese individuals appear willing and able to devote this much time and effort.

D. C. Nieman, PhD

Reference

1. Miller WC, Koceja Dm, Hamilton EJ: A meta-analysis of the past 25 years of weight loss research among diet, exercise or diet plus exercise intervention. *Int J Obes Relat Metab Disord* 21:941-947, 1997.

Prevalence of Attempting Weight Loss and Strategies for Controlling Weight

Serdula MK, Mokdad AH, Williamson DF, et al (Ctrs for Disease Control and Prevention, Atlanta, Ga)
JAMA 282:1353-1358, 1999

6–5

Objective.—Weight loss is an important consideration for many Americans. The prevalence of weight loss attempts has not been studied. Data from the 1996 state-based Behavior Risk Factor Surveillance System were used to determine the prevalence of attempts to lose or maintain weight and the factors associated with those attempts, what weight control strategies individuals use with regard to exercise and diet, what individuals attempting to lose weight report their weight to be, and what they want it to be.

Methods.—A random-digit telephone survey was conducted among adults aged 18 years or older in 49 states and the District of Columbia in 1996.

Results.—About half the responders were men (49.6%). Most were white (79.9%); 10.1% were black and 6.9% were Hispanic. There were 53.2% who had some college education and 23.7% who were at least 60 years of age. The prevalence of weight loss attempts was 28.8% for men and 43.6% for women. Among women with normal body mass index, 28.7% wanted to lose weight. Participants with more education and those who smoked were more likely to want to maintain weight rather than doing nothing about weight. Although 90% reported modifying their diet, 34.9% of men and 40.0% of women consumed less fat but not less food energy. Only about 20% of men and women dieted and engaged in exercise for 150 min/week. Men trying to lose weight had a median weight of 90.4 kg and wanted to weigh 81.4 kg. Women trying to lose weight had a median weight of 70.3 kg and wanted to weigh 59.0 kg.

Conclusion.—Most Americans trying to lose weight are not following the recommended strategy of reducing energy intake and participating in at least 150 min/week of physical activity.

▶ Physical activity is a critical component of programs for long-term control of obesity,[1-3] and it is disappointing (although not surprising) that while two thirds of obese people in the United States are trying to correct their problem, few are taking even the low minimum of physical activity recommended in current guidelines. It is unclear as yet how large a fraction of the total are so obese that they have genuine difficulty in meeting the required activity target. However, it seems likely that the main problems are a lack of motivation and a lack of understanding of how much exercise is required.

R. J. Shephard, MD, PhD, DPE

References

1. King AC, Tribble DL: The role of exercise in weight regulation of non-athletes. *Sports Med* 11:331-349, 1991.
2. Bouchard C, Després JP, Tremblay A: Exercise and obesity. *Obes Res* 1:133-147, 1993.
3. Brownell KD: Exercise and obesity treatment: Psychological aspects. *Int J Obes Relat Metab Disord* 19:122S-125S, 1995.

Weight Control in Wrestling: Eating Disorders or Disordered Eating?
Dale KS, Landers DM (Arizona State Univ, Tempe)
Med Sci Sports Exerc 31:1382-1389, 1999   6–6

Background.—Concern is increasing that adolescents and teenagers who participate in sports in which weight is important may exhibit the clinical symptoms of eating disorders. It is well known that the techniques that many junior high school and high school wrestlers use to make the desired weight are symptomatic of bulimia nervosa. Several studies of high school wrestlers have reported vomiting and bingeing used as weight control methods. In 1 investigation, 16% of wrestlers fit a pathologic Eating Disorder Inventory (EDI) profile. However, binge eating involves a sense of loss of control or an attempt to manage difficult emotions, which may not be present in the athlete. It is important to consider the emotional or psychological state of the athlete in question. Whether wrestlers' eating behaviors are transient, because such transient behavior is not characteristic of bulimia nervosa, was investigated as part of an attempt to address those concerns.

Methods.—A group of 85 male wrestlers from junior high schools and high schools in the Phoenix area were studied, with a group of 75 nonwrestlers used as a control. Average age of both groups was 15 years; the average weight was 136.7 pounds for the wrestlers and 147 pounds for the nonwrestlers. The EDI, which was used as a screening instrument for identifying subjects at risk of bulimia nervosa, was completed by both groups once during the wrestling season and again in the off-season.

Results.—Although there were no significant differences between the groups in the off-season in numbers of subjects classified as "at risk" for bulimia, the "Drive for Thinness" scale revealed significant differences both between wrestlers and nonwrestlers in-season and between in-season and off-season wrestlers. On the "Drive for Thinness" scale, 27% of in-season wrestlers scored "at risk" versus 15% of off-season wrestlers and 13% of nonwrestlers. Interviews with in-season wrestlers showed that their weight concerns centered almost entirely on the demands of their sport and the need to "make weight" for matches, rather than on concerns with body shape or appearance. Many of the wrestlers worried about body shape in the off-season, out of concern that they were getting out of shape for competition.

Conclusions.—Wrestling does not put athletes at a greater risk for eating disorders; although wrestlers are more weight conscious than non-wrestlers, this concern is transient and is caused by the demands of the sport. Transient behavior is not a characteristic of eating disorders, and the weight concerns and behaviors among the wrestlers in this study did not meet the severity level consistent with bulimia nervosa. However, some weight-loss practices among wrestlers are potentially dangerous to their health. Research should focus on educating wrestlers about safe weight loss and better ensuring their physical health.

▶ There is a growing concern that athletes in activities that emphasize leanness (eg, wrestlers, gymnasts, bodybuilders, runners, and ballet dancers) are exceptionally preoccupied with weight, tend to use unhealthy methods of weight control, are prone to eating disorders, and demonstrate poor nutrition practices.[1] The desire of the highly competitive wrestler to alter body weight without medical supervision has caused much concern among sportsmedicine professionals. A high percentage induce dehydration, using sauna baths, fluid restriction, and rubber or plastic suits. Some also resort to laxatives, diuretics, and vomiting. Such practices may endanger health, adversely affect performance, and affect a young person's growth potential.[2] The good news of this study is that participating in wrestling does not place these athletes at a higher risk than normal for developing bulimia nervosa. Interviews with in-season wrestlers revealed that their concerns with weight were caused entirely by the demands of wrestling.

D. C. Nieman, PhD

References

1. Sundgot-Borgen J: Risk and trigger factors for the development of eating disorders in female elite athletes. *Med Sci Sports Exerc* 26:414-419, 1994.
2. Oppliger RA, Case HS, Horswill CA, et al: American College of Sports Medicine position stand. Weight loss in wrestlers. *Med Sci Sports Exerc* 28:ix-xii, 1996.

The Effect of a Preexercise Meal on Time to Fatigue During Prolonged Cycling Exercise

Schabort EJ, Bosch AN, Weltan SM, et al (Sports Science Inst of South Africa, Newlands)

Med Sci Sports Exerc 31:464-471, 1999   6–7

Introduction.—Previous studies have found that carbohydrate (CHO) loading in the days before an endurance athletic event improves performance. The improvement is associated with increased CHO oxidation during exercise. However, many athletes refrain from eating breakfast before early-morning athletic events. Although a high-CHO breakfast should ensure optimal liver glycogen stores, it may also increase plasma insulin levels while reducing serum free fatty acid, which may reduce endurance. The effects of eating a CHO breakfast on endurance exercise performance were examined.

Methods.—Seven moderately trained male endurance cyclists were studied while performing cycle ergometer exercise to exhaustion at 70% of maximal oxygen uptake. On 1 occasion, the athletes ate a 100-g CHO breakfast 3 hours before exercise. On another occasion, they performed the exercise task after fasting overnight. Endurance performances were compared, along with blood hormone concentrations, muscle glycogen utilization, and carbohydrate oxidation.

Results.—Time to fatigue was 136 minutes after the CHO breakfast versus 109 min in the fasted state. There were no significant differences in muscle glycogen utilization, respiratory exchange ratio, CHO and fat oxidation, or lactate and insulin concentrations. In both trials, exercise was associated with a significant reduction in insulin concentration (from 4.7 to 2.8 µIU/mL in the fed state vs 6.6 to 3.7 µIU/mL in the fasted state) and a significant increase in free fatty acid concentration (from 0.09 to 1.4 mmol/L and 0.17 to 0.74 mmol/L, respectively).

Conclusion.—In endurance athletes, eating a CHO meal before exercise improves endurance performance. Preexercise CHO ingestion has no negative impact on insulin or free fatty acid concentrations. The mechanism of the improvement in endurance is unknown but does not appear to result from differences in hormonal control.

▶ Should athletes eat a high CHO pregame meal? This study indicates that there was a significant increase in time to fatigue for those who ingested this meal 3 hours before testing. There was no indication in this study that there was a negative effect on insulin or free fatty acid concentrations. Encourage athletes to eat a high CHO meal before competition; their performance may improve.

F. J. George, ATC, PT

Physical Activity and Preference for Selected Macronutrients
Tremblay A, Drapeau V (Laval Univ, Ste-Foy, Quebec)
Med Sci Sports Exerc 31:S584-S589, 1999   6–8

Background.—A significant factor in the increased risk for obesity in the industrialized world is the lack of physical activity and the increase in the number of sedentary individuals. Thus, an increase in regular aerobic exercise should result in substantive weight loss. However, studies have indicated that increased exercise alone does not always lead to substantive weight loss. This may be caused by the level of postexercise energy intake from a high-fat, macronutrient diet, which can lead to a positive energy balance that overcomes the energy cost of exercise. Other studies have indicated that a combination of physical activity and a low-fat diet leads to a substantial acute negative energy balance and subsequent weight loss. Thus, it is important for an active individual to make appropriate dietary choices to maintain or lose weight. Whether exercise influences dietary preferences for macronutrients was studied, with an aim to improving therapeutic and preventive strategies concerning obesity.

Method.—A review of the literature was conducted, specifically for references to the acute effects of physical activity and the chronic and short-term effects of exercise on macronutrient preferences.

Results.—There is no standardized measurement of macronutrient preferences. One way to measure macronutrient preference is by assessing the macronutrient content of the diet, while another is to use a buffet test meal with a variety of macronutrients offered. Results of 1 experiment offering a variety of macronutrient solutions found that obese subjects had a greater preference for lipids than lean subjects. Other studies have found an increase in preference for high-carbohydrate foods after prolonged exercise, as well as a preference for sucrose after exercise in a study of university students.

Conclusions.—The literature does not allow identification of any specific physical activity as having an acute effect on macronutrient preference. Nor is there any clear evidence of a specific effect of chronic training on macronutrient preference. Physical activity is not associated with a preference for any specific macronutrients; however, it may stimulate a general preference for foods high in fat, carbohydrates, proteins, or alcohol. As people who are active do not systematically select food with a low fat content, the intake of dietary fat needs to be controlled for exercise to create a negative energy balance and result in weight loss. Thus, it is important to provide nutritional guidelines to individuals who are using physical activity to control or reduce weight.

▶ A claim often made by highly fit individuals is that the initiation of regular exercise prompted them to eat better.[1] Do people who start moderate exercise programs alter the quality of their diet? In this study, no definitive relationship between acute and chronic exercise training and macronutrient preference could be established. A practical application is that instead of relying on the impact of physical activity to induce good food selection, exercise physiologists and dietitians should provide supportive nutrition counseling, especially to obese individuals adopting new exercise habits.

D. C. Nieman, PhD

Reference

1. Nieman DC, Butler JV, Pollett LM, et al: Nutrient intake of marathon runners. *J Am Diet Assoc* 89:1273-1278, 1989.

Diet, Physical Activity, and Gallstones–A Population-based, Case-Control Study in Southern Italy
Misciagna G, Centonze S, Leoci C, et al (State Univ of New York, Buffalo)
Am J Clin Nutr 69:120-126, 1999   6–9

Background.—Despite the high prevalence of gallstones, the nutritional and lifestyle risk factors of this disorder remain unclear. The association among diet, physical activity, and incident cases of gallstones detected by ultrasonography (US) was investigated in a population-based, case-control study.

Methods.—The patients were 100 persons with newly diagnosed gallstones and 290 persons without gallstones selected randomly. All participants completed a questionnaire about their usual diet and physical activity level for the year preceding US.

Findings.—In a multiple logistic regression analysis, the risk of gallstone formation was associated directly with body mass index and intake of refined sugars. Physical activity, dietary monounsaturated fats, dietary cholesterol, and dietary fibers from cellulose were correlated inversely with the risk of gallstone formation. Saturated fat intake was a risk factor for gallstone formation. This association appeared stronger for men than women. The odds ratios of gallstone risk for various energy-adjusted nutrient quartiles (with the lowest quartile used as the reference category) and the results of the linear trend analysis are shown in Table 3.

Conclusions.—Nutritional factors can play an important role in the etiology of gallstones. Most of these factors also play an important role in the pathogenesis of other chronic illnesses, such as cardiovascular disease and cancer. Preventive strategies designed to improve nutrition and energy imbalance can have a significant impact on a spectrum of pathologic conditions that cause major morbidity and mortality in Western society.

▶ When I was a medical student, the aphorism describing a typical patient with gallstones was a woman, fair, fat, and 40. We did not talk much about physical activity in those days, but an extension of the aphorism might imply protection against gallstones from exercise-induced leanness. This case-control study from Italy took the important precaution of basing a 10-item activity questionnaire on the known activity patterns of elderly people in rural areas,[1] finding a substantial protective effect in a multiple logistic regression model that included a wide range of dietary and nondietary risk factors. At least 2 other reports have noted a similar protective effect.[2,3] The mechanism is as yet unclear. Possibly, physical activity increases colonic motility or modifies insulin resistance.

R. J. Shephard, MD, PhD, DPE

References

1. Ferro-Luzzi A: *Time allocation and activity pattern of the elderly.* Rome: National Institute of Nutrition, 1987.

TABLE 3.—Odds Ratios (ORs) and 95% Confidence Intervals (CIs) of the Risk of Gallstone Formation, by Quartiles 1-4 (Q_{1-4}) of Nutrient Intakes*

Nutrients	OR (95% CI) Q_2	Q_3	Q_4	P^2
Protein				
Model 1	1.25 (0.64, 2.48)	1.54 (0.78, 3.06)	1.24 (0.62, 2.49)	0.45
Model 2	1.55 (0.66, 3.64)	2.29 (0.82, 6.41)	2.43 (0.73, 8.08)	0.13
Saturated fat				
Model 1	0.99 (0.50, 1.97)	1.37 (0.70, 2.64)	1.25 (0.64, 2.44)	0.37
Model 2	1.11 (0.43, 2.84)	2.65 (0.87, 8.06)	3.79 (0.86, 16.82)	0.03
Monounsaturated fat				
Model 1	0.89 (0.46, 1.72)	0.96 (0.50, 1.86)	0.47 (0.23, 0.96)	0.06
Model 2	0.73 (0.31, 1.70)	0.85 (0.31, 2.31)	0.30 (0.09, 1.04)	0.09
Polyunsaturated fat				
Model 1	0.77 (0.39, 1.50)	0.81 (0.42, 1.56)	0.68 (0.34, 1.33)	0.30
Model 2	0.68 (0.29, 1.62)	0.72 (0.26, 1.99)	0.77 (0.24, 2.52)	0.75
Cholesterol				
Model 1	0.96 (0.50, 1.83)	0.94 (0.48, 1.83)	0.75 (0.38, 1.49)	0.43
Model 2	0.53 (0.22, 1.25)	0.36 (0.13, 1.01)	0.24 (0.07, 0.82)	0.02
Refined sugar				
Model 1	1.34 (0.66, 2.71)	1.61 (0.80, 3.25)	2.10 (1.06, 4.16)	0.03
Model 2	1.91 (0.77, 4.74)	3.13 (1.05, 9.28)	6.34 (1.55, 25.98)	0.01
Glycogen				
Model 1	0.52 (0.26, 1.04)	0.83 (0.44, 1.59)	0.78 (0.41, 1.48)	0.73
Model 2	0.41 (0.18, 0.92)	0.71 (0.28, 1.84)	0.76 (0.21, 2.78)	0.62
Fiber from cellulose				
Model 1	1.03 (0.53, 2.0)	0.66 (0.33, 1.33)	1.2 (0.63, 2.32)	0.86
Model 2	0.85 (0.34, 2.10)	0.54 (0.16, 1.84)	0.76 (0.14, 4.02)	0.56
Fiber from noncellulose				
Model 1	0.69 (0.34, 1.36)	0.78 (0.40, 1.52)	1.14 (0.60, 2.17)	0.60
Model 2	0.42 (0.16, 1.09)	0.28 (0.08, 0.97)	0.33 (0.06, 1.85)	0.12
Calcium				
Model 1	1.17 (0.60, 2.27)	1.02 (0.52, 2.01)	1.35 (0.69, 2.63)	0.48
Model 2	0.77 (0.33, 1.80)	0.51 (0.20, 1.30)	0.40 (0.11, 1.43)	0.11
Alcohol[3]				
Model 1	0.66 (0.35, 1.25)	0.59 (0.31, 1.13)	0.38 (0.18, 0.78)	0.008
Model 2	0.83 (0.39, 1.78)	0.74 (0.32, 1.67)	0.42 (0.14, 1.28)	0.17
Energy				
Model 1[4]	0.92 (0.49, 1.73)	0.48 (0.24, 0.96)	0.58 (0.29, 1.16)	0.04
Model 2[5]	0.97 (0.44, 2.15)	0.33 (0.13, 0.81)	0.46 (0.18, 1.19)	0.03

*Quartile 1 (low) is the reference category. In model 1, age, sex, body mass index (BMI), and energy were controlled; in model 2, age, sex, BMI, energy, and all other nutrients were controlled for.

†Chi-square test for trend.

‡Reference category was "no drinking alcohol" and drinking quantities in tertiles.

§Controlled for age, sex, and BMI.

‖Controlled for age, sex, BMI, and all other nutrients.

(Courtesy of Misciagna G, Centonze, Leoci C, et al: Diet, physical activity, and gallstones—a population-based, case-control study in southern Italy. *Am J Clin Nutr* 69:120-126, 1999. Copyright Am. J. Clin. Nutr. American Society for Clinical Nutrition.)

2. Williams CN, Johnston JL: Prevalence of gallstones and risk factors in Caucasian women in a rural Canadian community. *Can Med Assoc J* 120: 664-668, 1980.
3. Kato I, Nomura A, Stemmermann GN, et al: Prospective study of clinical gallbladder disease and its association with obesity, physical activity, and other factors. *Dig Dis Sci* 37: 784-790 1992.

Insulin Action on Muscle Protein Kinetics and Amino Acid Transport During Recovery After Resistance Exercise

Biolo G, Williams BD, Fleming RYD, et al (Univ of Texas, Galveston; Shriners Burns Hosp, Galveston, Tex)
Diabete Metab 48:949-957, 1999   6–10

Objective.—Exercise stimulates insulin-induced glucose uptake in skeletal muscle. The interaction between the effects of insulin and exercise on the rates of muscle protein synthesis and breakdown, and amino acid transport was investigated in untrained healthy volunteers.

Methods.—Five healthy male volunteers who had not engaged in regular exercise training for at least 1 year ate a weight-maintaining diet of 15% to 20% protein for at least a month before testing. Blood was drawn in the postabsorptive state at rest and twice about 3 hours after heavy leg resistance exercise. Insulin was infused into the femoral artery to increase leg insulin levels to high physiologic concentrations. Radiolabeled amino acids were infused to assess the kinetics of intracellular free amino acids and the fractional synthetic rate of protein.

Results.—Glucose uptake at rest was significantly enhanced by insulin infusion. The rate of glucose uptake was significantly higher with insulin infusion after exercise than before exercise. Insulin infusion affected only leucine concentration, decreasing it significantly both at rest and after exercise. Protein synthesis and degradation rates at rest were 30 and 46 nmol/min/100 mL leg volume, respectively. Protein synthesis and degradations during recovery were 65 and 74 nmol/min/100 mL leg volume, respectively (Fig 3). Insulin infusion boosted protein synthesis at rest but not during recovery (51 vs 64 nmol/min/100 mL leg volume, respectively).

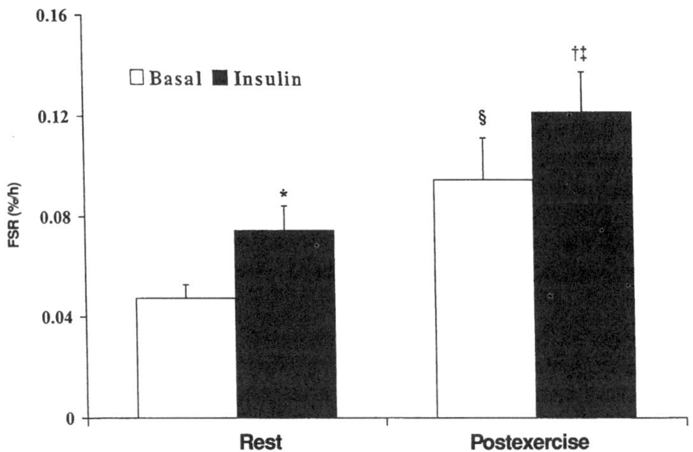

FIGURE 3.—Fractional synthetic rate (FSR) of muscle protein at rest and after exercise in the basal state and during insulin infusion. *$P<.05$ insulin versus basal; §$P<.05$ postexercise basal versus rest basal; ‡$P<.05$ postexercise insulin versus rest insulin. (Courtesy of Biolo G, Williams BD, Fleming RYD, et al. Insulin action on muscle protein kinetics and amino acid transport during recovery after resistance exercise. *Diabetes Metab.* 48:949-957, 1999.)

Although insulin infusion significantly decreased the rate of protein degradation after exercise, insulin infusion had no effect on protein degradation at rest (52 vs 48 nmol/min/100 mL leg volume, respectively). Compared with at rest values, insulin enhanced glucose uptake by a factor of 3 during postexercise recovery.

Conclusion.—Exercise enhances the ability of insulin to stimulate glucose uptake and alanine transport, and slows protein degradation but has little effect on protein synthesis.

▶ In recent years, the trend has been to use naturally occurring hormones as a method of stimulating anabolism that is difficult to detect. The effect of insulin on both the resting and postexercise protein balance of muscle seems substantial, and may be a further concern for those who police the doping of athletes.

R. J. Shephard, MD, PhD, DPE

Walking Compared With Vigorous Physical Activity and Risk of Type 2 Diabetes in Women: A Prospective Study
Hu FB, Sigal RJ, Rich-Edwards JW, et al (Harvard Med School, Boston; Univ of Ottawa, Ont, Canada)
JAMA 282:1433-1439, 1999   6–11

Background.—There is much evidence that the risk of type 2 diabetes can be reduced through physical activity. Recent prospective studies, although offering powerful support for the beneficial role of physical activity in preventing type 2 diabetes, have not distinguished between moderate-intensity and vigorous exercise. In addition, the majority of participants in these studies have been male. Controversies have arisen in these studies regarding the relationship between the risk of type 2 diabetes and the frequency and intensity of the exercise activity, and also concerning the effects of physical activity on persons at high risk versus those at low risk for type 2 diabetes. The dose-response relationship between total physical activity and incidence of type 2 diabetes in women was quantified, and the potential benefits of walking, a moderate-intensity activity, was compared with more vigorous forms of exercise.

Methods.—The subjects for this study were drawn from the Nurses Health Study. The group consisted of 70,102 female nurses aged 40 to 65 years without diabetes, cardiovascular disease, or cancer at the baseline survey conducted in 1986. The surveys were updated in 1988 and 1992. Nurses in 11 states completed questionnaires regarding their medical history and health practices. Participants were asked about the average time per week spent on a range of physical activities, including moderate activities, such as walking and also more vigorous activities, such as running, aerobics, lap swimming, and playing tennis, racquetball, or squash. Participants were also asked to classify their walking pace as easy or casual (less than 3.2 km/hr), normal or average (3.2-4.8 km/hr), brisk

(4.8-6.2 km/hr), or very brisk or striding (6.4 km/hr or faster). This information was used to calculate energy expenditure in metabolic equivalent task hours (MET-hours). Vigorous activities, such as jogging, running, aerobics, calisthenics, lap swimming, and playing squash, tennis, or racquetball required 6 or more METs. In contrast, walking, which required only 2 to 4.5 METs was considered a moderate-intensity physical activity. The main outcome measure was the risk of type 2 diabetes by quintile of MET score, on the basis of the time spent per week on the physical activities surveyed, including walking.

Results.—During the 8 years of follow-up, 1419 cases of type 2 diabetes were confirmed. This translated to an incidence of 265 per 100,000 person-years. After adjusting for covariates such as age, smoking, history of hypertension, alcohol use, and high cholesterol levels, the relative risk of developing type 2 diabetes decreased with increasing levels of exercise, from 1.0 (least-exercise quintile) to 0.77, 0.75, 0.62, and 0.54 (most-exercise quintile) (*P* for trend < .001). This trend was also evident after adjusting for body mass index (BMI). Among women who engaged in moderate physical activity (walking) the relative risk across quintiles, from least exercise to most exercise, was 1.0, 0.91, 0.73, 0.69, and 0.58 (*P* for trend < .001). This trend continued and remained statistically significant after adjusting for BMI. An independent association was noted between faster walking pace and decreased relative risk.

Conclusions.—A substantial reduction in risk of type 2 diabetes is associated with increased amounts of physical activity, even when the activity is of moderate duration and intensity.

▶ There is growing evidence that, at least in terms of metabolic health, the beneficial effect of physical activity depends on total energy expended, with a similar response to vigorous and moderate intensity effort. However, those who adopt vigorous rather than moderate activity usually fare better even in terms of metabolic conditions such as diabetes mellitus, because their total daily energy expenditure is greater than those who walk more slowly. A question that remains to be answered is whether the cardiovascular benefits of increased physical activity also depend on total energy expenditure rather than the intensity of effort. On theoretical grounds, one might anticipate that the reduction of cardiac work-rate (which is probably a major source of cardiovascular benefit) would require activity in the aerobic training zone.

R. J. Shephard, MD, PhD, DPE

Preexercise Medium-Chain Triglyceride Ingestion Does Not Alter Muscle Glycogen Use During Exercise
Horowitz JF, Mora-Rodriguez R, Byerley LO, et al (Univ of Texas, Austin)
J Appl Physiol 88:219-225, 2000   6–12

Objective.—Administration of long-chain triglycerides (LCTs) increases plasma free fatty acid concentration, increases fat oxidation, and decreases muscle glycogen oxidation. Unfortunately, LCTs have slow rates of gastric emptying and transport into the circulatory system. Whether medium-chain triglycerides (MCTs)—which are more rapidly hydrolyzed, absorbed, and transported—can perform functions similar to those of LCTs has not been studied. The rate of muscle glycogen use during high intensity exercise, after ingestion of MCTs, was measured.

Methods.—Test meals containing either 0.72 g/kg of sucrose or 0.36 g/kg of tricaprin plus 0.72 g/kg of sucrose were administered on 2 occasions to 7 well-trained male cyclists 1 hour before 30 minutes of cycling at 84% maximal oxygen uptake. Vastus lateralis biopsy specimens were taken before and after exercise for glycogen analysis. Blood was drawn every 10 minutes at rest and every 5 minutes during exercise for glucose analysis. Oxygen uptake and carbon dioxide production were monitored by open-circuit spirometry. Glycogen oxidation and glucose disappearance rates from plasma were measured by the isotope dilution technique.

Results.—Reduction in muscle glycogen concentration after exercise was similar in both diets (38.8 mmol/kg without MCTs and 42.0 mmol/kg with MCTs). The minimum rate of muscle glycogen oxidation was similar after exercise for the 2 diets.

Conclusion.—The addition of MCTs before exercise did not affect muscle glycogen utilization.

▶ At first inspection, one might anticipate that the ingestion of MCTs would spare IM glycogen; however, the present small-scale trial showed remarkably similar figures with and without triglycerides. There are at least 2 possible reasons for this finding: First, the duration of exercise (30 minutes) was not enough to deplete muscle glycogen reserves fully, and second, the triglycerides were administered on only 1 occasion. It is possible that with chronic administration, enzyme systems would be modified so as to shift metabolism from glycogen to triglycerides. Neverthless, it is interesting that some benefit was observed in terms of greater glucose uptake, probably because of more rapid gastric emptying.

R. J. Shephard, MD, PhD, DPE

Effect of Fluvastatin in Combination With Moderate Endurance Training on Parameters of Lipid Metabolism

Wittke R (Sports Medicine Inst, Bayreuth, Germany)
Sports Med 27:329-335, 1999   6–13

Objective.—Regular endurance training is known to confer a cardioprotective effect. Whether patients receiving fluvastatin can experience an additional benefit from such exercise was investigated in an observational study.

Methods.—Three groups of 6 sedentary dyslipidemic men, aged 38 to 65 years, participated in a regular exercise program only (control), took fluvastatin and participated in a regular exercise program, or took fluvastatin only. Weight, body mass index, and total cholesterol, high-density lipoprotein (HDL) cholesterol, low-density lipoprotein (LDL) cholesterol, and triglyceride levels were determined before and after the 3-month study.

Results.—There were no adverse events resulting from exercise. All groups lost a significant 2.59% to 3.23% of body weight. Maximum oxygen uptake increased significantly, by 12% to 13% as did power output, by 10% to 20%. Total cholesterol and LDL cholesterol levels were significantly decreased and HDL cholesterol levels were significantly increased in all 3 groups. The changes were greatest in the treatment group, with a reduction in LDL cholesterol of 30% to 40%. The differences between the control and pretreatment groups was not significant.

Conclusion.—Endurance exercise potentiates the benefit of fluvastatin in men with dyslipidemia.

▶ This study provides good evidence that endurance training, in combination with diet restrictions and fluvastatin, can improve lipid parameters. Endurance training alone and fluvastatin alone can improve these parameters somewhat. However, for risk associated with high blood lipid level, the combination of endurance training, diet restrictions, and fluvastatin is necessary to reach a target range of −30% to −40%.

F. J. George, ATC, PT

Relationship of Lipoprotein(a) Levels to Physical Activity and Family History of Coronary Heart Disease
Martín S, Elosua R, Covas M-I, et al (Institut Municipal d'Investigació Mèdica, Barcelona)
Am J Public Health 89:383-385, 1999   6–14

Introduction.—Increased plasma levels of lipoprotein(a) [Lp(a)] are independently associated with coronary heart disease (CHD) and a family history of CHD. The effects of exercise, commonly recommended to reduce CHD risk, on Lp(a) are unknown. The effect of physical activity on Lp(a) level was analyzed in subjects with and without a family history of CHD.

Methods.—The cross-sectional study included 332 healthy men: 202 marathon runners and 130 men randomly selected from the population. The men were grouped by level of physical activity as active (less than 1.25MJ [300 kcal]/d of physical activity, 106 men) and very active (1.25MJ [300 or more kcal]/d, 226 men). Serum Lp(a) levels were measured by an enzyme-linked immunosorbent assay. The effects of physical activity on serum Lp(a) were analyzed with stratification by family history of CHD.

Results.—The mean body mass index was 24.8 in the very active group versus 26.6 in the active group. Mean serum Lp(a) values were 0.033 and 0.063 g/L, respectively, although the difference was not significant. Serum Lp(a) was not correlated with physical activity level and only slightly

TABLE 1.—Serum Lipoprotein(a) Levels in 2 Physical Activity Groups Stratified by Family History of Coronary Heart Disease

	n	Active Group Lp(a) Median (Range)	n	Very Active Group Lp(a) Median (Range)	n	All Participants Lp(a) Median (Range)
FHCHD	20	0.112 (0-0.488)*	46	0.013 (0-0.708)	66	0.068 (0-0.657)
No FHCHD	65	0.045 (0-0.695)	155	0.037 (0-0.556)	220	0.044 (0-0.672)

Note: Reference intervals are as follows: active group, less than 1.25MJ (300 kcal/d) of physical activity; very active group, greater than or equal to 1.25MJ (300 kcal/d); all participants, 8-9250kJ (2-2210 kcal/d). Lipid levels are in grams per liter.
  *P less than .05 versus other groups (Mann-Whitney test).
  (Courtesy of Martin S, Elosua R, Covas M-I, et al: Relationship of lipoprotein(a) levels to physical activity and family history of coronary heart disease. *Am J Public Health* 89-383-385, 1999, copyright, American Public Health Association.)

correlated with age. However, serum Lp(a) was significantly higher for men in the active group who had a family history of CHD (Table 1). For men with a history of CHD, the odds ratio for an Lp(a) level above the median was 0.13 (95% confidence interval, 0.03 to 0.50) for the very active group compared with the active group.

Conclusion.—For men with a family history of CHD, the risk of having an elevated serum Lp(a) level is reduced 8-fold at a physical activity level of more than 1.25MJ (300 kcal)/d. Thus, exercise could be prescribed as a means of controlling Lp(a) levels for patients with a family history of CHD. The mechanism of this relationship should be studied further.

▶ There has been considerable recent interest in Lp(a) as a primary genetic risk factor for atherosclerosis.[1,2] Previous studies concerning the impact of physical activity upon lipoprotein levels have been inconclusive, and the report of Martin and associates likewise found no relationship between Lp(a) levels and reported physical activity in their sample as a whole. However, they reasoned that an association might be obscured by the great mass of individuals who entered the study with relatively normal Lp(a) levels.

Sorting out those with a high level of Lp(a) on the basis of a family history of CHD, they were able to show that in this high risk group, the chances of finding an Lp(a) level above the median value was reduced 8-fold with a habitual energy expenditure greater than 1.3 MJ (300 kcal) per day. This cut-off point was chosen to coincide with the energy expenditure of 8.4 MJ/week (2000 kcal/week), which was previously advocated for protection against heart attacks on the basis of a follow-up of Harvard alumni.[3]

R. J. Shephard, MD, PhD, DPE

References

1. Rosengren A, Wilhelmsen L, Eriksson E, et al: Lipoprotein (a) and coronary heart disease: A prospective case-control study in a general population sample of middle-aged men. *Br Med J* 300:1248-1251, 1990.
2. Boerwinkle E, Leffert CC, Lin J, et al: Apolipoprotein (a) gene accounts for greater than 90% of the variation in plasma lipoprotein (a) concentrations. *J Clin Invest* 90:52-60, 1992.

3. Paffenbarger R, Wing AL, Hyde RT: Physical activity as an index of heart attack risk in college alumni. *Am J Epidemiol* 108:161-175, 1978.

Predictors of Adipose Tissue Lipoprotein Lipase in Middle-aged and Older Men: Relationship to Leptin and Obesity, But Not Cardiovascular Fitness

Berman DM, Rogus EM, Busby-Whitehead MJ, et al (Univ of Maryland, Baltimore; Baltimore VA Med Ctr, Md; Johns Hopkins Univ, Baltimore, Md)
Metabolism 48:183-189, 1999   6–15

Introduction.—The enzyme lipoprotein lipase (LPL), which is involved in the catabolism of triglyceride-rich lipoproteins and production of high-density lipoprotein 2 cholesterol (HDL_2-C), occurs mainly in adipose tissue (AT) and skeletal muscle. The effects of exercise training on AT-LPL levels are unclear. This study assessed the effects of endurance exercise training and other variables on AT-LPL and lipid profile in middle-aged and older men.

Methods.—The study included 66 healthy men (mean age, 61 years). Nineteen men were classified as master athletes, with maximal oxygen intake ($\dot{V}O_2$max) of 40 mL/[kg·min] or greater. The remaining men were sedentary, with $\dot{V}O_2$max of less than 40 mL/kg/min; of these, 20 were classified as lean and 27 as obese, with body fat of greater than 27%. AT-LPL activity was measured in subcutaneous abdominal and gluteal fat. In a cross-sectional comparison, the relationship of AT-LPL activity to body composition and $\dot{V}O_2$max was assessed, along with the effects of AT-LPL on lipid profiles.

Results.—The athletic and lean sedentary men had comparable fasting insulin and leptin levels, although both values were lower in obese sedentary men. Fasting total cholesterol and low-density lipoprotein cholesterol were similar among the 3 groups. However, the athletic men had lower levels of triglyceride, high-density lipoprotein cholesterol (HDL-C), and HDL_2-C. Regional AT-LPL activity was similar between groups. Abdominal AT-LPL activity was 2.1 nmol/10^6 cells · min, compared with 0.8 and 0.5 nmol/10^6 cells · min in lean sedentary and athletic men, respectively, with similar differences in gluteal AT-LPL activity. Both AT-LPL measurements were positively correlated with percentage body fat, fasting insulin, and leptin, but not with $\dot{V}O_2$max (Table 4). Multivariate analysis revealed leptin as the main independent predictor of abdominal and gluteal AT-LPL. There was a positive correlation between abdominal AT-LPL and plasma triglyceride and a negative correlation between abdominal AT-LPL and HDL-C. These correlations became nonsignificant after controlling for percentage body fat or leptin.

Conclusion.—Obesity and the obesity-related hormones leptin and insulin are the major factors associated with AT-LPL activity in middle-aged and older men. However, AT-LPL does not appear to be associated with

TABLE 4.—Pearson Correlation Coefficients for Adipose Tissue Lipoprotein Lipase and Measurements of Body Fatness and Fitness in All Subjects

Parameter	ABD AT-LPL (nmol/10^6 cell · min)	GLT AT-LPL (nmol/10^6 cell · min)
Weight (kg)	.32†	.32†
BMI (kg/m^2)	.40*	.31*
Waist (cm)	.40*	.41*
Hip (cm)	.40*	.37†
WHR	.21	.18
Body fat (%)	.50*	.37†
Insulin (pmol/L)	.45*	.32†
Leptin (ng/mL)	.65*	.63*
$\dot{V}O_2$max (L/min)	−.19	−.16

*P less than .001.
†P less than .05.
Abbreviations: ABD, abdominal; *AT-LPL*, adipose tissue lipoprotein lipase; *GLT*, gluteal.
(Courtesy of Berman DM, Rogus EM, Busby-Whitehead MJ, et al: Predictors of adipose tissue lipoprotein lipase in middle-aged and older men: Relationship to leptin and obesity, but not cardiovascular fitness. *Metabolism* 48:183-189, 1999.)

cardiovascular fitness. The elevated HDL-C levels present in endurance-trained older men are unrelated to increased AT-LPL activity.

▶ In younger individuals, the activity-induced increase of HDL-C has been related to increases in AT-LPL activity.[1] However, the present report suggests that this explanation does not hold for older individuals. Those who are active have high HDL-C readings, but their AT-LPL activity does not differ from that of their sedentary but lean peers. AT-LPL readings are unrelated to $\dot{V}O_2$max and are unrelated to HDL-C after control of the data for body fatness.

The table suggests that the effect of $\dot{V}O_2$max was tested in terms of absolute oxygen consumption (liters per minute) but not in terms of the more usual measure of fitness (oxygen consumption per unit of body mass). It would, thus, be interesting to repeat the statistical analysis using the relative units. Other possible mechanisms for the effect of habitual activity on HDL-C include changes in the activity of skeletal muscle and hepatic lipases, and in cholesterol ester transfer protein.[2]

R. J. Shephard, MD, PhD, DPE

References

1. Nikkilä EA, Taskinen M-R, Rehunen S, et al: Lipoprotein lipase activity in adipose tissue and skeletal muscle of runners: Relation to serum lipoproteins. *Metabolism* 27:1661-1671, 1978.
2. Serrat-Serrat J, Ordóñez Llanos J, Serra-Grima R, et al: Marathon runners presented lower serum cholesterol ester transfer activity than sedentary subjects. *Atherosclerosis* 101:43-49, 1993.

Differential Effect of Resistance Training on the Body Composition and Lipoprotein-Lipid Profile in Older Men and Women

Joseph LJO, Davey SL, Evans WJ, et al (Pennsylvania State Univ, Univ Park; Univ of Arkansas, Little Rock)
Metabolism 48:1474-1480, 1999   6–16

Background.—There is a dearth of documentation regarding the effects of resistance training (RT) on the lipoprotein-lipid profile. In addition, the results that have been documented are not as consistent as those for aerobic training. The effects of RT on the lipoprotein-lipid profile in older men and women is little studied. Studies have shown a reduction in total and relative body fat stores in elderly men and women associated with RT. The hypothesis that, if there are any beneficial effects of RT on the lipoprotein-lipid profile, they would only be seen with a reduction in stores of body fat, was tested.

Methods.—The study group comprised 18 men and 17 women aged 54 to 71 years who were not actively participating in any physical training. All the subjects were weight-stable and moderately overweight. They participated in a 12-week resistance training program to assess the effects of RT on body composition and serum lipid concentrations. The RT program comprised a progressive, twice weekly set of resistance exercises with a minimum of 2 days of rest between sessions.

Results.—After 12 weeks of RT, the men showed a significant increase in fat-free mass and a decrease in both the percentage of body fat and fat mass. In contrast, the women demonstrated no change, which resulted in

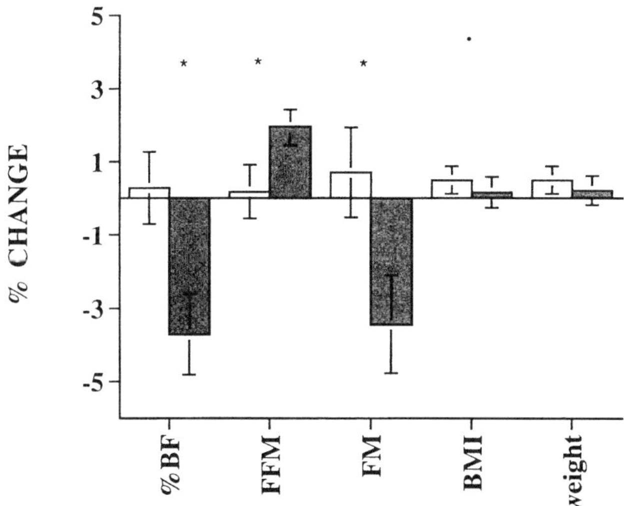

FIGURE 1.—Comparison of relative change in body composition measures after 12 weeks of RT. (□) Women; (■) men. *Significant time-by-sex interaction, *P* < .05. (Courtesy of Joseph LJO, Davey SL, Evans WJ, Campbell WW: Differential effect of resistance training on the body composition and lipoprotein-lipid profile in older men and women, *Metabolism* 48:1474-1489, 1999.)

significant time-by-sex interaction for fat-free mass, percentage body fat, and fat mass (Fig 1). RT did not alter the total cholesterol, low-density lipoprotein cholesterol, or triacylglycerol levels of the group. However, high-density lipoprotein cholesterol decreased in the men and increased in the women. In the combined group, the changes in high-density lipoprotein cholesterol and the ratio of cholesterol to high-density lipoprotein cholesterol were not associated with any changes in body fat stores.

Conclusions.—The implication in these findings is that RT may alter the lipoprotein-lipid profile in older, weight-stable men and women. The changes in the lipoprotein-lipid profile were small, but the men had significant increases in high-density lipoprotein cholesterol and decreases in cholesterol/high-density lipoprotein cholesterol ratio. Changes in the women were in opposition to changes in the men.

▶ The body of literature on the physiological adaptations to exercise in older women and men is growing, yet there have been relatively few studies of the sex dimorphism in such adaptations. It should not be assumed that the adaptations to exercise will be similar, as some may be mediated or potentiated by sex hormones, which decline earlier and more dramatically in women than in men. This study demonstrates a sex specificity for several of the adaptations to resistance exercise in older people. Resistance training is often recommended as a means of preventing the loss of muscle mass in old age, which is a more serious problem for women than for men, yet increases in lean mass were observed only in the older men in this study. It will be important to determine whether these adaptations to exercise are modulated by the replacement of sex hormones in women.

W. M. Kohrt, PhD

A Marathon Run Increases the Susceptibility of LDL to Oxidation In Vitro and Modifies Plasma Antioxidants
Liu M-L, Bergholm R, Mäkimattila S, et al (Helsinki Univ)
Am J Physiol 276:E1083-E1091, 1999   6–17

Background.—Oxygen free radicals may consume antioxidants and oxidize low-density lipoprotein. Oxidative modification of low-density lipoprotein (LDL) is considered a major component in the development of atherosclerosis. The production of oxygen free radicals increases during physical activity. This study investigated whether oxidation of LDLs and modification of plasma antioxidants occurs during strenuous aerobic exercise. Marathon running was selected as the form of exercise to be studied because it is an extreme form of physical activity.

Methods.—Eleven runners in the Helsinki City Marathon were studied, together with a control group of 10 healthy untrained subjects matched for age, sex, and body mass. Blood samples were collected before the marathon, immediately after, and then 4 days after the race. The samples were used to assay circulating antioxidants and LDL oxidizability. Determina-

TABLE 2.—Conjugated Diene Formation, Lipid-Soluble Antioxidants in Low-Density Lipoprotein, and Low-Density Lipoprotein Particle Size of Subjects Before, Immediately After, and 4 Days After the Marathon

	Before	Immediately After	4 Days After	P Value (ANOVA)
LDL oxidation				
Lag time, min	180 ± 7	152 ± 4*	155 ± 7*	<0.001
Diene, nmol/mg				
LDL	475.2 ± 20.7	477.3 ± 14.1	487.3 ± 23.9	NS
Rate, nmol · mg				
$LDL^{-1} \cdot min^{-1}$	3.87 ± 0.24	4.68 ± 0.23†	4.31 ± 0.27	<0.05
Antioxidants in LDL, nmol/mg LDL protein				
α-Tocopherol in LDL	10.1 ± 0.9	10.8 ± 1.0	11.0 ± 1.1	NS
β-Carotene in LDL	0.78 ± 0.10	0.77 ± 0.07	0.73 ± 0.10	NS
Retinol in LDL	0.06 ± 0.00	0.06 ± 0.00	0.063 ± 0.00	NS
LDL peak particle, size, nm	27.1 ± 0.3	27.5 ± 0.3	27.2 ± 0.2	NS

Note: Values are means ± standard error. Statistical comparisons among repeated measures of subjects were tested by 1-way analysis of variance for repeated measures followed by Bonferroni *t*-test.
*P < .001 compared with values before the marathon.
†P < .05 compared with values before the marathon.
Abbreviations: LDL, low-density lipoprotein; *NS,* not significant.
(Courtesy of Liu M-L, Bergholm R, Mäkimattila S, et al: A marathon run increases the susceptibility of LDL to oxidation in vitro and modified plasma antioxidants. *Am J Physiol* 276:E1083-E1091, 1999. Copyright, The American Physiological Society.)

tions were made of lipid-soluble antioxidants in LDL, plasma oxidants, concentrations of lipid and lipoproteins, maximal aerobic power, and body composition. Statistical analyses were crossed out with the SYSTAT statistical package.

Results.—The lag time for oxidation of LDL was longer in the marathon runners before the race than it was in the untrained subjects. Lag time, diene concentration, and propagation rate before and after the marathon run are given in Table 2. LDL samples taken after the marathon showed no significant changes in concentrations of α-tocopherol, β–carotene, or retinol compared with samples taken before the race. There were no significant changes in lipid-soluble antioxidants in LDL or in peak LDL particle size after the race. Increases in the total peroxyl radical trapping antioxidant capacity of plasma (TRAP) and uric acid concentrations were noted after the race, but these increases disappeared within 4 days.

Conclusion.—These data indicate that for up to 4 days afterward, strenuous aerobic exercise increases the susceptibility of LDL to oxidation in vitro. The increased concentration of plasma TRAP reflects increased plasma antioxidant capacity; however, the increase does not seem to be enough to prevent the increased susceptibility of LDL to oxidation in vitro.

▶ The potential problem of free radical production during prolonged vigorous exercise has long been recognized, and various authors have argued that the body counters this trend by an increase in the activity of antioxidant enzymes such as peroxidases. The report of Liu et al suggests that adjustments may be insufficient to counter oxidant production in really prolonged events such as a marathon run. If true, this could explain why there appears to be an increased susceptibility to upper respiratory infections after such events.[1] However, the proof of danger is less than complete, because oxidant trapping capacity before the event was 15% greater than in the sedentary population, with a corresponding advantage in resting LDL oxidation. Participation in the marathon event merely induced a temporary increase in oxidant load to that found in sedentary individuals.

R. J. Shephard, MD, PhD, DPE

Reference

1. Nieman DC, Johanssen LM, Lee JW, et al: Infectious episodes in runners before and after the Los Angeles marathon. *J Sports Med Phys Fitness* 30:316-328, 1990.

The Influence of Intermittent High-Intensity Shuttle Running and Fluid Ingestion on the Performance of a Soccer Skill
McGregor SJ, Nicholas CW, Lakomy HKA, et al (Loughborough Univ, England)
J Sports Sci 17:895-903, 1999   6--18

Background.—Several studies have demonstrated the adverse effects of dehydration on prolonged, continuous, moderate-intensity exercise. However, the effects of dehydration on the intermittent, high-intensity exercise characteristic of participation in team sports are unknown. A test that simulates the prolonged, intermittent physical demands of a sport such as soccer was used to measure the effects of diet, fluid intake, and environmental conditions on performance.

Methods.—The test was the Loughborough Intermittent Shuttle Test, a 105-minute test designed to simulate the performance demands placed on soccer players during a game (Fig 1). The research subjects were 9 semiprofessional soccer players (mean age, 20 years; body mass, 73 kg; maximal oxygen uptake, 59 mL/kg/min). In randomized, crossover fashion, the players performed the test on 2 occasions, once with and once without fluid ingestion. Fluid intake was 5 mL/kg immediately before the test and 2 mL/kg every 15 minutes thereafter. A soccer skill test and a mental performance test were administered before and after each trial. Heart rate, perceived exertion, and blood measurements were made as well.

Results.—The athletes showed a 5% decline in performance of the soccer skill test after the trial without hydration. In contrast, performance remained stable after the trial with fluid intake. There was no change in the mental performance test. The no-fluid trial was also associated with a higher mean heart rate, greater perceived exertion, and higher serum aldosterone levels, osmolality, and sodium and cortisol levels.

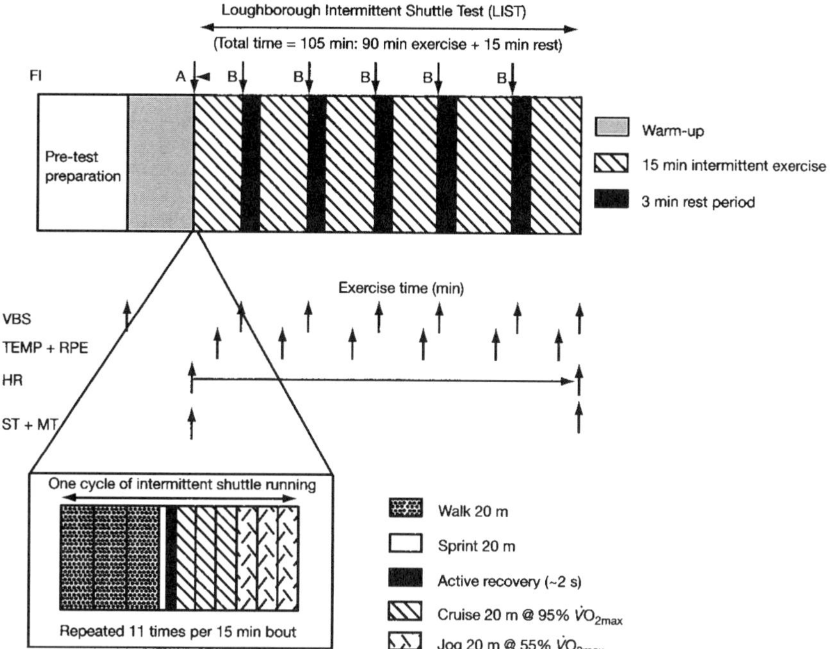

FIGURE 1.—Schematic representation of the Loughborough Intermittent Shuttle Test protocol. *Abbreviations*: *VBS*, Venous blood sample; *HR*, heart rate (measured every 15 seconds); *ST + MT*, skill and mental test; *FI*, fluid intake; *A*, 5 mL/kg body mass; *B*, 2 mL/kg body mass; *TEMP*, environmental temperature; *RPE*, rating of perceived exertion. (Courtesy of McGregor SJ, Nicholas CW, Lakomy HKA, et al: The influence of intermittent high-intensity shuttle running and fluid ingestion on the performance of a soccer skill. *J Sports Sci* 17:895-903, 1999. Published by Taylor & Francis, Ltd. at http://www.tandt.cc.uk/journals/jspihtm.)

Conclusions.—This study documents a significant reduction in sport-specific skill in athletes who do not receive adequate hydration during a prolonged, high-intensity exercise test. The results underscore the importance of drinking fluids throughout a game to maintain skill performance. Drinking fluids during exercise also helps to limit increases in heart rate and other physiologic responses.

▶ If there are still coaches and athletes out there who believe that fluid ingestion is not an important factor in athletic performance, they should read this article. Everyone seems to agree on the need for fluid replacement to prevent heat stress problems. Now we can agree that it is also important for athletic performance. These athletes drank a commercially available no-sugar-added concentrated lemon drink, diluted 1:4 with tap water (52 mOsm/-kg; J Sainsbury plc, London, England). The authors continually referred to this drink as water.

F. J. George, ATC, PT

Carbohydrate-Electrolyte Ingestion During Intermittent High-Intensity Running

Nicholas CW, Tsintzas K, Boobis L, et al (Loughborough Univ, England; Sunderland Gen Hosp, England)
Med Sci Sports Exerc 31:1280-1286, 1999   6–19

Background.—Previous research in trained athletes suggested that drinking a carbohydrate-electrolyte (CHO-E) solution significantly increased intermittent, high-intensity exercise endurance. However, it is possible that the observed differences in running times may have resulted from differing rates of muscle glycogen utilization when the athletes drank CHO-E solution. The effects of CHO-E solution on glycogen utilization during intermittent, high-intensity running were evaluated.

Methods.—The study included 6 trained college soccer, hockey, or rugby players with a mean maximal oxygen uptake of 56.3 mL/kg/min. The athletes performed two 90-minute exercise trials, 1 week apart, consisting of maximal sprinting alternating with less-intense running and walking. During the trial they drank either a 6.9% CHO-E solution or a noncarbohydrate placebo. They drank 5 mL/kg of the solution before exercise and 2 mL/kg every 15 minutes during exercise; the total mean volume was 1114 mL. Vastus lateralis muscle biopsy specimens were obtained before and after each exercise session to assess muscle glycogen utilization. Venous blood samples were taken for measurement of blood lactate and serum insulin.

Results.—Mean muscle glycogen utilization in mixed muscle samples was 192.5 mmol of glucosyl units during the CHO-E trials versus 245.3 mmol of glucosyl units during the control trials. On analysis of single muscle fibers from control trials, glycogen utilization was 18.2 mmol of glucosyl units in type I fibers versus 287.4 mmol in type II fibers. The control trials were associated with significantly higher blood lactate and serum insulin concentrations at 30 minutes after the start of exercise.

Conclusion.—Drinking a CHO-E beverage during intermittent high-intensity exercise reduces muscle glycogen utilization 22% in trained athletes. Glycogen utilization appears to be significantly reduced in both type I and type II muscle fibers. This change may account for the improved exercise endurance observed in athletes drinking CHO-E solution.

▶ This study indicated that a 6.9% CHO-E solution may improve endurance capacity of soccer, hockey, or rugby players when ingested before and during a game. The amount of muscle glycogen utilized was reduced by 22% in this study. This glycogen sparing occurred in both type I and type II muscle fibers.

F. J. George, ATC, PT

Gastrointestinal Mucosal Integrity After Prolonged Exercise With Fluid Supplementation

Peters HPF, Wiersma WC, Akkermans LMA, et al (Utrecht Univ, The Netherlands; Eemland Hosp, Amersfoort, The Netherlands)
Med Sci Sports Exerc 32:134-142, 2000

6–20

Objective.—Exercise produces alterations in the gastrointestinal (GI) tract, and many endurance athletes show GI blood loss after competitions. This and other GI symptoms may result from local gut ischemia. Previous studies assessing the effect of exercise on GI mucosal integrity have used occult blood tests, which are prone to false-positive results. The effects of exercise, as well as those of carbohydrate supplementation, on GI mucosal integrity were examined using more specific tests than those previously adopted.

Methods.—Twenty-two male triathletes were studied while performing two 150-minute exercise tests, including alternate bouts of running, cycling, and running at 70% to 75% maximal oxygen intake. VO_{2max}. The athletes performed 1 trial with a 7.0% carbohydrate drink and 1 with water only. The amount of fluid supplementation was up to 2.3 L. Fecal lysozyme levels, α_1-antitrypsin levels, and occult blood loss were measured. The presence of blood was assessed using 2 tests specific for human blood (ie, the Colon-Albumin and Monohaem tests). The 2 trials were also compared for GI symptoms.

TABLE 6.—Fecal Test Characteristics After Exercise (First/Second Bowel Movement) With Carbohydrate (CHO) or Water (W) as Supplement in 8 Research Subjects Who Showed 1 or More Deviating Data

Subject	Supplement	Haemoccult	Colon Albumin	Lysozyme (mg CEL-L^{-1} Feces)	α-1-Antitrypsin* (mg·L^{-1} Feces)
1	CHO	−/−†	−/−	55/41	12/97
	W	−/−	−/−	6/23	
2	CHO	−/−	+‡/−	11/<1	288/165
	W	−/−	−/−	5/6	
3	CHO	−/−	−/−	125/26	22/120
	W	−/−	−/−	<1/<1	
4	CHO	/	/	<1/4	
	W	−/−	+‡/−	<1/<1	63/<10
5	CHO	−/−	−/−	<1/3	
	W	+‡/+‡	−/−	<1/<1	
6	CHO	−/−	−/−	<1/3	
	W	−/−	+‡/−	<1/8	207/182
7	CHO	−/−	−/−	130/29	<10/<10
	W	−/−	−/−	<1/<1	
8	CHO	−/−	−/−	44/40	320/102
	W	−/−	−/−	1/17	

*α_1-Antitrypsin test was applied with either a fecal lysozyme concentration greater than 24 mg CEL/L feces or a positive colon albumin test.

†Negative test.

‡Negative Monohaem test.

Abbreviation: CEL, Chicken egg-white lysozyme.

(Courtesy of Peters HPF, Wiersma WC, Akkermans LMA, et al: Gastrointestinal mucosal integrity after prolonged exercise with fluid supplementation. *Med Sci Sports Exerc* 32(1):134-142, 2000.)

Results.—Three athletes had albumin only, with no hemoglobin, in their first stool after exercise. This happened in 2 trials with water supplementation and in 1 with carbohydrate supplementation. In 4 participants, lysozyme levels were elevated after exercise with carbohydrate supplementation but not with water supplementation. Of these 7 specimens—showing either elevation of albumin and/or lysozyme levels—3 showed elevated α_1-antitrypsin levels (Table 6). Ninety-five percent of research subjects experienced GI symptoms during exercise, generally more frequent and longer lasting during running than cycling. The occurrence of symptoms was no different with carbohydrate versus water supplementation and was unrelated to measures of mucosal integrity.

Conclusions.—Studies using tests specific for human blood suggest that exercise-associated GI blood loss is clinically insignificant. Some postexercise stool specimens show evidence of local mucosal damage and inflammation. Carbohydrate supplementation has no apparent effect on GI symptoms or other GI changes.

▶ Ischemic damage to the intestinal wall during very prolonged endurance exercise has been thought to be a contributing factor in exercise-related immunosuppression and sepsis-like reactions,[1,2] and damage has been reported in 8% to 23% of triathletes. Some of the earlier investigations have looked for bacterial lipopolysaccharides in the blood, and others have used somewhat nonspecific tests to look for blood in the feces. The present study used tests of blood loss that were specific to human albumin and hemoglobin rather than those based on the peroxidase reaction, which can generate false-positive results from plant and bacterial peroxidases in the gut. Although no evidence of blood loss was obtained in this study, there are 3 reasons for a cautious approach to the present data: (1) the feces showed increases in α_1-antitrypsin and lysozyme concentrations, which suggests a local inflammatory response, (2) the duration of activity (150 minutes) was less than a full triathlon or ultramarathon, and (3) the sample of 22 participants may have been a little small to detect a phenomenon affecting only 8% of participants.

R. J. Shephard, MD, PhD, DPE

References

1. Øktedalen O, Lunde OC, Opstad PK, et al: Changes in the gastrointestinal mucosa after long-distance running. *Scand J Gastroenterol* 27:270-274, 1992.
2. Shephard RJ: *Physical Activity, Training and the Immune Response.* Carmel, Ind, Cooper, 1997.

Shortening of Muscle Relaxation Time After Creatine Loading

Van Leemputte M, Vandenberghe K, Hespel P (Katholieke Universiteit Leuven, Belgium)

J Appl Physiol 86:840-844, 1999

6–21

Purpose.—High-dose creatine (Cr) supplementation can increase muscle Cr and phosphocreatine levels, which may enhance maximal high-intensity muscle contractions. However, the mechanisms underlying this effect of Cr loading remain unclear. The effects of short-term Cr supplementation on torque generation and relaxation during intermittent voluntary elbow flexion were examined.

Methods.—The study included 16 healthy young men who were randomized to receive Cr supplementation (5 g of creatine monohydrate 4 times/day for 5 days) or placebo. Before and after the supplementation period, the subjects performed 12 maximal, isometric, 3-second elbow flexions, alternating with 10-second rest periods. The group's performance

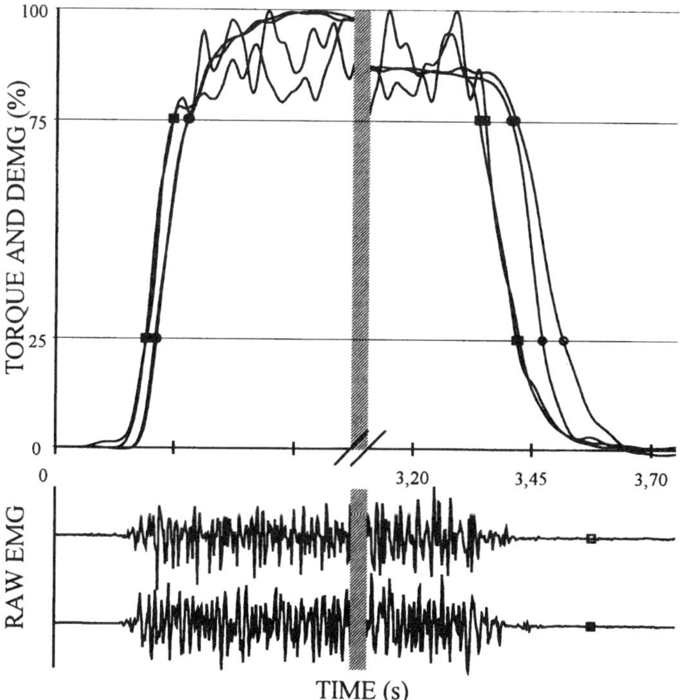

FIGURE 1.—Typical examples of raw time-series data for a 3-second maximal, static, elbow-flexion effort. Graph is interrupted for 2.2 seconds (*hatched bar*) Torque (*circles*), raw electromyogram (EMG) and quantified EMG (DEMG) (*squares*) of biceps of 1 subject before (*open symbols*) and after (*solid symbols*) creatine intake are shown. Torque and DEMG are given as percentage of maximum during contraction. Contraction and relaxation times and activation and deactivation times are defined as time of torque and DEMG change, respectively, between 25% and 75% of maximum. (Courtesy of Van Leemputte M, Vandenberghe K, Hespel P: Shortening of muscle relaxation time after creatine loading. *J Appl Physiol* 86:840-844, 1999.)

was compared in terms of maximal torque (Tmax), contraction time (CT) from 25% to 75% of Tmax, and relaxation time (RT) from 75% to 25% of Tmax (Fig 1).

Results.—All variables were similar between groups at baseline. After the supplementation period, Tmax and CT were still similar. However, subjects in the Cr group showed a consistent 20% reduction in RT after supplementation. The extent of their reduction in RT after Cr supplementation was positively correlated with their initial RT.

Conclusions.—The results suggest that a 5-day period of Cr loading can significantly reduce muscle RT during brief isometric contractions. This effect occurs with no change in torque production. Thus, the ergogenic effect of Cr supplementation may be attributable to shortening of muscle relaxation after maximal contractions.

▶ It is well known that Cr supplementation for several days may markedly increase muscle Cr and phosphocreatine levels, which are associated with enhanced capacity for high-intensity muscle contractions and increased performance. This study investigated the effect of Cr loading on the rate of torque generation and relaxation during intermittent maximal voluntary elbow flexions. The authors reported no increases in torque production but a shortened muscle relaxation time with Cr loading. This shortened relaxation time can enhance performance during brief isometric muscle contractions, but it is unclear whether these results also apply to performance of high-intensity sports performances that include extended eccentric and concentric contractions.

M. J. L. Alexander, PhD

Creatine Supplementation Increases Muscle Total Creatine but Not Maximal Intermittent Exercise Performance

McKenna MJ, Morton J, Selig SE, et al (Victoria Univ of Technology, Melbourne, Australia; Alfred Hosp, Prahran, Australia; Deakin Univ, Burwood, Australia)

J Appl Physiol 87:2244-2252, 1999 6–22

Purpose.—Previous studies have reported that creatine supplementation (CrS) can increase muscle total creatine content (TCr). Some but not all studies suggest that CrS improves maximal intermittent exercise performance (Table 3), possibly by increasing muscle Cr phosphate (CrP) content. If CrS does improve exercise performance, then the initial gain will be lost over time as muscle TCr decreases to normal. The effects of CrS on muscle TCr and CrP and on exercise performance, accounting for the rise and subsequent washout of muscle TCr, were examined.

Methods.—The study included 14 recreationally active young men and women. One group received 5 days of CrS, consisting of 30 g/d, whereas the other group received placebo. Before and at 0, 2, and 4 weeks after the start of their assigned supplementation, the research subjects performed

TABLE 3.—Effects of Creatine Supplementation on Resting Muscle Creatine Phosphate, Creatine, Total Creatine Content, and Maximal Exercise Performance in Humans

Study Design (Ref. No.)	n	Dose, g	CrP, %Δ	Cr, %Δ	TCr, Δ	TCr, %Δ	Performance Measurements	Performance Results
Ordered, single blind	6	100	22‡	7	18‡	15‡	Cycle: 4×1 min at $\sim$115% $V_{O_{2max}}$, then single bout to fatigue	NS time to fatigue
Ordered, nonblinded	7	120	10	29‡	23‡	18‡	Cycle: 5×6 s, 1×10 s, constant work (30-s rest) Vertical jump	Final bout ↓4% cadence decline‡ NS
Ordered, nonblinded	9	100	10‡	36‡	23‡	19‡	Cycle: 2×30-s sprint (4-min interval)	↑4% peak work *bouts 1* and 2§ ↑4% total work *bouts 1* and 2‡
Crossover, double blind	9	3*	4‡				Knee extension: isometric MVC	NS
							Knee extension: 3×30, 4×20, 5×10 MVC	NS fatigue index; ↑ mean torque
Crossover, double blind	9	60	NS†			13†‡	Cycle: 1×30-s sprint	NS peak power, fatigue index, work
Ordered, double blind	10	80	6‡				Arm flexion: 5×30 MVC	NS fatigue index; mean torque
Crossover, double blind	8	150	3	22‡	12‡	9‡	Cycle: 1×20-s sprint	NS peak power, fatigue index, work
Independent groups, four repeated measures, double blind (present study)	7	150	10‡	41‡	23‡	18‡	Cycle: 5×10s sprint (180-, 50-, 2×20-s intervals)	NS peak power, fatigue index, work

Note: Change (Δ) in TCr is expressed in millimoles per kilogram dry mass. Double-blind crossover studies are listed in order of trial washout period (3, 2, and 4 weeks, respectively). Studies cited are those that measured both muscle Cr status as well as performance; these have a single-drop design, except where indicated.

*Cr dose in grams per kilogram.
†Raw data are reported. CrP/ATP and TCr/ATP ratio.
‡$P < .05$.
§$P < .06$.

Abbreviations: ATP, Adenosine triphosphate; *Cr*, creatine; *CrP*, creatine phosphate; *TCr*, total creatine content; *n*, number of research subjects: $V_{O_{2max}}$, maximal O_2 consumption; *MVC*, maximal voluntary contraction; *NS*, not significant; ↑, increase; ↓, decrease.

(Courtesy of McKenna MJ, Morton J, Selig SE, et al: Creatine supplementation increases muscle total creatine but not maximal intermittent exercise performance. *J Appl Physiol* 87:2244-2252, 1999.)

five 10-second maximal cycle ergometer sprints, separated by rest intervals of 180, 50, 20, and 20 seconds. Resting vastus lateralis muscle biopsies were performed as well. The rise and fall of muscle TCr and CrP levels were measured and correlated with changes in performance after CrS.

Results.—At week 0, resting muscle TCr was increased by 22.9 mmol/kg dry mass, whereas the CrP level was increased by 8.9 mmol/kg and the Cr level was increased by 14.0 mmol/kg. Significant changes were still present at 2 weeks but not at 4 weeks. There were no changes in the placebo group. Both groups showed increased peak power and cumulative work after supplementation, which was an apparent placebo effect. However, CrS had no main effect on either performance variable.

Conclusions.—This study documents the increase and subsequent washout of muscle TCr and CrP after CrS. However, supplementation has no demonstrable effect on maximal intermittent exercise performance. The improvements in performance that occur in research subjects taking CrS are no different from those in research subjects taking placebo.

▶ Many teams in events such as soccer are now taking CrS in the belief that such a regimen enhances sprinting performance. However, the experimental data supporting such a practice are still far from conclusive (see Table 3). Some of the studies have failed to use an appropriate double-blind protocol, and others have not taken muscle samples to ensure that the treatment has enhanced local reserves of CrP. The present study took both of these precautions and used a small sample and a randomized, controlled design; the authors found no benefit from CrS in terms of peak power output, cumulative work production, or fatigue index. There remain 3 limitations to the present study: (1) because of the small sample size, experimental and control groups were not well matched in sex or in body mass (a crossover design would have been more appropriate for such a sample size); (2) participants were unfamiliar with maximal sprint exercise, and learning of the test protocol was incomplete; and (3) there was limited control over activity outside the experimental protocol. The question thus remains open to further investigation, and the data on washout times for CrS will be useful for anyone who wishes to repeat observations using a crossover design.

R. J. Shephard, MD, PhD, DPE

Performance and Muscle Fiber Adaptations to Creatine Supplementation and Heavy Resistance Training
Volek JS, Duncan ND, Mazzetti SA, et al (Pennsylvania State Univ, Univ Park; Ball State Univ, Muncie, Ind; Ohio Univ, Athens; et al)
Med Sci Sports Exerc 31:1147-1156, 1999   6–23

Purpose.—Previous studies suggest that 1 week of creatine supplementation increases creatine and phosphocreatine concentrations in skeletal

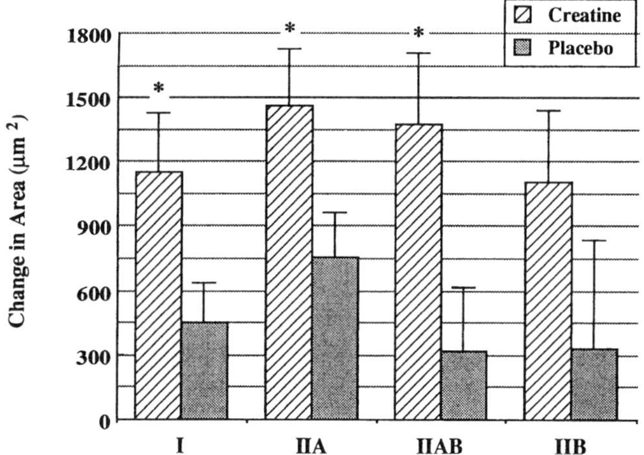

FIGURE 4.—Delta changes in cross-sectional areas of specific muscle fiber types after 12 weeks of heavy resistance training in creatine and placebo subjects. *P .05 or less from corresponding change in the placebo group. Values are mean ± SE. (Courtesy of Volek JS, Duncan ND, Mazzetti SA, et al: Performance and muscle fiber adaptations to creatine supplementation and heavy resistance training. *Med Sci Sports Exerc* 31:1147-1156, 1999.)

muscle and may increase body mass and resistance exercise performance. However, there are few data on the effects of creatine supplementation during prolonged training periods. The effects of creatine supplementation and resistance training on weight-training performance and other responses to training were examined.

Methods.—The study included 19 healthy resistance-trained men. One group was randomized to receive creatine supplementation—25 g/day for 1 week, then 5 g/day for the remainder of the 12-week training period—and the other to placebo. Training consisted of periodized heavy resistance training. After 12 weeks, the 2 groups were compared for physical performance, body composition, skeletal muscle morphologic findings, and creatine accumulation (Fig 4).

Results.—Body mass increased by 6.3% in the creatine group versus 3.6% in the placebo group. Increases in fat-free mass were 6.3% and 3.1%, respectively. The creatine group had a 24% increase in bench press performance, compared with 16% in the placebo group; squat performance increased by 32% and 24%, respectively. Creatine supplementation was associated with a greater increase in type I muscle fiber cross-sectional area (35% vs 11%), with similar increases in type IIA and IIB cross-sectional area. By the first week, the creatine group had a 22% increase in muscle creatine, which persisted throughout the 12-week study period. In contrast, the placebo group had no increase.

Conclusions.—Creatine supplementation during heavy resistance training significantly increases fat-free mass, exercise performance, and muscle morphology, compared with placebo. The creatine-enhanced responses appear to result from more intense training, producing accelerated physiologic adaptations. No adverse effects of creatine supplementation are observed.

▶ Creatine supplementation is now very popular with contestants in many types of sport; for example, it was used by many of the teams participating in the last World Soccer Cup competition. Although the group size is relatively small, these data demonstrate a clear creatine-induced enhancement in the hypertrophy of all types of muscle fiber relative to controls. It has been less clear whether creatine acts directly to enhance the synthesis of muscle protein[1] or whether it allows more vigorous resistance training. In the present study, those subjects who received creatine were able to use greater resistances, supporting the hypothesis that creatine supplementation enhances the resynthesis of phosphocreatine between sets.[2]

R. J. Shephard, MD, PhD, DPE

References

1. Ingwall JS, Morales MF, Stockdale FE: Creatine and the control of myosin synthesis in differentiating skeletal muscle. *Proc Natl Acad Sci* 69:2250-2253, 1972.
2. Greenhaff PL, Bodin K, Söderlund K, et al: Effect of oral creatine supplementation on skeletal muscle phosphocreatine resynthesis. *Am J Physiol* 266:E725-E730, 1994.

Long-term Oral Creatine Supplementation Does Not Impair Renal Function in Healthy Athletes
Poortmans JR, Francaux M (Université Libre de Bruxelles, Brussels, Belgium; Université Catholique de Louvain, Belgium)
Med Sci Sports Exerc 31:1108-1110, 1999   6–24

Objective.—Creatine is widely used by athletes to enhance performance and adaptations to training. In contrast to reports of renal dysfunction, the authors have found no detrimental effect of creatine supplementation on renal responses. However, creatine has a high nitrogen content, which could place a strain on the kidneys over the long term. The long-term effects of creatine supplementation on renal function in healthy athletes were studied.

Methods.—The study included 9 healthy, young, highly trained athletes who were regular users of creatine monohydrate. The athletes took creatine in doses of 1 to 80 g/day over a period of 10 months to 5 years. Renal function studies—including glomerular function, urea clearance, and protein excretion rates—were performed in the athletes and in 85 noncreatine users.

Results.—The 2 groups were similar in their plasma creatine, creatinine, urea, and albumin levels (Table 2). Both groups had normal urine creatine, urea, and albumin rates. The results were consistent with normal glomerular filtration rate, tubular resorption, and glomerular membrane permeability in both groups.

TABLE 2.—Mean Values (±SEM) of Plasma and Urine Contents of the Control and Creatine Groups

	Control Group (N = 85)	Creatine Group (N = 9)
Plasma		
Creatine (μmol·L^{-1})	50.3 ± 6.1	62.2 ± 11.0
Creatinine (μmol·L^{-1})	80.4 ± 5.3	72.5 ± 13.3
Urea (mmol·L^{-1})	2.51 ± 0.10	2.45 ± 0.15
Albumin (g·L^{-1})	42.4 ± 1.1	42.5 ± 1.2
Urine		
Output (mL·min^{-1})	0.96 ± 0.11	1.20 ± 0.16
Creatine (μmol·24 h^{-1})	288 ± 96	10,828 ± 3,264*
Creatinine (mmol·24 h^{-1})	16.4 ± 0.6	13.9 ± 1.1
Urea (mmol·24 h^{-1})	188 ± 15	205 ± 22
Albumin (μg·min^{-1})	6.9 ± 1.6	6.3 ± 1.1
Creatine/creatinine (μmol·mmol^{-1})	19.7 ± 2.0	1,108 ± 400*
Clearance		
Creatine (mL·min^{-1})	4.7 ± 1.5	156 ± 55*
Creatinine (mL·min^{-1})	145 ± 8	143 ± 11
Urea (mL·min^{-1})	64 ± 9	86 ± 8
Albumin (μL·min^{-1})	0.19 ± 0.05	0.15 ± 0.03

*$P < .001$ between the control group and the creatine supplementation group.

(Courtesy of Poortmans JR, Francaux M: Long-term oral creatine supplementation does not impair renal function in healthy athletes. *Med Sci Sports Exerc* 31:1108-1110, 1999.)

Conclusions.—Long-term use of creatine does not appear to adversely affect renal function in athletes. The results suggest that creatine may safely be used by healthy individuals for a period of months to years.

▶ Despite the growing popularity of creatine supplementation, a substantial additional load is imposed on the kidneys because of the high nitrogen content of this compound (32%). There have been persistent claims of renal dysfunction from various protein and amino acid supplements[1-3] and alarming press reports that creatine supplementation has caused death in American wrestlers. Certainly, we need to keep careful watch for adverse responses to any departure from our "natural" diet, but the present study shows that, at least over periods of use from 10 months to 5 years, there is no detectable difference in renal function between creatine users and a control group. Some athletes may continue to use creatine for longer than 5 years, and there is a need for even more extended studies before creative supplementation can be given a categorical clean bill of health.

R. J. Shephard, MD, PhD, DPE

References

1. Pritchard NR, Kalra PA: Renal dysfunction accompanying oral creatine supplements. *Lancet* 351: 1252-1253, 1998.
2. Coppo R, Porcellini MG, Gianoglio B, et al: Glomerular preselectivity to macromolecules in reflux nephropathy: Microalbuminuria during acute hyperfiltration due to amino acid infusion. *Clin Nephrol* 40: 299-307, 1993.
3. Tolins JP, Schultz PJ, Westberg G, et al: Renal hemodynamic effects of dietary protein in the rat: Role of nitric acid. *J Lab Clin Med* 125: 228-236, 1995.

7 Environment, Ergogenic Aids, and Doping

Rainfall, Evaporation and the Risk of Non-contact Anterior Cruciate Ligament Injury in the Australian Football League
Orchard J, Seward H, McGivern J, et al (Univ of New South Wales, Kensington, Australia; Australian Football League Med Officers Assoc, Melbourne, Australia)
Med J Aust 170:304-306, 1999   7–1

Background.—Tears of the anterior cruciate ligament (ACL) produce the most devastating consequences for athletes, whether professional or amateur. Risk of this type of injury was postulated to be affected by the weather conditions during play in the Australian Football League.

Methods.—Football matches were observed from 1992 through 1998 (total, 2280 matches), and a prospective analytic study was performed. The variables observed were rainfall amounts, degree of evaporation of water from the field, and surgically proven ACL injury that was not the result of a direct contact mechanism during a match.

Results.—A total of 59 ACL injuries for which no direct contact was responsible were noted during the observed matches. Injuries occurred more commonly in cities north of Melbourne, in senior grade matches, when there was high water evaporation during the 28 days before the match, and when rainfall was low during the preceding 365 days.

Conclusions.—High water evaporation during the month before a match and low rainfall during the year before the match were significantly correlated with an increased risk of ACL injuries that were not caused by direct contact. These associations may indicate that dry conditions produce friction and torsional resistance with football boots. If the grounds are consistently watered when rainfall is lacking and are covered when high degrees of evaporation are likely, the incidence of this type of injury may be decreased.

▶ What goes around comes around. In the early 1970s, Garrick and Requa[1,2] made similar observations about anterior cruciate ligament injuries that occurred in American football and about surface moisture. In fact, they implemented a program whereby the playing surface was wetted before games at the University of Washington. Of course, this and many other factors that relate to the shoe surface interface and knee injuries have been pretty much ignored by athletic administrators despite the fact that the literature clearly indicates the effect of ambient temperature, artificial versus a natural grass surface, shoe sole configuration, and sole material composition.

J. S. Torg, MD

References

1. Adkinson JW, Requa RK, Garrick JG: Injury rates in high school football. A comparison of synthetic surfaces and grass fields. *Clin Orthop* 99:131-136, 1974.
2. Bramwell ST, Requa RK, Garrick JG: High school football injuries: A pilot comparison of playing surfaces. *Med Sci Sports* 9:166-169, 1972.

Respiratory Energetics During Exercise at High Altitude

Cibella F, Cuttitta G, Romano S, et al (Istituto di Fisiopatologia Respiratoria del Consiglio Nazionale delle Richerche, Palermo, Italy; Istituto di Tecnologie Biomediche Avanzate del Consiglio Nazionale delle Richerche, Milan, Italy; McGill Univ, Montreal)
J Appl Physiol 86:1785-1792, 1999   7–2

Background.—Breathing is generally believed to be more difficult at altitude than at sea level because ventilation is greater at altitude than at sea level both for persons at rest and for a given intensity of exercise. The effects of high altitude on the work of breathing as well as external work capacity were assessed.

Methods.—The mechanical power of breathing was measured in 4 subjects during exercise at sea level and after they had spent 1 month at an altitude of 5050 m near the Mount Everest base camp in Nepal. All subjects were healthy men between the ages of 33 and 35 years, and all were also participants in a study of exercise endurance at altitude conducted at the Mount Everest base camp. The measurements were based on simultaneous records of esophageal pressure and lung volume. Two of the subjects were basically sedentary, whereas the other 2 were physically active. The same testing methods and equipment were used at sea level and at high altitude. Total body oxygen intake was measured by means of the open circuit method during incremental cycle ergometer exercise both at sea level and at altitude.

Results.—The maximal exercise ventilation was higher at altitude than at sea level in all subjects, and the maximal oxygen intake average was lower at altitude than at sea level. The relationship of the mechanical power of breathing to minute ventilation was the same at sea level and at altitude in 3 of the subjects, whereas in 1 subject (1 of the sedentary subjects), the mechanical power of breathing for any given minute ventilation was lower at altitude than at sea level.

Conclusion.—Increased ventilation in response to inadequate oxygenation is usually cost-effective; however, there is a point at which the oxygen cost of the additional work may exceed the increase in peak oxygen intake that accompanies the increased work. Normally, under sea level conditions this point is never reached, but, as this study demonstrates, this crossover point can be reached at high altitude when mechanical efficiency of ventilation is low. This increased work of breathing can significantly limit external work capacity at high altitude unless mechanical efficiency is high.

▶ One of the body's reactions to inadequate tissue oxygenation is an increase of ventilation. Although there is usually an efficacious response, there is at least a theoretical possibility that the oxygen cost of the additional respiratory work may exceed the resulting increase in peak oxygen intake.[1] Under normal, sea level conditions, the crossover point is rarely reached, but the zone of diminishing returns is reached when the mechanical efficiency of ventilation is low (as in some forms of chronic chest disease) and (as in the present example) at high altitudes. Some of the early pioneers of Mount Everest talk vividly of the struggle to breath and of taking 12 breaths for each upward step.

R. J. Shephard, MD, PhD, DPE

Reference

1. Shephard RJ: *Aerobic Fitness and Health.* Champaign, Ill, Human Kinetics Publishers, 1994.

Brain Magnetic Resonance Imaging (MRI) and Neurological Changes After a Single High Altitude Climb
Anooshiravani M, Dumont L, Mardirosoff C, et al (Hôpital des Enfants Reine Fabiola and Hôpital Brugmann, Brussels, Belgium; Hôpital Cantonal de Genève, Switzerland)
Med Sci Sports Exerc 31:969-972, 1999   7–3

Background.—Previous studies have reported neurologic impairment, mental dysfunction, and brain, imaging changes in high-altitude climbers. More and more recreational climbers are climbing peaks as high as 6000 m. These climbs often lead to acute mountain sickness (AMS), with associated brain hypoxia. MRI and neurophysiologic studies were used to examine the effects of a single high-altitude climb.

Methods.—The study sample comprised 8 men, age 31 to 48 years, who were planning trips to altitudes of over 6000 m. Before the climb and 5 to 10 days after returning to sea level, each subject underwent a MRI scan of the brain and a battery of neuropsychological tests. The AMS symptom score was assessed every day during the climb.

Results.—Assessed at an altitude of 5500 m, the mean AMS symptom score was 3. Headache was the major symptom; none of the patients experienced ataxia. Sinus disease developed in 2 climbers, and 4 had aggravation of past sinus disease. There were no significant changes in either the MRI scan of the brain or the neuropsychological tests. Some patients reported euphoria, whereas others had memory disturbances after returning to sea level.

Conclusions.—Mountain climbing to altitudes of 6000 m or higher is not associated with any changes in MRI brain scans or neuropsychological test performance. The neurologic symptoms experienced at high altitude do not appear to be associated with any permanent brain impairment. As always, smooth acclimatization is recommended as a precautionary measure.

▶ There have been disturbing reports that even a single climb to 8000 m is associated with abnormal MRI brain scans and neuropsychological abnormalities in as many as 50% of climbers.[1] It is unlikely that substantial numbers of climbers will ascend to such extreme altitudes, but more and more middle-aged individuals are going on hiking treks to the Himalayas, and the question thus arises as to whether the more modest altitudes encountered by such individuals will have an adverse effect, particularly in those who are older and unfit. It is difficult to be sure, from negative results, that no damage has occurred particularly when the authors themselves admit that the psychological test scores may have improved with practice. However, the data that show no change in MRI or psychological test scores after a group of men with an average age of 37 years (range, 31-48 years) had ascended to altitudes of 6200 to 7100 m is somewhat reassuring. One factor is that the alveolar oxygen pressure drops dramatically with the further climb from 6000 to 8000 m. It is also important that the present group took time for acclimatization to high altitude and took acetazolamide prophylactically to diminish the risk of the various manifestations of AMS (including cerebral edema).

R. J. Shephard, MD, PhD, DPE

Reference

1. Garrido E, Segura R, Capdevilla A, et al: New evidence from MRI of brain changes after climbs at extreme altitude. *Eur J Appl Physiol* 70: 477-481, 1995.

Radiographic Evidence of Interstitial Pulmonary Edema After Exercise at Altitude
Anholm JD, Milne ENC, Stark P, et al (Loma Linda Univ, Calif; Univ of California Irvine Med Ctr, Orange; Stanford Univ, Palo Alto, Calif; et al)
J Appl Physiol 86:503-509, 1999   7–4

Objective.—Prolonged endurance exercise can lead to reductions in vital capacity and gas exchange abnormalities, including decreases in diffusing capacity for carbon dioxide. Whether the latter changes are associated with pulmonary edema is not known. A radiographic study of

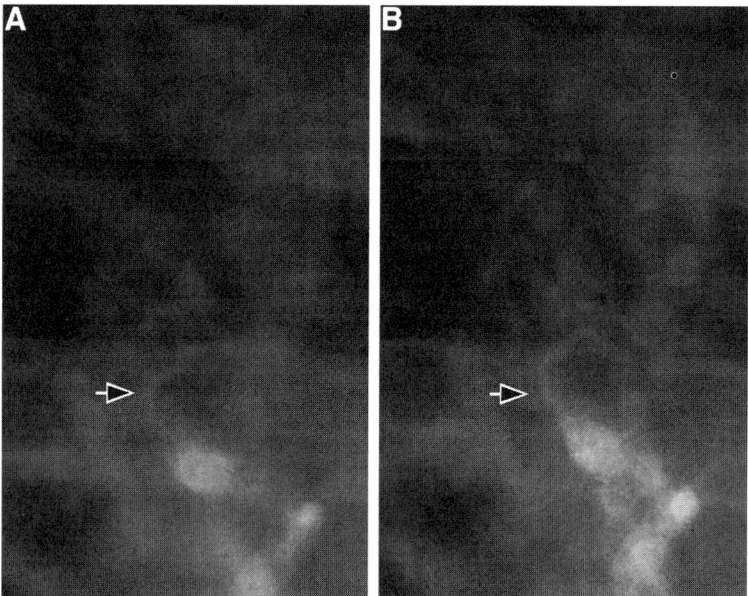

FIGURE 2.—Coned-down views of bronchus from subject shown in Figure 1. After exercise (**B**), bronchial wall demonstrates thickening ("cuffing") compared with same area before exercise (**A**). (Courtesy of Anholm JD, Milne ENC, Stark P, et al: Radiographic evidence of interstitial pulmonary edema after exercise at altitude. *J Appl Physiol.* 1999, 86:503-509.)

healthy well-trained cyclists with no prior history of altitude-related problems was performed to determine whether there is evidence of pulmonary edema after severe exercise at moderate altitude.

Methods.—On 5 occasions chest radiographs were obtained in 37 highly trained cyclists before and immediately after endurance cycling 5.3 to 131.5 km as rapidly as possible at altitude. Radiographs were interpreted by radiologists blinded to the sequence and the performance of the cyclist.

Results.—None of the cyclists had a productive cough after cycling, and all but 2 finished the courses. Cyclists maintained heart rates of greater than 80% of their peak heart values. Although all radiologists found subtle changes, there was no evidence of severe pulmonary edema. (Fig 2). Overall edema scores increased significantly, from 0.8 before exercise to 1.8 after exercise in 26 cyclists. Overall edema scores increased by 1 point or more in 18 (49%) cyclists and by 2 points or more in 9 (24%) cyclists. The altitude at which the cyclists lived did not affect occurrence of edema. Performance did not affect occurrence of edema.

Conclusion.—Radiographic evidence of pulmonary edema is present in endurance cyclists after exercise at altitude.

▶ Temporary changes in lung volumes and pulmonary diffusing capacity following a bout of prolonged endurance exercise are well recognized,[1-3] and although edema has been demonstrated in experimental animals (particularly racehorses and greyhounds), it has remained unclear whether the human changes should be attributed to pulmonary edema or whether factors such as respiratory muscle fatigue, changes in cardiac output, or the oral inhalation of large volumes of cold, dry, or polluted air were to blame. In this study, the likelihood of a positive response was enhanced by performing the activity at an altitude of up to 3000 m, but this was offset by a period of acclimatization to the high altitude. Changes in lung function were relatively slight, and only the decrease in forced expiratory volume in 1 second was statistically significant. Evaluation of the radiographs was exemplary, with 3 radiologists reading the plates in blinded fashion. Seven measures of fluid infiltration were assessed, but only vascular markings and the overall edema score increased significantly from before to after the exercise bout. Although it appears that some of the study participants developed edema, because the data were grouped and treated statistically, it is not clear what proportion of the study participants developed edema.

R. J. Shephard, MD, PhD, DPE

References

1. Gordon B, Levine SA, Wilmaers A: Observations on a group of marathon runners with special reference to the circulation. *Arch Intern Med* 33: 425-434, 1924.
2. Mahler DA, Loke J: Lung function after marathon running at warm and cold ambient temperatures. *Am Rev Respir Dis* 124: 154-157, 1981.
3. Manier G, Moinard J, Techoueyres P, et al. Pulmonary diffusion limitation after prolonged strenuous exercise. *Respir Physiol* 83: 143-153, 1991.

Exaggerated Endothelin Release in High-Altitude Pulmonary Edema
Sartori C, Vollenweider L, Löffler B-M, et al (Centre Hospitalier Universitaire Vaudois, Lausanne, Switzerland; Univ of Lausanne, Switzerland; F Hoffman-La Roche Ltd, Basel, Switzerland; et al)
Circulation 99:2665-2668, 1999   7–5

Objective.—The underlying causes of high-altitude pulmonary edema (HAPE) are unknown, but endothelin-1, a potent and long-lasting vasodilator, is thought to play a role. The effects of high-altitude exposure (4559 m) on endothelin-1 plasma concentration and pulmonary artery pressure were compared in mountaineers susceptible to HAPE and mountaineers resistant to HAPE.

Methods.—Endothelin-1 plasma levels and pulmonary artery pressure were measured in 16 mountaineers (3 women), average age 41 years, with documented HAPE within the last 4 years, and in 16 control mountaineers (5 women), average age 41 years, at 580 m and after 48 hours at 4559 m. Posteroanterior chest radiographs were obtained every morning.

Results.—Pulmonary edema developed in 8 of the HAPE mountaineers and in none of the control subjects after 18 to 36 hours (Fig 1). At high altitude, endothelin-1 plasma levels were significantly related to systolic pulmonary artery pressure and inversely related to arterial oxygen saturation. Endothelin-1 plasma levels were 33% higher in HAPE mountaineers than in control mountaineers (22.2 vs 16.8 pg/mL) at high altitude. At

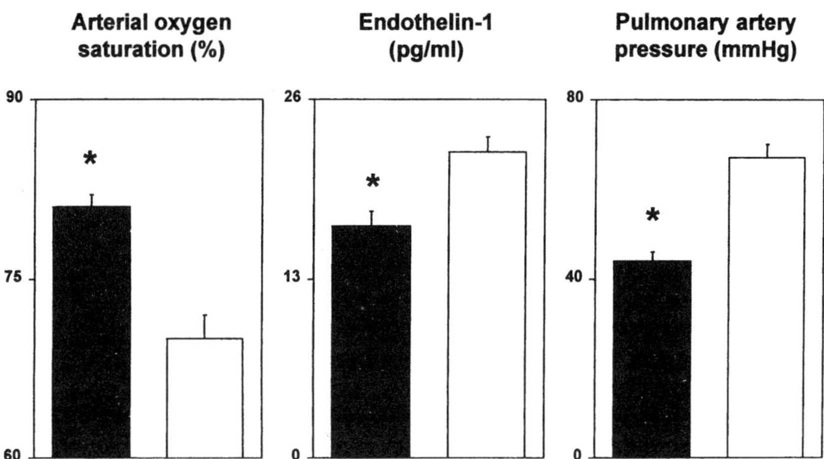

FIGURE 1.—Mean ± SE values at high altitude (4559 m) for arterial oxygen saturation (Sa_{O_2}), venous endothelin-1 plasma concentration and systolic pulmonary artery pressure in 16 mountaineers prone to high-altitude pulmonary edema (*open bars*) and 16 control subjects resistant to this condition (*filled bars*). *$P<.05$, patients versus control subjects. (Courtesy of Sartori C, Vollenweider L, Löffler B-M, et al: Exaggerated endothelin release in high-altitude pulmonary edema. *Circulation* 99:2665-2668, 1999.)

low altitude, pulmonary artery pressure and arterial oxygen saturation were similar in both groups, but endothelin-1 levels were higher in HAPE mountaineers than in control mountaineers (14.5 vs 11.8 pg/mL).

Conclusion.—Mountaineers susceptible to HAPE have higher plasma endothelin-1 levels than nonsusceptible mountaineers.

▶ Although the subject sample is relatively small, this article makes a good case for the involvement of an excessive production of endothelin-1 as a possible etiological factor in individuals who are unusually susceptible to HAPE. Not only could this hypothesis be tested by the administration of oral endothelin receptor antagonists, but such agents may offer a possible preventive therapy in the future.[1]

R. J. Shephard, MD, PhD, DPE

Reference

1. Chen SJ, Chen YF, Meng QC, et al: Endothelin-receptor antagonist bosentan prevents and reverses hypoxic pulmonary hypertension. *J Appl Physiol* 79:2122-2131, 1995.

High-Altitude Retinopathy and Altitude Illness
Wiedman M, Tabin GC (Harvard Med School, Boston; Univ of Vermont, Burlington)
Ophthalmology 106:1924-1927, 1999   7–6

Background.—Altitude illness consists of acute mountain sickness, high-altitude retinopathy (HAR), high-altitude cerebral edema (HACE),

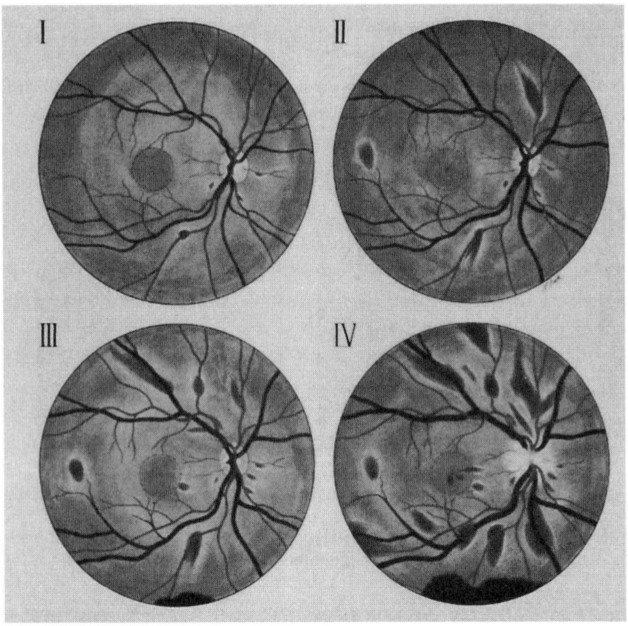

FIGURE 1.—Classification of high-altitude retinopathy. **Grade I:** A. Dilated retinal veins, B. Hemorrhages up to 1 disc area; **Grade II:** A. Moderately dilated retinal veins, B. Hemorrhages up to 2 disc areas; **Grade III:** A. Advanced dilated veins, B. (1) Hemorrhages up to 3 disc areas, (2) paramacular hemorrhage, or (3) vitreous hemorrhage, minor; **Grade IV:** A. Engorged retinal veins, B. (1) Hemorrhages over 3 disc areas, (2) macular hemorrhage, (3) vitreous hemorrhage, major, or (4) papilledema. (Courtesy of Wiedman M, Tabin GC: High-altitude retinopathy and altitude illness. *Ophthalmology* 106:1924-1927, copyright 1999 by Elsevier Science Inc.)

and high-altitude pulmonary edema. The relationship of HAR to other altitude-related illnesses was investigated, and a classification for HAR was established.

Methods.—Forty climbers in 3 Himalayan expeditions ascending to altitudes between 5000 and 8850 m feet above sea level were assessed. All participants had dilated fundus examinations before the climb, and intermittent fundus and medical examinations during the climb. Dilated fundus and medical examinations were repeated within 2 days of attaining the highest altitude.

Findings.—HAR developed in 19 of 21 climbers ascending to more than 7600 m. Fourteen of 19 climbers reaching 5000 to 7600 m had retinopathy. A grading system for HAR based on retinopathy severity was developed (Fig 1). When retinopathy was correlated with other altitude illness, acute mountain sickness was found to be endemic. In addition, HAR was significantly associated with HACE.

Conclusions.—On the basis of the proposed classification of HAR, empirical treatment with oxygen, steroids, diuretics, and immediate descent may be initiated to prevent HAR progression, macular involvement, or potentially fatal HACE. HAR is a significant component and predictor of progressive altitude sickness.

▶ HAR seems to be a very common problem in those climbing to extreme altitudes. Although in itself it is relatively benign, HAR can be an early harbinger of the much more dangerous condition of HACE.

R. J. Shephard, MD, PhD, DPE

Snorkelling Deaths in Australia, 1987-1996
Edmonds CW, Walker DG (Diving Med Ctr, St. Leonards, NSW, Australia; Project Stickybeak, Narrabeen, NSW, Australia)
Med J Aust 171:591-594, 1999   7–7

Introduction.—Snorkeling is an increasingly popular sport in Australia. There are few data on deaths related to snorkeling or breath-hold diving in any country. Australian deaths from snorkeling from 1987 to 1996 were analyzed.

Methods.—Data were gathered from a continuing study of diving fatalities and from coroners' offices. Additional information was obtained from police reports, members of the diving industry, and other sources to analyze the cause of death and the associated circumstances.

Results.—There were 60 snorkeling-related deaths during the period studied. The most frequent causes of death were drowning (27 cases) and cardiac events (18 cases). The remaining 12 research subjects died of hypoxia with breath-holding after hyperventilation and/or during ascent, leading to unconsciousness and, thus, to drowning. The average age was 45 years overall—57 years in divers who died of cardiac events versus 35 years in those who died of hypoxia. Fifteen of the deaths occurred in women. Drowning often occurred in overseas tourists, and most of the divers who died of cardiac events were middle-aged men. Young Australian men were most likely to die of breath-holding hypoxia. Except for the latter group, many of the deaths occurred in inexperienced divers. Only 4 deaths occurred in the presence of a "buddy" diver. Many of the research subjects who died of drowning or cardiac events were not wearing flippers. Fourteen deaths were related to adverse environmental conditions.

Conclusions.—Hyperventilating to increase breath-holding time is a dangerous practice than can lead to death from hypoxia. Recommended measures to prevent snorkeling deaths include wearing flippers and diving using a buddy system.

▶ Simple analysis of case or autopsy reports can sometimes provide very useful information. Our group[1] has long emphasized the importance of hypoxia subsequent to hyperventilation, originally described by Craig,[2] as a problem of snorkeling. Hypocapnia leads to apnea and a fall of oxygen pressure; not only does this confuse even an experienced diver but also gas expansion causes an even more dramatic drop in oxygen pressure if the diver attempts to surface. The high proportion of casualties among those lacking experience in local conditions and unable to communicate effectively with instructors is another important observation.

R. J. Shephard, MD, PhD, DPE

References

1. Shephard RJ: *Physiology and Biochemistry of Exercise.* New York, Praeger, 1982.
2. Craig AB: Causes of loss of consciousness during underwater swimming. *J Appl Physiol* 16:583-586, 1961.

Effect of Ambient Temperature on Human Skeletal Muscle Metabolism During Fatiguing Submaximal Exercise
Parkin JM, Carey MF, Zhao S, et al (Victoria Univ, Australia; Univ of Melbourne, Australia)
J Appl Physiol 86:902-908, 1999   7–8

Objective.—Fatigue during prolonged submaximal exercise results from glycogen depletion. Inosine 5'-monophosphate (IMP) has been shown to accumulate at fatigue during prolonged exercise when glycogen stores are low but not when they are high. Because exercise in heat increases intramuscular glycogen utilization, IMP accumulation would be expected to be low during prolonged submaximal exercise to fatigue in the heat. The effect of temperature on glycolytic rate during prolonged submaximal exercise to fatigue was investigated.

Methods.—Blood samples, rectal and muscle temperature, oxygen uptake, and respiratory exchange ratio were obtained from 8 male endurance athletes, average age 22.6 years, before and after exercising to exhaustion on a friction-braked cycle ergometer in 3 sessions at least 1 week apart. Each session was conducted at different temperatures, 3°C (cool, group CT), 20°C (thermoneutral, group NT), and 40°C (hot, group HT).

Results.—Oxygen uptake and respiratory exchange ratio were similar at all 3 temperatures. CT exercise time was significantly longer than NT exercise time, which was significantly longer than HT exercise time. Muscle temperatures were the same for all 3 trials at rest, but were significantly higher at fatigue compared with rest values. Muscle temperature at fatigue was significantly higher in HT than in NT or CT. Plasma epinephrine levels were similar at rest but were significantly higher after 20 minutes of exercise in the HT group compared with the NT or CT group and significantly higher in the NT group compared with the CT group. Muscle lactic acid levels, similar at rest in all 3 protocols, were significantly higher at fatigue in all trials and significantly higher in the HT group than in the CT group. Muscle ammonia concentrations were also significantly higher at fatigue than at rest in all trials. Muscle glycogen content at fatigue was significantly lower than at rest in all groups but was significantly greater in the HT protocol than in either the NT or CT protocol. The longer the exercise period, the greater the glycolytic rate. IMP concentrations at rest were not significantly different from those at fatigue, but there was a significant effect for exercise for this metabolite (Fig 4).

Conclusion.—IMP accumulates at fatigue after submaximal exercise when adequate glycogen stores are present. Fatigue during heat is appar-

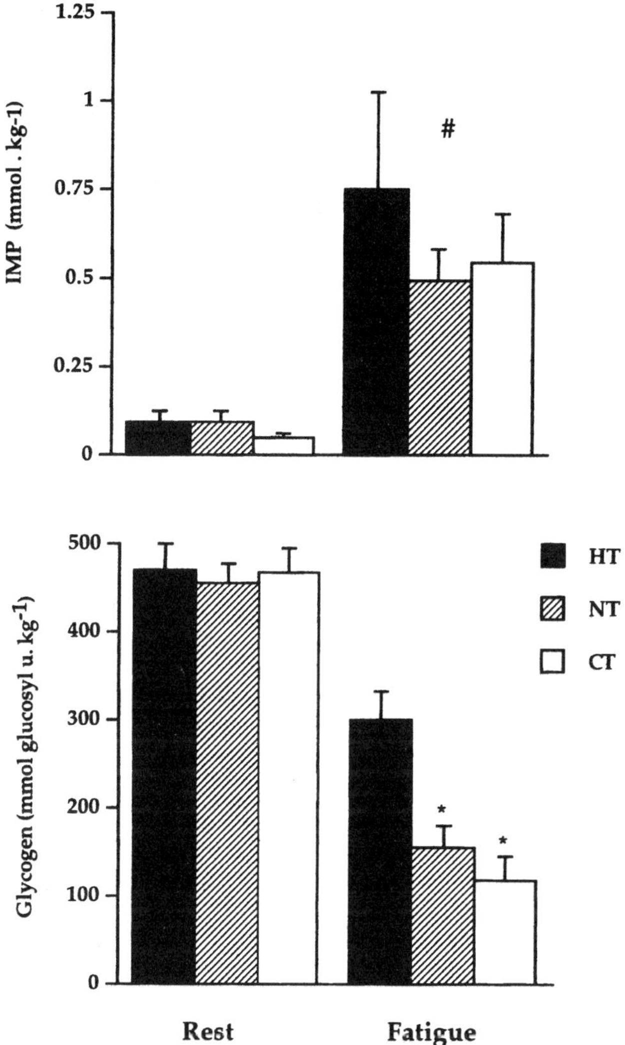

FIGURE 4.—IMP (*top*) and glycogen (*bottom*) before (Rest) and after (Fatigue) cycling exercise at 70% peak pulmonary oxygen uptake in hot temperatures (HT), thermoneutral temperatures (NT), and cool temperatures (CT). Values are means ± SE for 8 men. *Significantly different from HT, *P* less than .05. #Main effect for exercise, *P* less than .05. (Courtesy of Parkin JM, Carey MF, Zhao S, et al: Effect of ambient temperature on human skeletal muscle metabolism during fatiguing submaximal exercise. *J Appl Physiol* 86:902-908, 1999.)

ently caused by a metabolic perturbation that lowers the glycolytic rate and, therefore, the availability of energy.

▶ This study reported a reduction in exercise performance in the heat as compared with normal or cold temperatures. Muscle glycogen concentration was found to be higher at fatigue in high-temperature exercise than in exercise in colder temperatures. The results of this study suggest that fatigue during prolonged exercise in hot conditions is not related to carbohydrate availability. The increased endurance in cold temperatures as compared with normal temperatures is likely caused by a reduced rate of usage of glycogen. Fatigue under conditions of heat stress could indicate a temperature-induced metabolic perturbation that may include mitochondrial disruption. This disruption in mitochondrial function appears to decrease the rate of carbohydrate breakdown and the production of energy for exercise.

M. J. L. Alexander, PhD

Exertional Heat Illness and Hyponatremia in Hikers

Backer HD, Shopes E, Collins SL, et al (Kaiser Permanente Med Ctr, Hayward and Walnut Creek, Calif; Tucson Veterans Administration Med Ctr, Ariz; Dept of Emergency Med Service, Grand Canyon Natl Park; et al)
Am J Emerg Med 17:532-539, 1999   7–9

Background.—Heat exhaustion and heatstroke are the illnesses usually associated with exercise in hot environments. Because exercise-associated hyponatremia is also being identified in people who develop heat illnesses, the study was designed to clarify its characteristics, outline its clinical course, and provide a basis for differentiating it from heat exhaustion and heatstroke in a population of hikers in the Grand Canyon.

Methods.—Patients were chosen from among those who sought and required medical treatment from the emergency medical services provided at the Grand Canyon or the Grand Canyon Clinic. Serum samples were collected from 44 patients and analyzed for several parameters, including sodium, potassium, glucose, and urea nitrogen levels.

Results.—Hyponatremia was identified in 7 patients who had clinically significant symptoms (Table 2). Identifying characteristics included subtle altered mental status or seizures, without fever or hypoglycemia; other symptoms were nausea, vomiting, headache, and dizziness. Alterations in mental status and seizures tend to develop or progress after halting exercise. In this study, hyperhydration may have produced the low sodium levels, with hyponatremic patients drinking significantly more fluids than patients whose serum sodium levels were normal.

Conclusions.—It is possible that hyponatremia is a fairly common exercise-induced illness associated with hot environments. Because it is only later that the characteristic seizures and mental status changes occur, early hyponatremia may be mistakenly diagnosed as heat exhaustion.

▶ There is growing recognition that heat casualties include people with hyponatremia. However, there is less solid evidence that the patient should be blamed for an excessive fluid intake. In this study, those individuals with hyponatremia do appear to have drunk rather more than those with normal or increased sodium ion concentrations. But the volume of fluid ingested by the hyponatremic group, on average, 7.4 L/d, does not seem excessive in a

TABLE 2.—Hyponatremia Cases Identified Among Hikers in Grand Canyon, Arizona, 1993

No	Age	Sex	Medical/Exercise History	Onset of Major Symptoms/ Signs, GCS, Vital Signs	NA, K, Cl	Basis for Hydration Estimate	Treatment
1	50	F	Untrained, diabetes (glipizide as needed), levothyroxine sodium, conjugated estrogens	Day 2 in canyon after ascent: weak, shaky, vomiting; few hours later, after medical evaluation and 2 L IV NS: seizure; GCS = 9; BP = 120/90; P = 68; RR = 28	117, 3.9, 84	Clinically hydrated, urine SG 1.005, urine 609 mOsm/kg, urine Na 115 mmol/L	500 mL 3% NaCl; D/C day 3
2	64	F	No medical problems	Day 2 in canyon, 9-mi hike: vomiting, diarrhea; few hours after return to hotel: obtunded, seizures; GCS = 9; BP = 100/50; P = 96; RR = 24	109, 2.5	Drank "large amounts water," urine 476 mOsm/kg, urine Na 120 mmol/L; moderate diuresis day 2 in hospital	3% NaCl, then NS with KCl; D/C day 4
3	19	F	Untrained, no medical problems	1 day in canyon to river, on ascent halfway up: dizzy, nausea, vomiting; lethargic, disoriented; GCS = 9; BP = 116/78; P = 70; RR = 35	117, 2.8, 83	Estimates 10.5 L water; urine 569 mOsm/kg, urine Na 95 mmol/L; marked diuresis in hospital	NS with KCl; D/C day 4
4	21	F	Regular exercise, no medical problems	During full day of hiking in canyon: headache, dizzy, nausea, vomiting; at least 6 hours after return to cabin: seizure (lab after partial correction) GCS = 10; BP = 130/88; P = 88; RR = 16	127, 4.8	Estimate 4-6 L water; urinated 4-6 times in afternoon; frequent urination in clinic; urine SG 1.003	NS; D/C next day from clinic

(Continued)

TABLE 2 (cont.)

No	Age	Sex	Medical/Exercise History	Onset of Major Symptoms/ Signs, GCS, Vital Signs	NA, K, Cl	Basis for Hydration Estimate	Treatment
5	52	F	Migraines, sumatriptan taken morning prior to episode	1 day in canyon to river, on ascent 1.5 miles from top: chest pain, dizzy, nausea, lethargic; GCS = 14; BP = 107/74; P = 88; RR = 20	124, 4.3	Rest and 1.5 L fluid before evaluation; urine SG 1.005	2 L NS given in field; D/C day 2
6	45	F	No medical problems	Day 2 in canyon ascending from river, walked to clinic on rim: dizzy, nauseated, anxious, "disoriented"; GCS = 15; BP = 116/76; P = 76; RR = 16	127, 3.8	Forced fluids, about 8-9 L mostly sports drink; urine SG maximally dilute	Fluid restriction, salty snacks; D/C from clinic
7	23	M	Good health	1 day in canyon to river, on ascent 1.5 mi from top (14 h after starting); vomiting, diarrhea, dizzy, uncoordinated; while awaiting evacuation: combative, disoriented, muscle rigidity; GCS = 11; BP = 140/116; P = 85; R = 10	122, 2.9	Estimate 4 L water, 2 L sports drink; urine 518 mOsm/kg, urine Na 36 mmol/L; diuresed >3,200 mL, in hospital	NS with KCl; D/C day 2

Abbreviations: GCS, Glasgow coma score; *NS*, normal saline solution; *BP*, blood pressure; *P*, pulse rate; *RR*, respiratory rate; *SG*, specific gravity; *D/C*, discharge from treatment.
(Courtesy of Backer HD, Shopes E, Collins SL, et al: Exertional heat illness and hyponatremia in hikers. *Am J Emerg Med* 17:532-539, 1999.)

situation where sweat production may well have been as high as 2 L/hr. The methods section of this report suggests that "serum samples were consistently drawn from the sicker patients, who had. . .symptoms which *did not resolve rapidly with rehydration*" [italics added]. As in other reports of hyponatremia, one is left with the uncomfortable suspicion that, in at least some of these individuals, the problem may have arisen from injudicious administration of excessive quantities of IV fluid. It is quite difficult to drink to excess while exercising, but overhydration with an IV needle occurs all too quickly. The recent findings on the prevalence of hyponatremia underline the importance of obtaining serum sodium concentrations *before* IV therapy is instituted.

R. J. Shephard, MD, PhD, DPE

Sodium-Free Fluid Ingestion Decreases Plasma Sodium During Exercise in the Heat
Vrijens DMJ, Rehrer NJ (Otago Univ, Dunedin, New Zealand)
J Appl Physiol 86:1847-1851, 1999   7–10

Objective.—Exercise-induced hyponatremia can have serious consequences in athletes participating in prolonged endurance events. Its cause is unknown. Whether plasma sodium concentration was lowered by replacing sweat losses with a sodium-free beverage during exercise in the heat was assessed, and the change in plasma sodium was compared between water (W) and a sodium-containing sports drink.

Methods.—Maximal aerobic power and fluid needs were determined in 10 trained men, average age 24.8 years, during 1 hour using a cycle ergometer at 34°C and 65% relative humidity and during two 3-hour experimental periods during which the athletes exercised to voluntary exhaustion. Exercise intensity was geared to 55% of maximal oxygen intake. In a randomized crossover design, W or Gatorade (G) was provided every 15 minutes at a rate to equal fluid loss. Glucose, lactose, aldosterone, and plasma volume were determined from venous blood samples drawn after 15 and 30 minutes of exercise and at half-hour intervals thereafter.

Results.—Four participants completed the W trial, and 6 completed the G trial. The rate of plasma sodium change was significantly greater with W than with G (-2.48 vs -0.86 mmol/L/h) and was significantly and inversely correlated with exercise time (Fig 1). The rate of plasma sodium change and sweat rate were not correlated, but the rate of plasma sodium change and the rate of urine production were significantly and inversely correlated. Plasma glucose levels, but not lactate levels, decreased significantly with time in both trials, but the change was significantly greater during the W trial. Plasma aldosterone levels, heart rate, thermal response, and subjective rating of exertion increased similarly in both trials. Rate of perceived exertion and exercise time were significantly correlated.

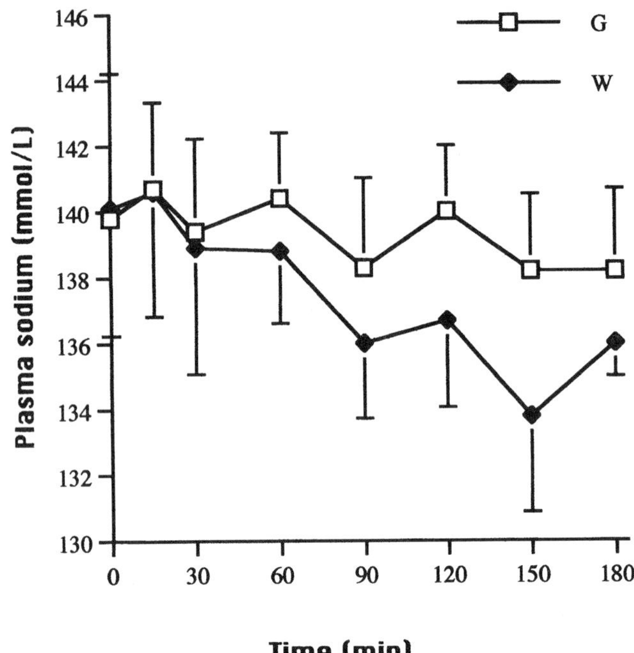

Time (min)

FIGURE 1.—Plasma sodium concentration during exercise in the heat in which fluid replacement was with either water (W) or a sodium-containing sports drink, Gatorade (G). Analysis of variance demonstrated a significantly greater decrease with W (P=.0007). (Courtesy of Vrijens DMJ, Rehrer NJ: Sodium-free fluid ingestion decreases plasma sodium during exercise in the heat. *J Appl Physiol* 86:1847-1851, 1999.)

Conclusion.—The risk of hyponatremia is increased when fluids lost during prolonged endurance exercise are replaced with sodium-free fluids.

▶ This article seemingly provides convincing evidence that plasma sodium falls over the course of 3 hours of vigorous exercise under hot and humid conditions (Fig 1). The data are at variance with the normal hypotonic sodium ion concentration in sweat. One possible explanation could be that the ingestion of water draws sodium ions into the gut.[1] However, closer inspection of the article suggests that the fall in plasma sodium had an iatrogenic origin; subjects drank water ad libitum prior to the trial, were then weighed, and given fluid at a rate to compensate for the decrease in weight seen in a 1-hour pretrial. They probably began the trial somewhat hyperhydrated and, with a likely depletion of glycogen reserves over the 3 hours of exercise, the observed 0.6 kg weight loss would have been equivalent to a further 1.4 L excess of fluid intake, because of a mobilization of the water reserves associated with the glycogen molecule.[2] Plainly, there is a need for caution in urging water upon long-distance exercisers, as in some cases people ingest excessive amounts.

R. J. Shephard, MD, PhD, DPE

References

1. Noakes, TD: The hyponatremia of exercise. *Int J Sport Nutr* 2: 205-228, 1992.
2. Shephard, RJ: *Physiology and Biochemistry of Exercise*. New York, Praeger, 1982.

Keeping Sports Participants Safe in Hot Weather
Sparling PB, Millard-Stafford M (Georgia Inst of Technology, Atlanta)
Physician Sportsmed 27:27-34, 1999   7–11

Objective.—Hot-weather event planning is important to prevent heat-related illness in athletes. Metabolic heat is dissipated primarily through the skin at rest and primarily by sweating during exercise. When the temperature is high, cutaneous blood flow is increased and blood supply to working muscles is decreased lowering performance. In high humidity, vaporizing of sweat is greatly diminished. Acclimatization periods of 10 to 14 days for athletes are important. Fluid-replacement programs using formulated electrolyte rehydration solutions, hyperhydration before exercise, and postexercise rehydration are necessary.

Hot-Weather Event Planning: The Atlanta Olympic Experience.—Endurance events were scheduled when heat stress (measured using the wet bulb globe temperature) would be lowest. Spectators and volunteers accounted for most medical visits. Heat tolerance problems were the result of poor fitness, poor acclimatization, dehydration, improper clothing, obesity, physical exertion, and prolonged heat exposure in most patients. Few spectators and athletes needed treatment, probably because most people heeded warnings and took precautions.

Conclusion.—Acclimatization and drinking of formulated electrolyte solutions before and after exercise can avoid heat-related illness in athletes.

▶ The authors stress the important role that conditioning plays in heat acclimatization. They state that "regular vigorous training induces 'internal heat stress,' which enhances the physiologic adaptations that are similar to acclimatization." They also state that "the old rule that only water or a dilute sports drink should be consumed in the heat is not justified by current research." For postexercise rehydration, they state that sodium replacement maximizes rehydration.

F. J. George, ATC, PT

Exercise in the Heat: I. Fundamentals of Thermal Physiology, Performance Implications, and Dehydration
Casa DJ (Univ of Connecticut, Storrs)
J Athletic Train 34:246-252, 1999   7–12

Introduction.—Exercise in the heat produces physiologic changes in many body systems, including the circulatory, thermoregulatory, and en-

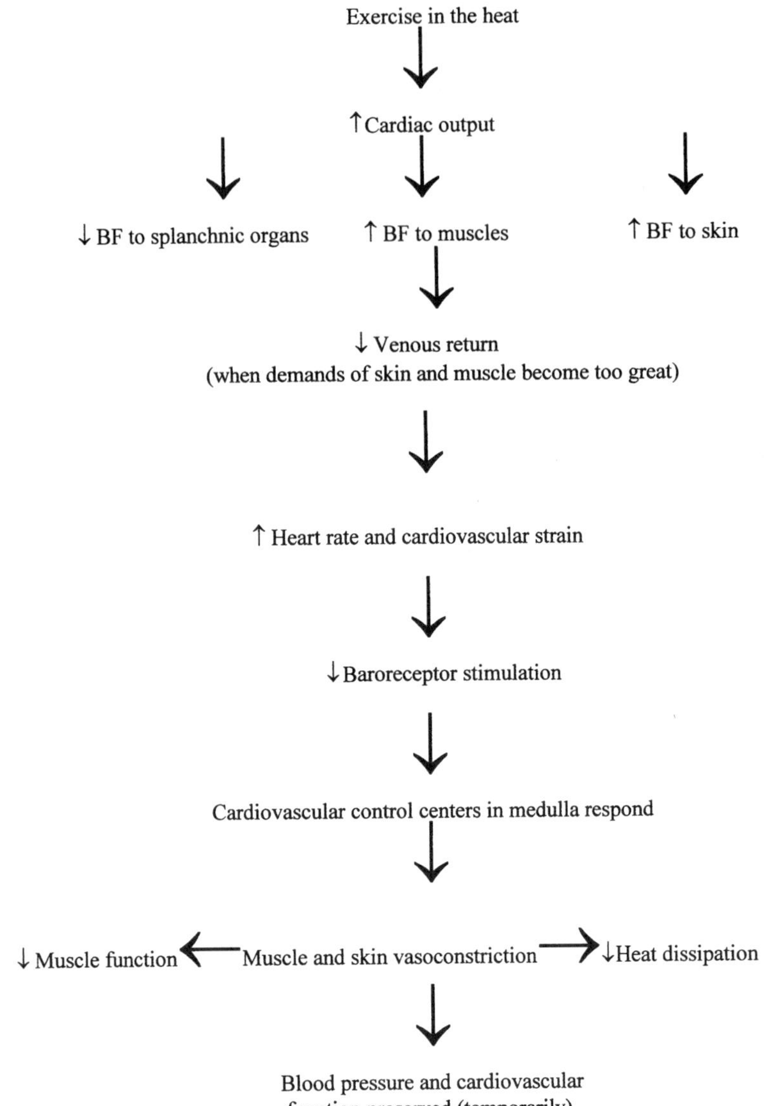

FIGURE 1.—Potential circulatory responses to exercise in the heat. *Abbreviation*: **BF**, blood flow. (Courtesy of Casa DJ: Exercise in the heat: I. Fundamentals of thermal physiology, performance implications, and dehydration. *J Athletic Train* 34:246-252, 1999.)

docrine systems. In a hot environment, the body is prone to overloading its ability to respond to stress, resulting in hyperthermia, dehydration, reduced physical and mental performance, and exertional heat illness. The physiologic principles of the body's response to exercise in the heat were reviewed.

Responses to Exercise in the Heat.—During intense exercise in the heat, the cardiovascular system cannot simultaneously meet the demands of the skin to reduce thermal load and the demands of muscle to increase blood supply. As a result, maintenance of blood pressure takes precedence over other needs (Fig 1). This can lead to hyperthermia and metabolic inefficiency. The circulatory and thermoregulatory responses are closely linked. Heat gain must be matched by heat dissipation if exercise is to continue. The ability to dissipate heat decreases as the ambient temperature increases. In a warm humid environment, heat dissipation cannot occur by any means: convection, radiation, or evaporation. This leads to dehydration with a rapid rise in core temperature.

Effects of Heat on Performance.—All of these stresses combine to impair exercise performance. Previous studies suggest that heat stress and dehydration act independently to compromise physiologic function, ultimately limiting the supply of oxygenated blood to the body. Reduced performance and thermal strain result from the combination of excess heat and decreased muscle performance. Dehydration produces fluid redistribution, ultimately leading to hypervolemic hyperosmolality. The precise means by which hyperosmolality affects the thermoregulatory system is unknown, but it is likely that both hyperosmolality and hypovolemia contribute to disturbed body fluid regulation. Reductions in muscle strength seem to occur when dehydration exceeds a 5% reduction in body weight. Endurance may decline at a dehydration level of 3% to 4% and maximal aerobic power at 2% to 3%.

Discussion.—This information on the basic physiologic and performance responses to exercise in the heat will be useful in supervising athletes who exercise in hot environments.

▶ Athletes exercising in heat and high humidity are subject to numerous physiologic changes, some of which may be serious. It is essential that coaches and athletic trainers understand these changes and how best to cope with them. These changes may affect performance as well as safety.

F. J. George, ATC, PT

Exercise in the Heat II. Critical Concepts in Rehydration, Exertional Heat Illnesses, and Maximizing Athletic Performance
Casa DJ (Univ of Connecticut, Storrs)
J Athletic Train 34:253-262, 1999   7–13

Objective.—Numerous factors contribute to rehydration of athletes who exercise in hot environments, including the specific environment, the timing of rehydration, and the type of rehydration.

Rehydration and Exercise.—Physiologic stress, psychologic variables, characteristics of the rehydration fluid, mood, and degree of concentration influence rehydration. The athlete should be well hydrated with properly balanced electrolytes before beginning exercise. Hyperhydration appears

TABLE 4.—When Athletes Exercise in the Heat: A Checklist for the Athletic Trainer

1. Pre-event preparation
——Am I challenging unsafe rules (eg, a 10K track runner may not be able to receive fluids; can these rules be changed to maximize safety?)?
——Am I encouraging athletes to drink before the onset of thirst?
——Am I familiar with which athletes have a history of a heat illness?
——Am I discouraging alcohol, caffeine, and drug use before and during exercise?
——Am I encouraging proper acclimatization procedures?
2. Checking hydration status
——Do I know the pre-exercise weight of the athletes I work with (to allow percentage of dehydration to be determined during and after practice or competition)?
——Are the athletes familiar with how to assess urine color? Is a urine color chart accessible?
——Do the athletes know their sweat rates so they know how much to drink during exercise?
——Is a refractometer present to double-check hydration status?
3. Environmental assessment
——Am I regularly checking the wet-bulb globe temperature (WBGT) during the day?
——Am I knowledgeable about the risk categories of a heat illness based on the WBGT?
——Are alternate plans made in case a high WBGT forces a rescheduling of events or practices?
4. Coaches' and athletes' responsibilities
——Are the coaches and athletes educated about the signs and symptoms of heat illnesses?
——Are athletes properly prehydrated for the activity?
——Am I double-checking to make sure coaches are allowing ample rest and rehydration breaks?
——Are modifications being made to reduce risk in the heat (eg, decrease in intensity, change practices to morning or evening, more frequent breaks, elimination of double sessions, reduction or change in equipment, clothing requirements, etc)?
——Are rapid weight-loss practices in weight-class sports adamantly disallowed?
5. Event management
——Have I checked to make sure proper amounts of fluids will be available and accessible?
——Are carbohydrate-electrolyte drinks available at events and practices lasting longer than 50 to 60 minutes and those that are extremly intense in nature?
——Am I aware of the factors that may increase the likelihood of a heat illness?
——Am I promptly rehydrating athletes to pre-exercise weight after an exercise session?
——Are shaded or indoor areas used for practices when possible, to minimize thermal strain?
6. Treatment considerations
——Am I familiar with the most common early signs and symptoms of a heat illness?
——Do I have the proper field equipment and skills to assess a heat illness?
——Is an emergency plan in place in case an immediate evacuation is needed?
——Is a kiddy pool available in situations of high risk in order to initiate immediate cold/ice-water immersion of heatstroke patients?
——Are ice bags available for immediate cooling when ice-water immersion is not possible?
——Have shaded, air-conditioned, and cool areas been identified to use when athletes need to cool down, recover, or receive treatment? Are fans available to assist evaporation when cooling?
——Am I properly equipped to assess high core temperatures?
7. Other situation-specific considerations

(Courtesy of Casa DJ: Exercise in the heat. II. Critical concepts in rehydration, exertional heat illnesses, and maximizing athletic performance. *J Athletic Train* 34:253-262, 1999.)

to reduce thermal strain and cardiovascular strain and increase exercise time and plasma volume. Rehydration during exercise enhances heat dissipation, limits plasma hypertonicity, maintains perfusion of working muscles, limits the degree of hyperthermia, and maintains athletic performance. Rehydration during exercise depends on rates of gastric emptying and intestinal absorption. Fluid intake should ideally be matched with sweating rate and urine volume.

Intravenous Rehydration and Exercise.—IV rehydration after exercise is standard treatment to restore physiologic function. IV rehydration before exercise has been shown to reduce cardiovascular and thermoregulatory strain and improve heart rate, core temperature, forearm blood flow, and plasma volume.

Exertional Heat Illnesses.—These illnesses include heat cramps (least serious), heat exhaustion (most common), and exertional heat stroke. Respective symptoms include spastic cramping; headache, weakness, dizziness, vertigo, heat sensations, nausea, vomiting, sweating, syncope, elevated pulse rate, and high blood pressure; and thermoregulatory failure and mental impairment. These illnesses can be prevented by knowledge in athletes, coaches, and medical staff, regular use of rehydration fluids and cooling equipment, modification of practice schedules, and an action plan in case of illness.

Maximizing Athletic Performance in the Heat.—A checklist is presented (Table 4).

Conclusion.—Proper hydration/rehydration for maximizing performance and minimizing risks of athletes exercising in the heat requires a coordinated plan that educates athlete trainers and athletes alike and focuses on safety first and performance second.

▶ Exertional heat illness is a problem we encounter every summer and early fall. Table 4 should help us prepare for and prevent this emergency from occurring. Mandatory hyperhydration before an event is a must. Rehydrating during and after the event is essential. It takes a great deal of effort and cooperation between coach, athlete, and athletic trainer to conquer this problem.

F. J. George, ATC, PT

Physiological Responses of Exercised-Fatigued Individuals Exposed to Wet-Cold Conditions

Tikuisis P, Ducharme MB, Moroz D, et al (Human Protection and Performance, Toronto)
J Appl Physiol 86:1319-1328, 1999
7–14

Objective.—Vasoconstriction and shivering protect cold-exposed individuals against hypothermia. Ability to produce heat through shivering has an important impact on survival time, particularly if the ability to exercise is limited. Exercise fatigue could impair shivering response. The effects of exercise fatigue on shivering response and the resultant heat debt during a very stressful sedentary wet-cold exposure were tested with pre-exposure exercise (fatigue) and without (control) to compare shivering responses using a repeated-measures design.

Methods.—Thirteen fit, nonsmoking, male volunteers performed cycling, rowing, and treadmill walking for 1 hour each separated by additional 1-hour sessions of resistance exercises for a total of approximately 5 hours. Immediately after exercise (fatigue group) or rest (control group), individuals, wearing only T-shirts and shorts, were exposed to calm air at 10°C for 30 minutes. Then their backs were exposed to 6 km/h wind and a 10°C water shower at about 920 mL/min for the rest of the time up to an additional 4 hours. Venous blood samples were analyzed for energy metabolites, hormones, indices of hydration, neurotransmitters, and thyroid hormones.

Results.—Individuals had more complaints during fatigue exposure and more requests for termination, but there was no significant difference in exposure between the control and fatigue groups (197 vs 172 minutes). Duration of exposure was significantly correlated to body fatness ($r=0.653$) and body mass index but not to oxygen consumption. The fatigue group was more dependent on fat metabolism for shivering thermogenesis than was the control group. Other studies have shown that prolonged exercise increases fat metabolism. The fatigue group and the control group shivered at the same intensity because of the body's ability to utilize available energy-producing substrates. There were no differences in metabolic variables and core temperature during cold stress between rested and recently fatigued individuals. There was no evidence of shivering fatigue despite muscle fatigue or muscle damage from exercise. Although a high metabolic rate is needed to prevent or delay hypothermia, lack of body fat makes it more difficult to contain this heat. Low body fat rather than rapid core cooling contributes to hypothermia after exercise fatigue, although the impact of exercise fatigue on the shivering response cannot be ruled out. Subject 12 had a metabolic rate during fatigue cold exposure that was 35% higher than during the control phase.

Conclusion.—The rate of core cooling appears to be related to low body fat and low shivering intensity. The latter cannot be related necessarily to exercise fatigue but may simply be the result of a lack of shivering drive in certain individuals. This may explain why some individuals survive cold exposure conditions that others do not.

► Hypothermia is defined as an abnormal and dangerous condition in which the temperature of the body is below 35°C. According to most textbooks, the people most likely to experience hypothermia are those who are very old, very young, or very lean; those who have heart or circulation problems; and people who are hungry, tired, or under the influence of alcohol or other drugs. Common causes include: falling overboard from a boat into cold water, being outside with an uncovered head in winter, wearing wet clothing for a prolonged period of time in windy weather, heavy exertion, or poor fluid or food intake.

In this study of 13 healthy and fit men, Tikuisis et al challenge the assumption that exercise fatigue impairs the shivering response and ability to withstand wet-cold conditions. Despite 5 hours of exertion prior to cold exposure, research subjects were able to shiver at the same intensity as measured when individuals avoided exercise. The wide subject variability in the rate of core cooling was best explained by low body fatness and a low shivering intensity, the latter apparently unrelated to exercise fatigue. The authors speculated that some individuals simply lack the shivering "drive" necessary to combat cold exposure.

D. C. Nieman, PhD

Recognizing and Treating Common Cold-induced Injury in Outdoor Sports

Sallis R, Chassay CM (Kaiser Permanente Med Ctr, Fontana, Calif; Univ of Texas, Austin)
Med Sci Sports Exerc 31:1367-1373, 1999   7–15

Objective.—Although core body temperature must remain between 25° and 40.5°C (75° to 105°F), body temperature may fluctuate widely. Participation in outdoor winter sports can lead to cold-induced injuries because of cold-weakened and slowed muscle contractions and delayed nerve conduction times. Sports physicians need to be able to recognize and know how to treat cold-induced injuries.

Cold-induced Injuries.—Hypothermia is most likely to occur in infants and the elderly and is worsened by drugs that act on the CNS. Because clinical thermometers can overestimate core temperature, rectal or esophageal readings should be obtained. A shivering patient will probably have a core temperature >32°C (>90°F), but a nonshivering patient or a patient with impaired consciousness usually has a lower core temperature. Basic life support techniques should be instituted. Endotracheal intubation should be performed carefully. CPR should be instituted in patients with nonperfusing cardiac rhythm only after the pulse is monitored for 1 minute to avoid inappropriate chest compression that can result in a lethal cardiac rhythm. In patients with ventricular fibrillation, core temperature should be >30°C (86°F) before defibrillation is attempted. Oxygen and fluids should be warmed. Active external rewarming can be used to supplement passive rewarming. Because hypothermic patients have decreased oxygen requirements, the usual criteria for death do not apply. Resuscitation efforts should be ongoing until the patient is completely rewarmed. Frostbite occurs in 4 phases: pre-freeze, freeze-thaw, vascular stasis, and ischemic phase. Rewarming should be rapid (Table 2) but should be avoided during transport. Débridement of blisters or débridement and amputation of gangrenous areas may be necessary, although gangrene may not appear for months.

Nonfreezing Cold-induced Injuries.—Treatment for immersion (trench) foot, and chilblains or cold sores is conservative. Raynaud syndrome is an idiopathic disorder that results in a decrease in digital artery diameter on cold challenge. If conservative treatment fails, prophylaxis with vasodilators, reserpine, or calcium channel blockers may be necessary. Some patients may require sympathectomy. Urticaria or anaphylaxis that is cold-induced is treated by prevention and prophylaxis. Cold-induced asthma is treated with β-agonist inhalants.

Adverse Effects of Cryotherapy.—Cryotherapeutic treatment of soft tissue injury and inflammation should be used cautiously.

Prevention of Cold-induced Injury.—Wear layers of loose-fitting clothing, avoid overheating, and avoid cotton clothing. Wear wool, treated polyesters, and blends of wool and synthetics. Wear several pairs of socks

---

TABLE 2.—Protocol for Rapid Rewarming Treatment of Frostbite

1. Admit frostbite patients to specialized unit if possible.
2. Retain victims of acute frostbite requiring hospitalization unless transfer to other facility is necessary for specialized care. Protect victims from cold exposure during transfer.
3. At admission, rapidly rewarm affected areas in warm water (4°-42°C; 104°-108°F) for 15 to 30 minutes or until thawing is complete.
4. After rewarming:
   Debride white blisters, apply aloe vera topically every 6 hours.
   Leave hemorrhagic blisters intact, apply aloe vera topically every 6 hours.
   Elevate affected part(s), splint as needed.
   Administer antitetanus proplylaxis.
   For analgesia, administer morphine or meperidine intravenously or intramuscularly as needed.
   Administer 400 mg ibuprofen orally every 12 hours.
   Administer 500,000 IV penicillin G intravenously every 6 hours for 48 to 72 hours.
   Give hydrotherapy daily for 30-45 minutes at 40°C (104°F):
   a. For large (425-gal) tank capacity, fill with 285 gal water containing 9.7 kg NaCl and 95 mL calcium hypochlorite solution.
   b. For medium (270-gal) tank capacity, fill with 108 gal water containing 3.7 kg NaCl and 36 mL calcium hypochlorite solution.
   c. For small (95-gal) tank capacity, fill with 72 gal water containing 2.5 kg NaCl, 71 g KCl, and 24-mL calcium hypochlorite solution.
5. To document, photograph affected areas at admission, at 24 hours, and serially every 2 to 3 days until patient is discharged.
6. At discharge, give patients specific instructions to protect injured areas, avoid reinjury, and follow up weekly until wounds are stable. If no exposed lesions, instruct patient to wear wool socks, a hat, and mittens instead of gloves to decrease interdigital heat loss. Explain that patients are more susceptible to refreezing and so should avoid exposure to cold and wear warm clothing, shoes, or boots if outdoor activity is necessary. Similarly, instruct patients who have exposed lesions at discharge, and instruct to keep affected extremity elevated and take 400 mg ibuprofen orally every 12 hours. For all patients, aloe vera should be applied to affected areas; if open areas are small, scarlet red ointment should be used instead.

(From Sallis R, Chassay CM: Recognizing and treating common cold-induced injury in outdoor sports. *Med Sci Sports Exerc* 31:1367-1373, 1999.)

---

and several pairs of gloves. Wear ski caps to protect ears and nose, and goggles to protect eyes.

Conclusion.—The best way to protect athletes against cold-induced injuries is to counsel them about avoiding injury and to wear appropriate clothing.

▶ Clinicians should be aware that cryotherapy should be used properly, especially when applied over the ulnar or peroneal nerves. Many clinicians use a thin layer of wet toweling over those areas to avoid nerve palsy.

The authors recommend several loosely fitting layers of insulation, including polypropylene, wool, treated polyesters, water repellant fabric, and blends of wool and synthetics. They also state that cotton fabrics should be avoided.

F. J. George, ATC, PT

Circulating Venous Bubbles in Recreational Diving: Relationships With Age, Weight, Maximal Oxygen Uptake and Body Fat Percentage

Carturan D, Boussuges A, Burnet H, et al (Faculté des Sciences du Sport, Luminy, Marseille, France; Hôpital Salvator, Marseille, France; CNRS, Marseille, France; et al)
Int J Sports Med 20:410-414, 1999   7–16

Objective.—Intravascular bubbles are thought to be the cause of decompression sickness in recreational scuba divers. Age, body mass, body fat weight, and fitness affect the grade of bubbles detected during decompression. With continuous Doppler monitoring, the effects of these variables on grades of bubbles were investigated in male recreational scuba divers.

Methods.—Forty male recreational divers, who had not dived in 48 hours, descended to 35 m in sea water for a total bottom time of 25 minutes. Decompression was performed during an ascent rate of 9 m/min according to the COMEX 1987 decompression table, with decompression

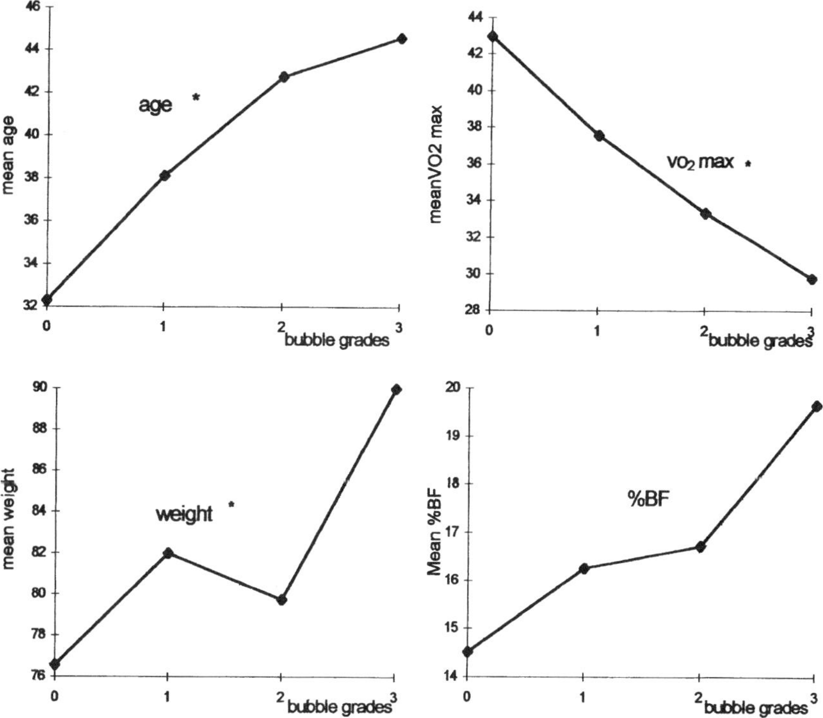

FIGURE 1.—Relationships between bubble grades and variables: the difference between the average values of age, weight, and maximal oxygen uptake ($\dot{V}O_2max$) is significant ($P < .05$) at grade 0 and grade 3 (*asterisk*). *Abbreviation: BF,* body fat. (Courtesy of Carturan D, Boussuges A, Burnet H, et al: Circulating venous bubbles in recreational diving: Relationships with age, weight, maximal oxygen uptake and body fat percentage. *Int J Sports Med* 20:410-414. Copyright 1999, Georg Thieme Verlag.)

stops at 6 m for 3 minutes and at 3 m for 15 minutes. Ascent and decompression stops were not included in bottom time. Bubble detection was performed 60 minutes after surfacing. The relationship of age, body mass, maximal oxygen intake, and percentage of body fat to bubble grades was evaluated.

Results.—Age, body mass, and maximal oxygen intake significantly affected bubble grade, particularly between grades 0 and 3 (Fig 1). Spearman correlation coefficients with respect to bubble grade were $P = .486$ for age, $P = .463$ for body mass, and $P = -.481$ for maximal oxygen intake.

Conclusion.—The probability of decompression sickness can be reduced if decompression tables take individual risk factors into account.

▶ The adverse impact of age, obesity, and a poor level of physical fitness on the risk of decompression sickness[1,2] was certainly well recognized when I was serving in the Royal Air Force almost 50 years ago. However, the formation of IV bubbles has been regarded as a chaotic phenomenon, with no obvious predisposing factors.[3] This report shows that given a substantial sample of divers, with an adequate dispersion of ages, body fat content, and fitness levels, these variables show significant correlation with bubble formation, thus opening up the possibility of developing individualized diving tables. The best preventive tactic remains to decrease body fat and to maximize physical fitness, but individualized tables may be a further method of reducing the incidence of clinically significant decompression sickness.

R. J. Shephard, MD, PhD, DPE

References

1. Dembert ML, Jekel JF, Mooley LW: Health risk factors for the development of decompression sickness among US Navy divers. *Undersea Biomed Res* 11:395-406, 1984.
2. Mebane GY, McIver NKI: Fitness to dive, in Bennett PB, Elliott DH (eds): *The Physiology and Medicine of Diving*, ed 4. London, WB Saunders, 1993, pp 52-76.
3. Powell M: The chaotic nature of decompression. *Aquacorps J* 5:12-14, 1993.

Randomized Trial of Physical Exercise Alone or Combined With Bright Light on Mood and Health-related Quality of Life
Partonen T, Leppämäki S, Hurme LJ, et al (Univ of Helsinki; Natl Public Health Inst, Helsinki)
Psychol Med 28:1359-1364, 1998   7–17

Objective.—Approximately 10% to 15% of primary care patients experience atypical prolonged depressive symptoms in the winter, including carbohydrate craving, prolonged sleep, weight gain, and increased appetite as a result of low light levels. The effect on mood and health-related quality of life of winter exercise alone or combined with bright light was tested in a randomized controlled trial of employees in southern Finland.

Methods.—Between November and January, 120 indoor employees in southern Finland were randomly allocated to supervised fitness training in bright (2500-4000 lux) light (group A), fitness training in ordinary (400-600 lux) room light (group B), or relaxation training (group C) for 1 hour 2 or 3 times weekly for 8 weeks. Participants completed the Seasonal Pattern Assessment Questionnaire at baseline, the revised version of the Structured Interview Guide for the Hamilton Depression Rating Scale - Seasonal Affective Disorders Version Self-Rating Format (SIGH-SAD-SR) and the RAND 36-item Health Survey 1.0 (RAND) at weeks 4 and 8, and the RAND and the SIGH-SAD-SR at 4 months' follow-up.

Results.—Of the 115 participants who entered the study, 82 completed it. Physical exercise in bright light was significantly more effective at elevating mood than physical exercise in ordinary room light or relaxation training alone. Physical training alone was only slightly more effective than relaxation exercises alone. The beneficial effects had disappeared at the 4-month follow-up assessment.

Conclusion.—Supervised physical exercise in bright light may be an effective intervention for treating individuals with seasonal affective disorder. The effectiveness of the intervention wears off quickly after the exercises are stopped.

▶ This important study from a group of researchers in Finland shows that atypical depressive symptoms can be reduced in employees who exercise in a gym with bright lights. Although the researchers utilized a control group of subjects who took part in relaxation sessions in a dimly lit room for 1 hour per week, it would have been useful to include a fourth group exposed to bright lights only (without exercise). Previous research has shown that bright lights alone (ie, phototherapy) can diminish symptoms associated with seasonal affective disorder.[1]

D. C. Nieman, PhD

Reference

1. Kasper S, Rogers SLB, Yancey A, et al: Phototherapy in individuals with and without subsyndromal seasonal affective disorder. *Arch Gen Psychiatry* 46:837-844, 1989.

Is Sleep Disturbed by Vigorous Late-Night Exercise?
Youngstedt SD, Kripke DF, Elliott JA (Univ of California, San Diego)
Med Sci Sports Exerc 31:864-869, 1999   7–18

Objective.—Whether vigorous exercise before bedtime impairs sleep is controversial. Most individuals who exercise in the late evening report improved ability to fall asleep (65%), improved depth of sleep (62%), and feeling better in the morning (60%). Exercise close to bedtime may reduce anxiety and cool the core body temperature. The influence of prolonged, exhaustive presleep exercise on sleep was investigated.

Methods.—Baseline sleep data were collected for 1 week from 16 highly fit competitive male cyclists, aged 22 to 36 years. The participants completed two 60-hour laboratory protocols, separated by 2 to 4 weeks, consisting of a baseline night (NIGHT 1), exercise and bright light or bright light only (NIGHT 2), and a recovery night (NIGHT 3). The exercise plus bright light protocol consisted of cycling at 65% to 75% of heart rate for 3 hours under 3000 lux light. Under the bright light only protocol, volunteers were exposed to 3000 lux light for 3 hours while reading and/or watching TV. Both 3-hour treatments were scheduled 6 hours before the volunteer's usual wake time. After the treatments, the volunteers showered for 5 to 10 minutes and went to bed exactly 30 minutes after completing exercise. Volunteers were wakened at their usual time. The duration of sleep on NIGHT 2 was 4 hours.

Results.—Sleep onset latency, wakefulness after sleep onset, and total sleep time were similar for exercise plus bright light and bright light only.

Conclusion.—Vigorous exercise before bedtime does not disturb sleep, at least in the physically fit. Fitness allows quick recovery of sympathetic nervous system arousal after exercise.

▶ According to the Better Sleep Council:
"Exercise enhances sleep by burning off the tensions that accumulate during the day, allowing both body and mind to unwind. Although the fit seem to sleep better and deeper. . .you don't have to push to utter exhaustion. A 20- to 30-minute walk, jog, swim, or bicycle ride at least 3 days a week. . .should be your goal. But don't wait until too late in the day to exercise. In the evening, you should be concentrating on winding down rather than working up a sweat. . .The ideal exercise time is late afternoon or early evening, when your workout can help you shift gears from daytime pressures to evening pleasures."[1]

It now appears that this long-held assumption may be wrong. In the study by Youngstedt et al, the addition of an intense 3-hour cycling bout to bright light exposure 30 minutes before bedtime failed to alter sleep compared with bright light alone. Thus, late-night exercise may not disturb sleep, allowing people who travel or work late to squeeze in a healthful workout before they go to bed.

D. C. Nieman, PhD

Reference

1. Better Sleep Council: *The Sleep Better, Live Better Guide.* Washington, D.C., Better Sleep Council, 1990.

Stability, Precision, and Near–24-Hour Period of the Human Circadian Pacemaker
Czeisler CA, Duffy JF, Shanahan TL, et al (Harvard Med School, Boston; Harvard Univ, Cambridge)
Science 284:2177-2181, 1999   7–19

Objective.—Endogenous circadian rhythm exists in almost all organisms, usually lasts 24 hours, and varies little within a given species. An age-related shortening of circadian rhythm is thought to be responsible for the early-morning wakening in the elderly. Attempts of quantification of the circadian period have led to results that vary from 13 to 65 hours, whereas the average free-running circadian period of the human body temperature varies between 24.2 and 25.1 hours. The free-running circadian period in humans can be influenced by activity, knowledge of the time of day, and exposure to ordinary indoor light. The intrinsic period of the circadian pacemaker was determined in 24 individuals living for 1 month in an environment free of time cues under conditions of controlled exposure to the light-dark cycle on a forced desynchrony protocol.

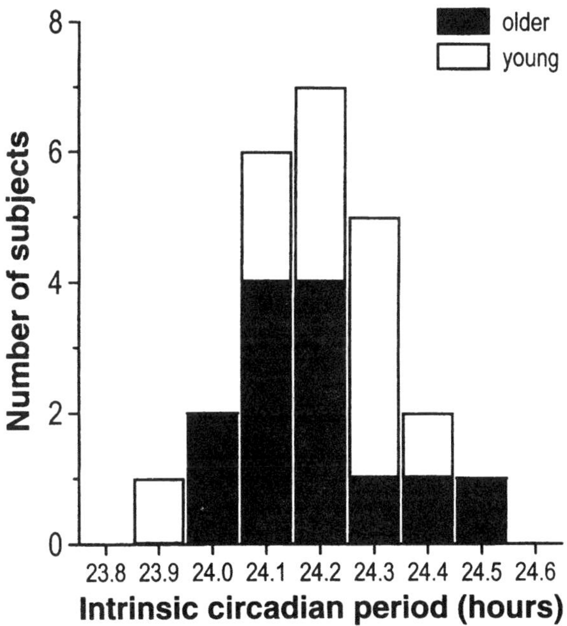

FIGURE 2.—Histogram of intrinsic circadian period (τ) estimates derived from young and older subjects. Intrinsic circadian period estimates of older subjects are indicated by *solid bars*, those of young subjects by *open bars*. Each subject's estimated intrinsic circadian period is reported as the average of the estimated periods from the individual's core body temperature, melatonin, and cortisol rhythms. (Reprinted with permission from *Science*, courtesy of Czeisler CA, Duffy JF, Shanahan TL, et al: Stability, precision, and near–24-hour period of the human circadian pacemaker. *Science* 284:2177-2181, 1999, copyright 1999, American Association for the Advancement of Science.)

Methods.—Eleven men (average age, 23.7 years) and 13 individuals (4 women), with an average age of 67.4 years, lived for 29 to 38 days on a 28-hour day. Core body temperature and plasma melatonin and plasma cortisol levels were measured.

Results.—Core body temperature and plasma melatonin and plasma cortisol levels were significantly correlated for each individual. Circadian periods varied between 24.00 and 24.35 hours and averaged 24.18 hours for 90% of individuals (Fig 2). The intrinsic periods for the 20- and 28-hour cycles were 24.29 and 24.38 hours, respectively.

Conclusion.—The human circadian pacemaker is as accurate as that of other mammals and involves a similar molecular regulating mechanism.

▶ Do humans have a different circadian period than other living organisms? Is the circadian period different in young and old humans? This study indicates that the answers to both of these questions is "No." Little variance was measured in the intrinsic circadian period estimates from the 24 subjects, with nearly 90% between 24.00 and 24.35 hours. The average circadian periods for the young and old subjects were nearly identical, negating the hypothesis that an age-related shortening of the circadian period accounts for the early-morning awakening observed frequently in the elderly.

D. C. Nieman, PhD

Evaluation of the Ergogenic Properties of Ginseng: An Update
Bahrke MS, Morgan WP (Human Kinetics, Champaign, Ill; Univ of Wisconsin-Madison)
Sports Med 29:113-133, 2000

7–20

Objective.—Although animal studies have demonstrated the effectiveness of ginseng to prolong survival and to reduce physical or chemical stress, there is a lack of controlled studies of ginseng's effectiveness in humans: The physiological and behavioral effects of ginseng in animals, the physiologic and psychological effects in humans, the purity and content of ginseng preparations, athletic doping regulations pertaining to ginseng use, methodologic issues involved in assessing the psychological and behavioral effects.

Varieties.—There are 3 Panax medicinal species of ginseng and Siberian or Russian ginseng, which is a different plant. The main active ingredients of the Panax species are saponins, whereas the main active constituents of Russian ginseng are eleutherosides.

Effects in Animals.—The Panax species may produce an anxiolytic effect in mice, may boost energy by altering lipid and carbohydrate mobilization, and may increase endurance by increasing muscle mass. Short-term use may improve spatial cognitive impairment and response to stressors in rats.

Effects in Humans.—Ginseng appears to have little or no effect on the cognitive, physical, or subjective responses of individuals with neurasthenic complaints. Adverse effects included dizziness, somnolence, and increased frequency of urination. Studies do not support any effects of ginseng on psychologic function and mood. Red ginseng may be effective when used as an adjunct to antihypertensive medication. The results do not support ginseng's supposed enhancement of aerobic exercise performance. Studies of maximal work capacity have yielded inconsistent results.

Adverse Effects.—There have been no reports of acute toxicity from high doses of ginseng.

Purity and Content of Preparations.—Labeling frequently does not reflect content. The contents of preparations need to be regulated. Many preparations are contaminated with other active ingredients and many contain alcohol. Dosages vary widely. The International Olympic Committee and the US Olympic Committee bans the use of ginseng.

Methodologic Considerations.—There are few controlled studies of the efficacy of ginseng in humans. Many suffer from methodologic flaws.

Future Research.—Rigorous, well-controlled, methodologically sound studies need to be conducted.

Conclusion.—The efficacy of ginseng has not been substantiated.

▶ This is the second review performed by the authors attempting to determine the efficacy of ginseng. In the first review[1], they pointed out that there was a lack of controlled research regarding its effect on performance in fatigued humans. This current review with 98 citations similarly concludes that "there is an absence of compelling research evidence regarding the efficacy of Ginseng use for the purpose of improving physical performance in humans." Considering the widespread use of this agent, an agent that is not under the control of the Federal Drug Administration, I would agree that there is a need for more rigorous research dealing with it.

J. S. Torg, MD

Reference

1. Bahrke MS, Morgan WP: Evaluation of the ergogenic properties of ginseng. *Sports Med* 18:229-248, 1994.

Sports Haematology
Shaskey DJ, Green GA (Univ of Utah, Salt Lake City; Univ of California Los Angeles)
Sports Med 29:27-38, 2000   7–21

Objective.—The optimum hematologic parameters in athletes are not known. Anemia, sickle cell trait, and hematologic manipulation for the purposes of ergogenic improvement are reviewed.

Anemia in Athletes.—Dilutional pseudoanemia caused by plasma volume expansion is common in athletes. Average hemoglobin concentration is lower in individuals who exercise than in those who do not. Those who exercise the hardest have the greatest plasma volume increase. Dilutional pseudoanemia should not affect hemoglobin level or cause symptoms. Hemolysis, linked to the mechanical trauma associated with running, is present in many athletes, particularly elite endurance runners but is seldom clinically significant. Measurement of serum haptoglobin, serum free hemoglobin, or hemoglobinuria is definitive. Treatment includes reducing footstrike forces. Iron deficiency with or without anemia is more common in nonathletes and is typically related to blood loss or nutritional deficits. Clinicians should check for gastrointestinal bleeding. Most studies have not linked nonanemic iron deficiency to exercise deficits. Iron screening or routine iron supplementation in the absence of anemia is not recommended. Nutritional anemia is common among weight-restricted athletes. A differential diagnostic approach is required.

Sickle Cell Trait (SCT).—There is a significant association between exercise, SCT, and sudden death and nonfatal exertional collapse. Individuals with SCT have normal or near normal exercise capacity but should avoid overexertion.

Hematologic Manipulation.—Blood doping works but can lead to bleeding, infection, and transfusion reactions. Use of recombinant erythropoietin can raise hematocrit to dangerous levels, resulting in death, deep venous thrombosis, pulmonary emboli, coronary thrombosis, or cerebral thrombosis.

Conclusion.—Sports hematology is a growing field that needs to perform additional investigations of athletic anemias and hematologic manipulation.

▶ A comprehensive documentation of the 3 areas of sports haematology: (1) anemia and pseudoanemia; (2) sickle cell trait; and (3) haematologic manipulation or blood doping. The original article is recommended reading for those intimately involved in the care of the athlete.

J. S. Torg, MD

Hematocrits of Triathletes: Is Monitoring Useful?
O'Toole ML, Douglas PS, Hiller WDB, et al (Univ of Tennessee-Campbell Clinic, Memphis; Harvard Med School, Boston; Univ of Hawaii, Honolulu)
Med Sci Sports Exerc 31:372-377, 1999   7–22

Objective.—Endurance training causes plasma volume expansion and creates pseudoanemia. Blood flow and thermoregulation improve, but oxygenation is limited by low hematocrit. Although endurance athletes are interested in reversing this "sports anemia," most commonly by altitude training, the optimal hematocrit has not been determined. Hematocrit greater than 50% results in an increase in blood viscosity and peripheral resistance that reduces blood flow rate. Hematocrit increases of more than 55% may result in encephalopathy, seizures, vascular distention, impairment of blood flow, pulmonary embolism, myocardial infarction, and

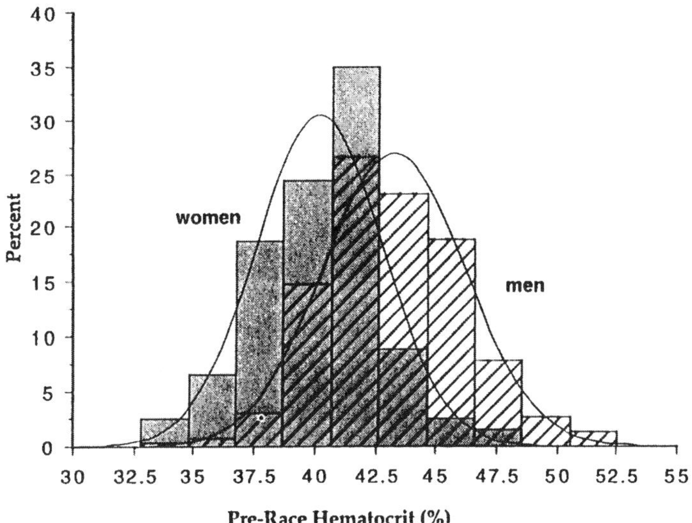

FIGURE 1.—Pre-race hematocrits, normal distributions overlayed from all 3 race distances (N = 289 men, 123 women triathletes). (Courtesy of O'Toole AL, Douglas PS, Hiller WDB, et al: Hematocrits of triathletes: Is monitoring useful? *Med Sci Sports Exerc* 31(3)372-377, 1999.)

stroke. Safe cutoffs for hematocrit levels in triathletes and background data for possible medical control regulations were provided.

Methods.—Prerace and postrace hematocrit levels were determined in 412 triathletes (123 women) involved in Olympic (n = 118), half-Ironman (n = 87), and Ironman (n = 207) competitions.

Results.—Average training distances varied significantly but were similar for men and women except for Olympic distance races which were significantly longer for men than for women. Prerace hematocrits were normal and normally distributed for both men and women (Fig 1). None had a hematocrit of greater than 55%, and all would fall into a prerace hematocrit cutoff for competition of 52% for men and 48% for women. Postrace hematocrits were significantly higher for men but not for women, although individual variability was substantial as were results for different race distances. Low hematocrits probably resulted from hemodilution, with hematocrits becoming progressively lower as competitive and training distances lengthened. Some women may also have been iron deficient. Some athletes had large changes in hematocrit (-7.1% to $+10\%$) on race days. Some athletes appeared to hemoconcentrate whereas others appeared to hemodilute. Fluid dynamics, fluid intake, sodium loss, intravascular/extravascular protein movement, intensity of exercise, and exercise mode may contribute to these response differences.

Although venipuncture sampling was used in this study, the practice may be unwieldy for large numbers of athletes. Finger-stick hematocrits may be a solution, although results have been reported to be 4% lower or 3% higher. Although there appears to be little danger from transiently elevated hematocrit, 18 deaths have been reported among Dutch cyclists receiving erythropoietin.

Conclusion.—Prerace hematocrit cutoffs for competition of 52% for men and 48% for women have been suggested, but these cutoffs do not address overall safety or the ability to detect rules violations.

▶ Although this study provides useful descriptive data on the variance in hematocrits in male and female triathletes before and after competition, it is doubtful that measurement of hematocrits by governing bodies will be used to detect rules violations or safety thresholds. The factors underlying different responses among individual athletes are unclear, and the logistics and cost of using venipuncture sampling are overwhelming. Although the data suggest a cutoff value of 52% for men and 48% for women, many questions underlying these values must be answered before they can be used for safety and medical control.

D. C. Nieman, PhD

Syncope and Atypical Chest Pain in an Intercollegiate Wrestler: A Case Report
Myers JB, Guskiewicz KM, Riemann BL (Univ of North Carolina, Ch˒ l Hill)
J Athletic Train 34:263-266, 1999 7–23

Introduction.—Wrestlers often go to extreme measures to maintain a lower weight class for competition. These may include the use of over-the-counter metabolic stimulants containing so-called natural ingredients like the Chinese herbal extract ma huang, a derivative of ephedrine. A case of a wrestler who had syncope and other symptoms associated with the use of ma huang is reported.

> *Case Report.*—Man, 20, a college wrestler, exhibited severe substernal chest pain, tachycardia, hyperventilation, and loss of consciousness during practice. Emergency medical services were called, and the patient was taken to the emergency department. He admitted taking a metabolic stimulant (Ripped Fuel) containing caffeine and ma huang. He had been taking the supplement for 2 months and had done so that day without eating or drinking anything. The patient was hospitalized for testing during 2 days, but no significant abnormalities were found. His symptoms were ascribed to dehydration, physical stress, and stimulant use. The team physician advised the athlete to avoid metabolic stimulants and other excessive weight-loss techniques.

Conclusions.—Although stimulants such as Ripped Fuel are marketed as natural and safe, they may contain ingredients that carry a significant risk of side effects (Table). Wrestlers and other athletes should be advised to avoid the use of such unregulated stimulants as an aid to weight loss.

TABLE.—Possible Adverse Effects of Ma Huang Use

Nervousness	Acute hepatitis
Diaphoresis	Renal failure
Blurred vision	Seizures
Insomnia	Arrhythmia
Headaches	Chest pain
Dizziness	Tachycardia
Paranoia	Palpitations
Psychosis	Hypertension
Tremors	Coronary spasm
Convulsions	Myocardial infarction
Syncope	Mortality

(Courtesy of Myers JB, Guskiewicz KM, Riemann BL: Syncope and atypical chest pain in an intercollegiate wrestler: A case report. *J Athletic Train* 34:263-266, 1999.)

▶ Legislation passed by the National Collegiate Athletic Association in 1998 should help prevent cases such as this on the collegiate level. The new legislation states that artificial weight loss practices such as the use of laxatives, emetics, steam rooms, and hot practice rooms are banned. Weight classes are established at the beginning of the season by a physician or athletic trainer. The athlete must be hydrated (specific gravity of urine must be checked with a refractometer), and a body fat assessment is done. Wrestlers may reduce their weight class between October 1 and December 7. They may not lose more than 1.5% of their original body weight per week. They may not wrestle in a class below their established body weight. Wrestlers must weigh in 1 hour before a dual match. The lowest collegiate weight class is now 125 lbs.

All athletes must be aware of the ingredients in the supplements they use. Some ingredients may be dangerous, and some may render athletes ineligible for participation if they have positive test results for a banned substance.

F. J. George, ATC, PT

Effect of Oral Androstenedione on Serum Testosterone and Adaptations to Resistance Training in Young Men: A Randomized Controlled Trial
King DS, Sharp RL, Vukovich MD, et al (Iowa State Univ, Ames; Experimental and Applied Sciences, Golden, Colo)
JAMA 281:2020-2028, 1999   7–24

Background.—The testosterone precursor androstenedione is being sold as a natural alternative to anabolic steroids. It is not clear whether androstenedione actually increases testosterone concentrations or produces anabolic-androgenic effects. The effects of short- and long-term androstenedione use on testosterone levels, response to resistance training, and blood lipids and liver function markers were examined.

Methods.—The study included 30 healthy men aged 19 to 29 years. At baseline, all subjects had normal testosterone levels, were not taking any nutritional supplements or androgenic-anabolic steroids, and were not engaged in resistance training. Twenty men engaged in 8 weeks of whole-body resistance training; at weeks 1, 2, 4, 5, 7, and 8, they were randomized to receive either androstenedione, 300 mg/d, or placebo. The remaining 10 subjects were studied to assess the effects of a single 100-mg dose of androstenedione on serum testosterone and estrogen levels.

Results.—Neither single-dose nor 8-week androstenedione treatment caused any change in serum free or total testosterone concentration. After a few weeks of treatment, the androstenedione group had significant increases in serum estradiol and serum estrone concentrations, compared with baseline. The androstenedione and placebo groups had similar and significant increases in knee extension strength and in the mean cross-sectional area of type 2 muscle fibers. Both groups had a significant increase in lean body mass and a significant decrease in fat mass. Serum high-density lipoprotein cholesterol decreased significantly in the androstenedione group.

Conclusions.—This randomized trial found that oral androstenedione does not increase testosterone levels or the response to resistance training in normal healthy young men. Androstenedione does increase serum estradiol and estrone concentrations and reduce high-density lipoprotein cholesterol levels. Thus, androstenedione supplementation is not only ineffective; it may have adverse health effects.

▶ A German patent for androstenedione has claimed that it will increase testosterone levels by 237% within 15 minutes,[1] but the only published report showing an increase in testosterone levels is based on the response of 2 healthy women.[2] The study by King and associates on healthy young men showed no increase in testosterone over 8 weeks of treatment with the heavy dose of 300 mg of androstenedione, apparently because the compound was converted to estrone rather than to testosterone. Further, the treatment did not enhance the response to resistance training, and it did lead to a substantial drop in HDL-cholesterol concentrations. The authors cautiously point out that some body builders may rashly take an even larger dose of the drug and that a testosterone and muscle-building response might be obtained in women or older men.

R. J. Shephard, MD, PhD, DPE

References

1. Hacker R, Mattern C: German Patent DE 42 14953 A1, 1995.
2. Mahesh VB, Greenblatt RB: The in vivo conversion of dehydroepiandrostenone to testosterone in the human. *Acta Endocrinol* 41: 400-406, 1962.

The Infectious Complications of Anabolic-Androgenic Steroid Injection
Rich JD, Dickinson BP, Feller A, et al (Miriam Hosp, Providence, RI; Brown Univ, Providence, RI)
Int J Sports Med 20:563-566, 1999
7–25

Objective.—About 25% of adolescent anabolic-androgenic steroid (AS) users who share needles are at increased risk of infection. The world literature was reviewed for reports of infections attributable to AS use.

Methods.—MEDLINE (1966-1998) and AIDSLINE (1980-1998) database searches were conducted for infections attributable to AS injection.

Results.—Three cases of HIV transmission were documented in male heterosexual bodybuilders who shared needles used for injecting AS. One of these individuals also was diagnosed with hepatitis B infection. Another bodybuilder contracted hepatitis C. Two semiprofessional weightlifters (1 male, 1 female) had thigh abscess from injecting a veterinary preparation of stanozolol contaminated with *Mycobacterium smegmatis*. Two young bodybuilders were diagnosed with staphylococcal gluteal abscesses. Another bodybuilder had a staphylococcal thigh abscess from reusing needles for AS injection. Another patient had pectoral and deltoid abscesses from *Staphylococcus* or *Streptococcus* contamination of his multidosage vial. A deep gluteal abscessing developed in an AS injector who used a counterfeit *Pseudomonas*-contaminated depo-testosterone product. Abscesses developed in 3 bodybuilders who used a product from Mexico, contaminated with *Mycobacterium chelonae* and *Mycobacterium fortuitum*. *Candida albicans* endophthalmitis developed in an athlete, probably as a result of immunosuppression secondary to long-term AS use.

Conclusion.—Shared needles, nonsterile technique, and contaminated supplies increase the risk of infection in AS injectors. Although the risk of transmitting HIV or hepatitis infection is low, the consequences of such infection is catastrophic. Additional prevalence and incidence studies need to be conducted.

► The importance of documenting these infectious complications associated with anabolic-androgenic steroid injection is acknowledged. However, it must be pointed out that the degree of risks or infectious rate cannot be determined. On the other hand, we can presume that many similar infections have occurred but not been reported.

J. S. Torg, MD

8 Muscle Function, Biomechanics and Injury, and Training and Rehabilitation

Effects of 4-Wk Training Using V_{max}/T_{max} on VO_{2max} and Performance in Athletes
Smith TP, McNaughton LR, Marshall KJ (Univ of Tasmania, Launceston, Australia; Kingston Univ, Surrey, England)
Med Sci Sports Exerc 31:892-896, 1999   8–1

Introduction.—Several different approaches to achieving physiologic and performance-related improvements have been suggested, although the physiologic significance or rationale for these approaches is not always clear. Many authors have proposed using the peak flow velocity (V_{max}) to prescribe training intensity to achieve the longest possible running time at maximal oxygen intake (VO_{2max}). An important related variable is the time of maximum concentration (T_{max}), which is the time that the V_{max} can be maintained. The effects of a V_{max}/T_{max}-based training program on athletes' VO_{max} were evaluated.

Methods.—The study included 5 male middle-distance runners: mean age, 23 years; height, 181 cm; weight, 74 kg; 5-skinfold thickness, 36; and VO_{2max}, 61.5 mL O_2/kg/min. At baseline, each athlete performed a 3000-m time trial as well as 3 trials each of the VO_{2max}/V_{max} and T_{max} tests. They then performed a 4-week treadmill exercise training program, in which the exercise intensity was defined as the V_{max}, and the exercise duration was set as 60% to 75% of the T_{max}. Each week, the athletes performed 2 high-intensity, interval-training sessions and 1 recovery session. At the end of the training period, the research subjects were retested.

Results.—The average V_{max} increased from 20.5 to 21.3 km/h from before to after the training program. At the same time, the T_{max} increased from 225.5 to 300.9 seconds, and the VO_{2max} increased from 61.5 to 64.5

mL O_2/kg/min. Performance on the 3000-m time trial improved from 616.6 to 599.6 seconds.

Conclusions.—This study demonstrates the effectiveness of a 4-week, V_{max}/T_{max}-based exercise program for middle-distance runners. The study program significantly improved running times. The improvement in T_{max} prolongs the time to fatigue, thus allowing athletes to maintain their top speed for a longer time and improving their personal performance. Improvements can be achieved across a wide range of pretraining performance levels.

▶ If runners can prolong the onset of fatigue and maintain their top speed for a longer period, then running times can be improved. In this study, participants used a 4-week training program of 2 high-intensity interval-training sessions and 1 recovery session per week. When between 60% to 75% of the runner's T_{max} was used as the exercise duration and the V_{max} was used as the exercise intensity, all the runners improved their times in a 3000-m run.

F. J. George, ATC, PT

Comparison of Two Abdominal Training Devices With an Abdominal Crunch Using Strength and EMG Measurements

Demont RG, Lephart SM, Giraldo JL, et al (Univ of Pittsburgh, Pa; Chulalongkorn Univ, Bangkok, Thailand)
J Sports Med Phys Fitness 39:253-258, 1999   8–2

Objective.—Strengthening abdominal muscles is believed to reduce back pain. The training effects of the Ab-Flex, the Ab-Roller, and the standard crunch on EMG production, isometric maximum voluntary contraction (MVC), and isokinetic average peak torque at 30 degrees/s (ISO) were prospectively compared.

Methods.—Recreationally active volunteers (21 women, 5 men) were randomly assigned to the control group (standard crunch), the Ab-Flex group, or the Ab-Roller group (Fig 3). Volunteers performed 18 sessions of progressively increasing repetitions over a 3-week period. Pretest and posttest MVC, ISO peak torque, and EMG for the upper rectus (UR), lower rectus (LR), internal oblique (IO), and external oblique (EO) muscles were compared by 1-way analysis of variance. Pretest and posttest skinfold measurements were compared using a t test.

Results.—The pretest-posttest mean differences per group were not significantly different. Ab-Flex device users had a posttest increase of 16.5% in the ISO test. EMG results and pretest-posttest body fat percentages were similar for all groups.

Conclusion.—Abdominal crunches are as effective as the Ab-Flex and Ab-Roller for strengthening abdominal muscles, reducing body fat, and improving EMG results.

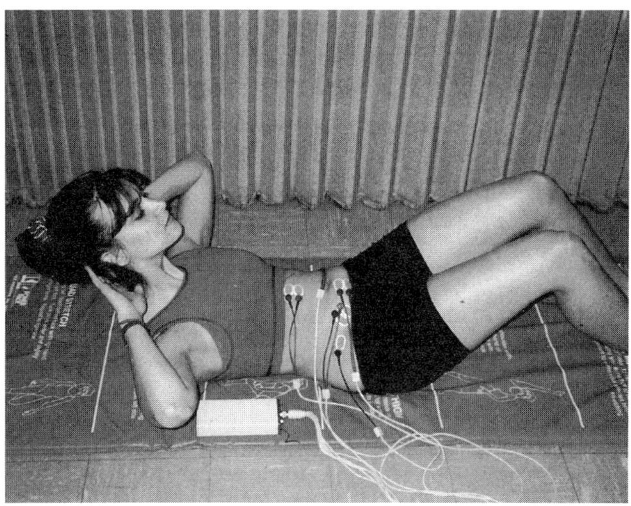

FIGURE 3.—Standard crunch. (Courtesy of Demont RG, Lephart SM, Giraldo JL, et al: Comparison of two abdominal training devices with an abdominal crunch using strength and EMG measurements. *J Sports Med Phys Fitness* 39:253-258, 1999.)

▶ The results of this study indicate that the abdominal crunch exercise is equally as effective as the 2 abdominal training devices tested. The devices were no more effective in developing abdominal strength, improving neuromuscular input, or reducing body fat.

F. J. George, ATC, PT

Eversion Strength Analysis of Uninjured and Functionally Unstable Ankles

Kaminski TW, Perrin DH, Gansneder BM (Univ of Florida, Gainesville; Univ of Virginia, Charlottesville)
J Athletic Train 34:239-245, 1999   8–3

Objective.—Ankle injuries are common among athletes. Repeated ankle injuries can result in functional ankle instability (FAI). Weak concentric muscle strength has been implicated as a cause of FAI. Concentric and eccentric isokinetic and isometric eversion ankle strength was compared in individuals with unilateral FAI and in individuals with no history of inversion ankle sprain.

Methods.—Eversion ankle motion was tested in 21 men (average age, 19.3 years) with unilateral chronic FAI and in 21 control subjects matched for height, weight, age, body type, and activity level. Eversion ankle concentric and eccentric strength was tested in both ankles in a dynamometer chair at 0, 30, 60, 90, 120, 150, and 180 degrees/s. The highest peak torque from 3 maximal repetitions was recorded.

Results.—There were no significant differences in concentric or eccentric strength measures between groups supporting the suggestions of Fiore and Leard that muscle mechanoreceptors may control the instantaneous and qualitative muscle contractions required for foot control.

Conclusion.—Eversion strength deficits do not appear to be the cause of FAI.

▶ A rehabilitation program for functional ankle instability must include progressive functional exercises. Range-of-motion and strengthening exercises alone will not solve this problem. Many factors, including balance, proprioception, and agility, must be addressed.

F. J. George, ATC, PT

The Role of Passive Muscle Stiffness in Symptoms of Exercise-induced Muscle Damage

McHugh MP, Connolly DAJ, Eston RG, et al (Univ of Wales, Bangor; Lenox Hill Hosp, New York; Univ of Vermont, Burlington)
Am J Sports Med 27:594-599, 1999   8–4

Background.—Predominantly eccentric exercise can cause muscle damage and delayed-onset muscle soreness. Such muscle damage is more likely to occur in some individuals than in others, although the reasons for this are unclear. Lack of flexibility, or muscle stiffness, may be an important factor. The contribution of passive hamstring stiffness to subsequent muscle damage after a bout of eccentric exercise was assessed.

Methods.—An instrumented straight-leg stretch was performed in 20 subjects to measure passive hamstring muscle stiffness. On the basis of the results, 7 subjects were classified as "stiff," 6 as "normal," and 7 as "compliant." The degree of stiffness was 78% greater in the stiff group compared with the compliant group. Each subject then performed eccentric hamstring muscle exercise, consisting of 6 sets of 10 isokinetic submaximal eccentric actions. The subjects were then followed up for symptoms of muscle damage, assessed as changes in isometric hamstring muscle strength, pain, muscle tenderness, and creatine kinase activity.

Results.—In the days after exercise, the stiff group had significantly more signs of muscle damage—including strength loss, pain, muscle tenderness, and creatine kinase activity—than the compliant group.

Conclusion.—The results suggest that subjects with stiffer hamstring muscles experience more muscle damage in response to eccentric hamstring exercise. The findings appear to reflect differences in sarcomere mechanics during eccentric actions in stiff versus compliant muscles. Muscle stiffness, and thus static flexibility, appears to be a risk factor for more severe muscle damage after eccentric exercise.

▶ Is good flexibility important to prevent muscle damage? This study indicates that the subjects with stiffer hamstrings suffered more muscle damage than their flexible counterparts. The study did not address whether stretching to improve flexibility, or warming up, would limit muscle damage.

Clinically, flexibility exercises and warming-up should play a significant role in an athlete's conditioning program.

F. J. George, ATC, PT

A Preliminary Examination of Cryotherapy and Secondary Injury in Skeletal Muscle

Merrick MA, Rankin JM, Andres FA, et al (Indiana State Univ, Terre Haute; Univ of Toledo, Ohio; Grand Valley State Univ, Grand Rapids, Mich)
Med Sci Sports Exerc 31:1516-1521, 1999   8–5

Objective.—The use of cryotherapy in acute musculoskeletal injury is based on the secondary injury model where injury is believed to occur after a period of hypoxia and posttrauma enzymatic activity. Hypoxia diminishes mitochondrial enzymatic activity and decreases the amount of reduction of triphenyltetrazolium chloride (TTC) that occurs during the oxidative phosphorylation process. Whether injured tissues have less TTC reduction than controls and whether more TTC reduction occurs in cryotherapy-treated tissues were investigated in rats.

Methods.—After injuries to the triceps surae muscles, rats were randomly assigned to a cryotherapy group (n = 10) or a control group (n = 9). The cryotherapy group was treated with an ice pack. After 5 hours, the triceps surae were removed and the TTC content determined.

Results.—The rate of TTC reduction was significantly greater in control limbs than in injured limbs. Control tissue showed a significantly greater reduction of TTC than did injured tissue treated with ice. Injured limbs treated with ice showed a significantly greater reduction of TTC than did injured limbs not treated with ice (Fig 3).

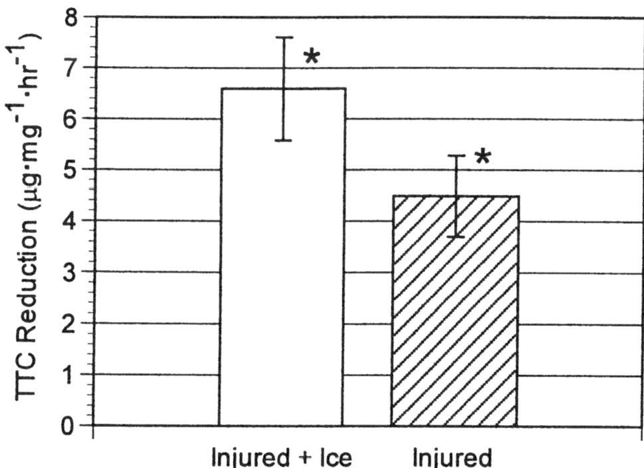

FIGURE 3.—Mean ± SEM TTC reduction for injured and ice-treated injured tissues. (Courtesy of Merrick MA, Rankin JM, Andres FA, et al: A preliminary examination of cryotherapy and secondary injury in skeletal muscle. *Med Sci Sports Exerc* 31:1516-1521, 1999.)

Conclusion.—The existence of secondary injury in muscle tissue is verified. Cryotherapeutic treatment of such injuries is effective at the molecular level.

▶ The authors did prove the hypotheses they tested, ie, that "secondary injury occurs after acute musculoskeletal trauma, that injured tissues would have less TTC reduction than controls (injured tissue), and that cryotherapy-treated injured tissues would have more TTC reduction than untreated injured tissues." They were able to answer some of "how" it works. Research still needs to be completed as to the duration and frequency of cryotherapy that is needed in the clinical setting to bring about desired results.

F. J. George, ATC, PT

Effects of Velocity on Upper to Lower Extremity Muscular Work and Power Output Ratios of Intercollegiate Athletes
Charteris J (Rhodes Univ, Grahamstown, South Africa)
Br J Sports Med 33:250-254, 1999   8–6

Background.—Peak torque expresses a point output that is only sometimes well correlated with full-range output measures such as work or power, especially in a rehabilitating muscle. Isokinetic performance variables were assessed to determine how speeds of 30 and 180 degrees per second influence agonist to antagonist ratios for torque, work, and power and to determine the effects of these speeds on upper to lower limb flexor (F), extensor (E), and combined (F + E) ratios as a guide to rehabilitation protocols and outcomes after injury.

Methods and Findings.—Twenty-seven healthy, athletic men were tested isokinetically at slow and moderate speed likely to be encountered in the early stages of rehabilitation after injury. At the speeds tested, all torque responses showed velocity-related decrements at rates that kept the F/E ratios and upper to lower extremity ratios constant for work and power. Regardless of speed, upper extremity relative torque, work, and power flexion responses were equal to extension responses. Conversely, all relative measures of torque, work, and power of flexors in the lower extremities were lower than extensor responses. Work and power F/E ratios were unaffected by speed in both upper and lower extremities. Increasing speed from 30 to 180 degrees per second did not affect upper to lower extremity work and power ratios.

Conclusions.—Peak torque responses may not sufficiently reflect tension development through extensive range of motion. However, total work produced and mean power generated are highly relevant performance measures. Expressed as F/E ratios, these measures are unaffected by speeds of 30 and 180 degrees per second in upper and lower extremities.

▶ This study provided a critical view of the use of peak torque as the key variable in evaluating muscle function, which is commonly done in muscle strength evaluation. The use of average work or power as a measure of muscle function after an injury may be more useful in reflecting tension development through an extensive range of motion. Results from testing torque outputs of the elbow and knee flexors and extensors revealed that both upper and lower limbs have constant F/E work and power output ratios. The elbow F/E work and power ratio is 1.05 and that for the knee is 0.66. These ratios are useful in establishing rehabilitation goals after upper or lower limb musculoskeletal injury

M. J. L. Alexander, PhD

Muscle Activity in the Slalom Turn of Alpine Skiing and In-line Skating
Zeglinksi CM, Swanson SC, Self BP, et al (Orthopedic Specialty Hosp, Salt Lake City, Utah; Orthopedic Biomechanics Inst, Salt Lake City, Utah)
Int J Sports Med 19:447-454, 1998   8–7

Background.—As in-line skating has increased in popularity among the general public, it has also become popular as a training and rehabilitation exercise for skiers. Many skiers believe that movements associated with in-line skating, particularly the turning motion, mimic the movements used in alpine skiing. However, the validity of this assumption was not known, as no studies had examined the muscle activities associated with in-line skating. In this study, the activity of 7 muscles is examined by use of electromyography (EMG) during a slalom turn by in-line skaters and alpine skiers.

Methods.—EMG telemetry and qualitative video analysis were used to record the muscle activity and correlate the EMG findings to specific movement patterns in 7 muscles, all on the right side of the body: the peroneals, anterior tibialis, gluteus maximus, biceps femoris, vastus medialis, adductors, and erector spinae. Five male masters-level skiers were selected as subjects for the study. All of these subjects had also used in-line skating as part of their training regimen. Before each activity, standard isometric contractions were measured for each muscle. Each subject completed 4 downhill runs of approximately 10 seconds' duration, and the movements of each subject through turn 6 were videotaped (Fig 2). Four days later, each subject completed 4 runs on a downhill in-line skating slalom course. Again, the subject's movements through turn 6 were videotaped for correlation with EMG data collected during the runs. To minimize the effects of fatigue on the subjects during the testing, all were given between 4 and 7 minutes to rest between skiing runs and as much time as they needed between in-line skating runs.

Results.—The EMG analysis showed significant levels of activity for all muscles during both skiing and in-line skating; however, the EMG readings for the erector spinae were significantly higher during the turn in the ski runs. There was little difference between in-line skating and downhill

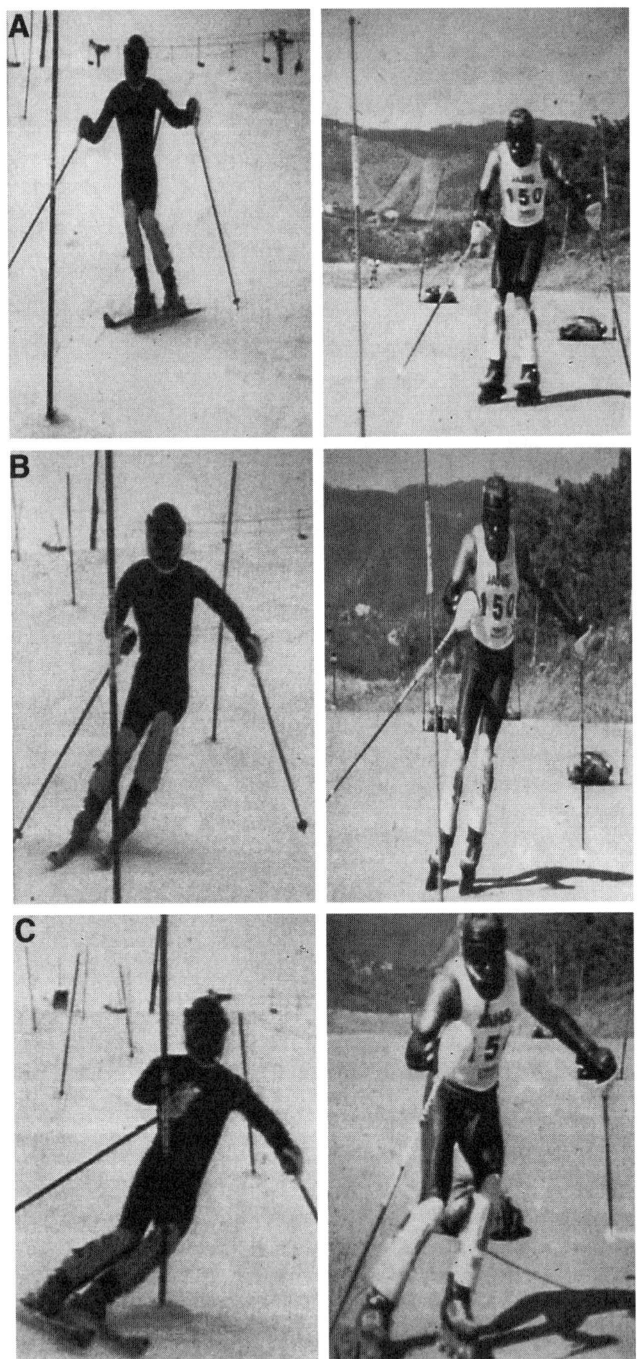

FIGURE 2.—Representative general body positions of one subject at the boundaries of the initiation and turning phases of both slalom skiing (left) and in-line skating (right). A illustrates the initiation phase; B illustrates the beginning of the turning phase; and C illustrates the end of the turning phase. (Courtesy of Zeglinski CM, Swanson SC, Self BP, et al: Muscled activity in the slalom turn of alpine skiing and in-line skating. *Int J Sports Med* 19:447-454, 1998. Georg Thieme Verlag.)

skiing in the EMG readings for the other muscles examined in the study. The initiation phase for the turn was of similar duration in both in-line skating and downhill skiing, but the turning phase was shorter and the speed greater during the skiing tests as compared with the in-line skating runs. The greater speed of downhill skiing may account for this difference.

Conclusion.—Overall, study findings indicate that in-line skating can be satisfactory as a training exercise for alpine skiing. The muscle activity patterns in alpine skiing and slalom in-line skating are similar, although the slower speeds of in-line skating may necessitate the use of steeper grades in order to decrease turning-phase time and increase activity in the muscles during the turn.

▶ Few studies have examined the muscle activity in an in-line skating turn, which was found to be similar to an alpine ski turn. EMG data were collected from 6 muscles during the turns with telemetry, and normalized to standard isometric contractions. Five lower extremity muscles and the erector spinae were examined for activity levels during the skills. Activity levels were found to be similar in the leg muscles, but the erector spinae were found to be significantly more active in the slalom skiing trial. This may have been caused by the higher turning speeds and the faster turns seen in alpine skiing. These results suggest that in-line skating may be a satisfactory dry land training modality for alpine skiing, although the relative energy requirements of the 2 activities were not measured.

M. J. L. Alexander, PhD

Effects of Chronic Anterior Cruciate Ligament Deficiency on Muscle Activation Patterns During an Abrupt Deceleration Task

Steele JR, Brown JMM (Univ of Wollongong, Australia)
Clin Biomech 14:247-257, 1999

8–8

Purpose.—Some patients with anterior cruciate ligament deficiency (ACLD) have a distinct syndrome associated with symptoms of progressive knee dysfunction and deterioration, whereas others have minimal impairment after complete ACL rupture. It has been suggested that the ACLD group may have compensatory adaptations to their injuries, arising from subconscious protection against excessive anterior tibial rotation. There are few data on the functional adaptations of ACLD patients in response to tasks known to load the ACL excessively. The muscle activation patterns of ACLD patients in response to abrupt deceleration, a task known to stress the ACL, were assessed.

Methods.—The study included 11 patients with unilateral, functional, chronic, isolated ACLD and 11 matched controls. Testing was performed a mean of 8 years after initial ACL injury. Kinematic data were collected while the subjects performed a dynamic, abrupt deceleration task (ie, landing on the injured limb and stabilizing their position without raising the landing foot). Muscle activation patterns were analyzed relative to the

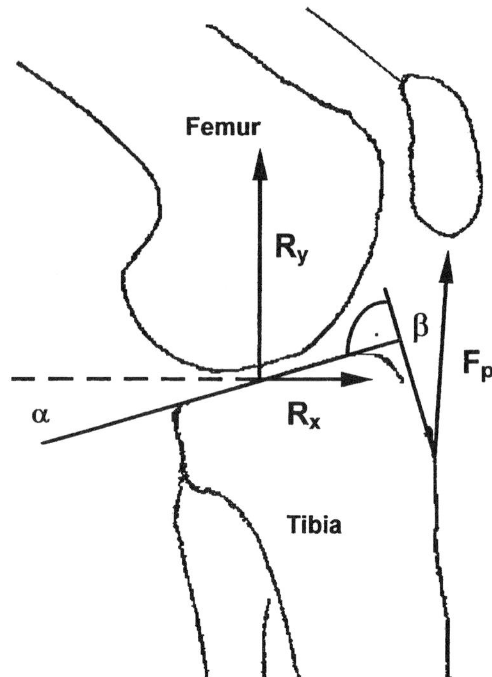

FIGURE 1.—Free body diagram of the knee joint. The tibiofemoral shear force (F_s) can be calculated from the joint reaction force R_x and R_y, the angle α of the tibial plateau to the horizontal plane, the patellar tendon force (F_p), and its angle β to the tibial plateau. (Adapted from Kuster M, Wood GA, Sakuria S, et al: Downhill walking: A stressful task for the anterior cruciate ligament? A biomechanical study with clinical implications. *Knee Surg Sports Trauma Arthoscopy* 2:2-7, 1994. Courtesy of Steele JR, Brown JMM: Effects of chronic anterior cruciate ligament deficiency on muscle activation patterns during an abrupt deceleration task. *Clin Biomech* 14:247-257, copyright 1999, with permission from Elsevier Science.)

timing of tibiofemoral shear forces (F_s) generated by the deceleration task (Fig 1).

Results.—Hamstring activation was delayed in the ACLD group, compared with the control group. As a result, peak hamstring activity in ACLD patients was more synchronous with initial contact and with the high F_s occurring thereafter.

Conclusions.—The injured limbs of subjects with chronic ACLD show changes in synchronization of hamstring onset and peak hamstring activity during an abrupt deceleration task. These appear to be the major functional compensations used in ACLD patients to withstand the high tibiofemoral forces generated by the study task. Achieving more synchronous activation of the hamstrings with the peak F_s would help to stabilize the knee by increasing joint compression at a time of enhanced vulnerability to anterior subluxation.

▶ It has been suggested that ACLD may alter muscle activation patterns because of decreased proprioceptive feedback from the injured limb. In normal subjects, the hamstring muscle group will fire before contact during a landing task, providing a posterior shear force to prevent anterior translation of the tibia and ACL strain on contact. Subjects with a chronic ACL injury were found to have a delay in hamstring activity, so that it occurred closer to the instant of peak anterior forces at contact. It was recommended that training activities be designed to produce better synchrony of hamstring activation, but no examples of such activities were provided. There still appears to be some controversy regarding the effects of ACL injury on muscle activation patterns.

M. J. L. Alexander, PhD

Relationship Between Static and Dynamic Foot Postures in Professional Baseball Players
Donatelli R, Wooden M, Ekedahl SR, et al (Physiotherapy Associates, Alpharetta, Ga; Physiotherapy Associates, Lilburn, Ga; Physiotherapy Associates, Memphis, Tenn; et al)
J Orthop Sports Phys Ther 29:316-330, 1999   8–9

Background.—In professional baseball, running, cutting, and sprinting activities may cause overuse injuries. An observational study of static and dynamic foot postures in professional baseball players was reported.

Methods.—Seventy-four male professional baseball players participated. Foot postures were examined at rest and during gait. Static foot posture was measured with a goniometer. The FootTrak motion analysis system was used to measure dynamic foot posture during the stance phase of gait. Men who had previous lower extremity injuries also completed a questionnaire.

Findings.—The forefoot varus and calcaneal valgus in standing was significantly correlated with maximum pronation in the stance phase of gait. Forty-three percent of the 65 men demonstrating excessive pronation had had a previous lower extremity injury. However, previously injured and uninjured players did not differ in mean values of static or dynamic foot posture (Fig 2). Foot postures were unrelated to a player's position.

Conclusions.—Selected measures of static rearfoot and forefoot postures may be useful for predicting dynamic rearfoot movement during the stance phase of gait. In the current series of professional baseball players, excessive pronation was not a significant contributing factor in the development of overuse injuries.

▶ Abnormal subtalar joint pronation has often been observed in runners with overuse injuries of the lower extremity. Excessive pronation in this study is rearfoot movement greater than 4 to 6 degrees; however, this value is controversial and not universally agreed on. This group of 74 baseball players underwent several measurements of static foot posture, 2 of which

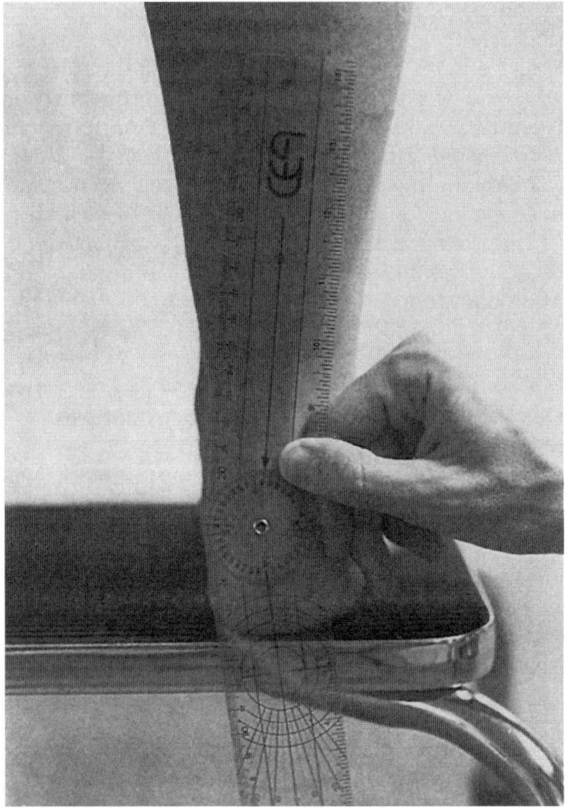

FIGURE 2.—Static compensated calcaneal valgus position measured with a goniometer. The stationary arm of the goniometer is aligned with the line bisecting the lower leg, and the moving arm is aligned on the bisecting line of the calcaneus. (Courtesy of Donatelli R, Wooden M, Ekedahl SR, et al: Relationship between static and dynamic foot postures in professional baseball players. *J Orthop Sports Phys Ther* 29:316-330, 1999, with permission of the orthopaedic and sports sections of the American Physical Therapy Association.)

were related to maximum pronation during the stance phase of gait. There were significant relationships between 2 measures of static foot posture and maximum pronation during gait. However, there were no differences between injured or noninjured players' foot postures or maximum pronation. Thus, the relationship between overuse injuries and excessive pronation remains unclear.

M. J. L. Alexander, PhD

Changes in Muscle-Tendon Length During the Take-off of a Running Long Jump

Hay JG, Thorson EM, Kippenhan BC (Univ of Iowa, Iowa City)
J Sports Sci 17:159-172, 1999   8–10

Background.—In the running long jump, the most important phase is the take-off. At this phase, the athlete generates the velocity to propel his or her body vertically. Little attention has been paid to how the body moves and how the involved muscles operate during takeoff. This study

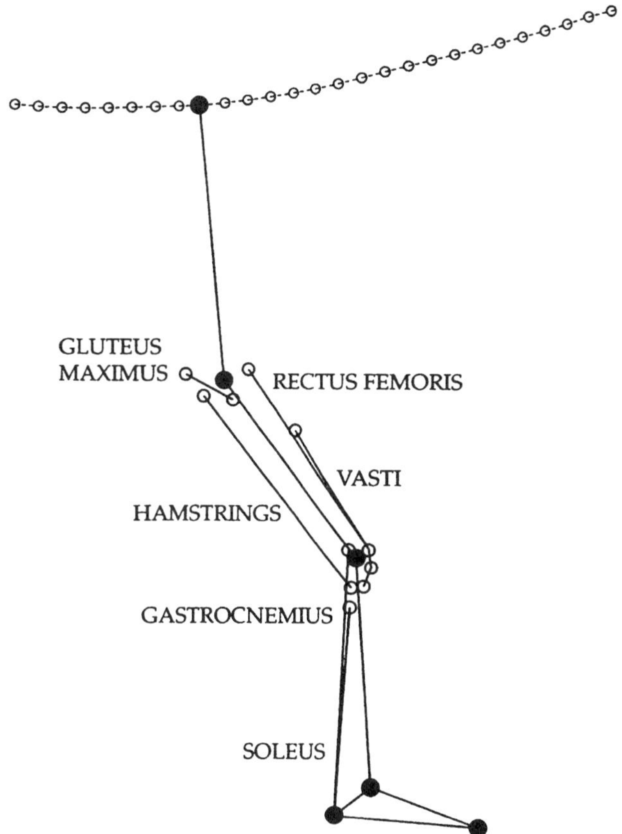

FIGURE 1.—Four-segment model of the trunk and jumping leg. Segments were the trunk (represented by a straight line from the midpoint of the trunk at the level of the suprasternal notch to the midpoint of the hips), thigh (from the hip joint to the knee joint), shank (from the knee joint to the ankle joint), and foot (from the heel to toe). Attachment points of muscles shown were based on values reported by Dostal and Andrews (1981: gluteus maximus, hamstrings, and rectus femoris), Hoy et al (1990: vasti), and Seirig and Arvikar (1989: soleus and gastrocnemius). The 3-line-segment representation of the vasti and rectus femoris muscles was developed by the method of Pierrynowski (1995, Appendix B). The *curved line* and the associated *circles* show the path followed by the suprasternal notch from the instant of touchdown to the instant of takeoff. (Courtesy of Hay JG, Thorson EM, Kippenham BC: Changes in muscle-tendon length during the take-off of a running long jump. *J Sports Sci* 17:159-172, 1999, published by Taylor & Francis, Ltd. at http://www.tandf.cc.uk/journals/jsp.htm

attempted to determine the actions of specific muscles in the supporting leg during takeoff; whether the moment of maximum knee flexion is a true indicator of the moment of a change in the actions of those specific muscles, from eccentric to concentric; and the nature of the relationship between those specific muscles and the change in velocity as the athlete executes the takeoff.

Methods.—The study group comprised 11 female elite long jumpers whose best distances in competition during a 2-year period before the study were between 6.3 and 6.82 meters. For the purposes of this study, all jumpers used the same runway and force platform. Two motion-picture cameras, synchronized with an external clock, were used to record the actions of the muscles, and an S-VHS camcorder recorded the position of the takeoff foot during the takeoff. Jumps during which the takeoff foot crossed the "foul" line were not used in the study. Each athlete made 6 jumps from a full approach. The best jump for each athlete was used for data analysis. The motion pictures of each of these 6 jumps were then digitized, and 21 body landmarks were defined (Fig 1). The digitization of the images allowed the elaboration of a 14-segment model of selected muscles to estimate the muscle-tendon lengths from various segment positions.

Results.—Although it was assumed before this study that all of the muscles under consideration were active during takeoff, analysis of the data showed that a lengthening-shortening sequence occurred in only half of the muscles. In addition, the moment that maximum knee flexion was recorded turned out to be a poor indicator of the moment that the muscles changed their mode of action from eccentric to concentric.

Conclusion.—It has been a common notion that the stretch-shortening cycle contributes significantly to vertical velocity during takeoff. However, the results of this study indicate that fast eccentric actions of the muscles in the early part of the takeoff are responsible for most of the force and vertical velocity during takeoff.

▶ Forceful muscle contraction is required to produce the high vertical forces required for takeoff in the long jump event. It was assumed that these muscles studied were active throughout the takeoff. For all 11 subjects studied, the length of the gluteus maximus remained almost constant for the first 30% to 50% of the takeoff, then decreased to takeoff, while the length of the hamstrings decreased in linear fashion from touchdown to takeoff. This study reported that only half of the muscles studied exhibited a stretch-shortening cycle of activity and that, contrary to popular belief, there was not a significant enhancement of performance during the stretch-shortening cycle.

M. J. L. Alexander, PhD

Muscle Activation During the Tennis Volley

Chow JW, Carlton LG, Lim Y-T, et al (Univ of Illinois at Urbana-Champaign)
Med Sci Sports Exerc 31:846-854, 1999   8–11

Objective.—Few studies have examined muscle activation during the volley in tennis. Activation of key muscles of the stroking arm and shoulder, as well as muscles related to postural support, were examined during the tennis volley under various ball placement and speed conditions.

Methods.—Seven skilled male tennis players participated in the study. They performed volley strokes under a wide range of experimental conditions, including forehand and backhand strokes; high, middle, and low ball contact height; and fast, medium, and slow ball speed. Surface elec-

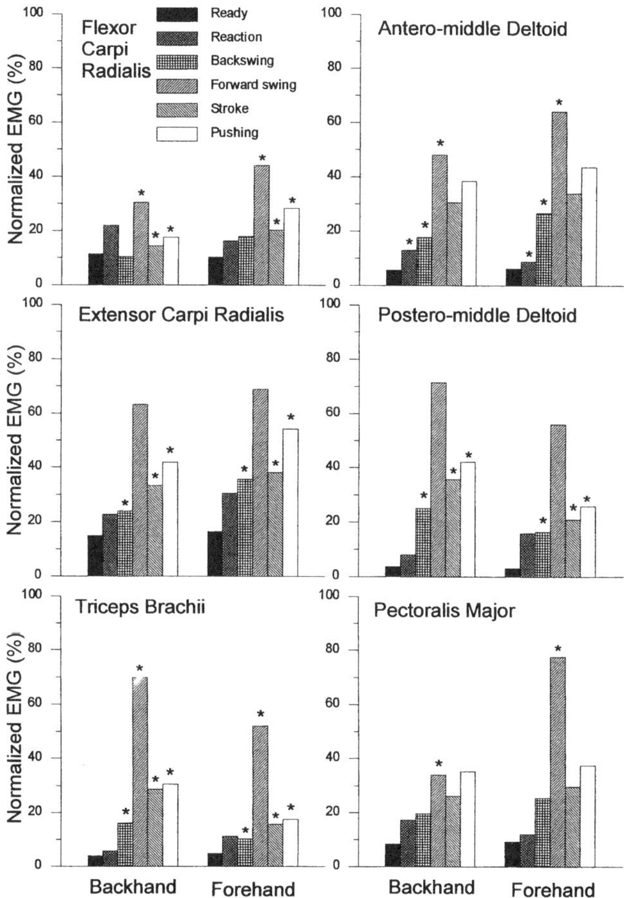

FIGURE 1.—Average normalized electromyographic levels of selected upper body muscles during different phases of a tennis volley for forehand and backhand trials. *Significant differences between forehand and backhand locations ($P \le .05$). (Courtesy of Chow JW, Carlton LG, Lim Y-T, et al: Muscle activation during the tennis volley. *Med Sci Sports Exerc* 31:846-854, 1999.)

tromyography (EMG) was used to detect activity of the flexor carpi radialis, extensor carpi radialis, triceps brachii, deltoids, and pectoralis major, as well as the left and right external oblique, lumbar erector spinae, and gastrocnemius muscles. Force platforms and high-speed video were used to capture the critical instants of the volley, and EMG values were calculated for different phases of the volley.

Results.—Faster ball speeds were generally associated with greater muscle activity. Both the forehand and backhand strokes were associated with greater activity of the extensor carpi radialis than of the flexor carpi radialis, consistent with the importance of wrist extension/abduction and grip strength. Activity of the forearm muscles showed an increase just before ball impact, suggesting that the grip and wrist were not tightened until that time (Fig 1). Flexor and extensor carpi radialis activity was greater during the forehand than during the backhand. Triceps brachii activity was greatest during the forward and swing phases. Throughout most phases of the stroke, both the anteromiddle and the posteromiddle deltoids were activated. Erector spinae activity increased from the ready to reaction phases and decreased at lower ball heights.

Conclusions.—The activities of the arm and shoulder muscles and of selected postural muscles during the tennis volley under varying conditions are reported. The deltoid muscles appear to be active through most phases of the volley stroke, although their role cannot be fully appreciated without information on the actions of the other muscles of the shoulder joint.

▶ Skilled tennis players will have high levels of EMG activity in the muscles of the upper limb and trunk during a high speed skill such as the volley. In this study, faster ball speeds required greater muscle activity from all muscles tested and muscle activity increased as ball height decreased. The extensor carpi radialis was more active than the flexor carpi radialis during the volley, probably because of the need for wrist extension and abduction for grip strength and stabilization of the wrist joint. The triceps muscle was active during the forward swing phase in both the forehand and the backhand, emphasizing its distinct importance during this punching-type skill. Knowledge of the most active muscles in this skill will assist in suggesting specific training exercises for the sport.

M. J. L. Alexander, PhD

Use of EMG Analysis in Challenging Kinetic Chain Terminology

Blackard DO, Jensen RL, Ebben WP (Northern Michigan Univ, Marquette; Marquette Univ, Milwaukee, Wis)
Med Sci Sports Exerc 31:443-448, 1999   8–12

Purpose.—Closed kinetic chain (CKC) activities are thought to be safer than open kinetic chain (OKC) activities for rehabilitation of certain conditions, such as knee problems. However, the lack of a standardized definition of CKC has led to vague applications of the term. It is generally accepted that, whereas the end segment is free to move during OKC activities, it is fixed and restricted from moving during CKC activities. Three classifications of activity have been proposed, based on the presence or absence of a moveable or fixed boundary condition and a load on the end segment: fixed external load (FEL) , the extreme CKC activity; moveable no load (MNL), the extreme OKC activity; and moveable external load (MEL), the gray area between the 2 extremes. Mean integrated electromyography (EMG_{int}) values were compared between biomechnically comparable CKC/FEL, OKC/MNL, and MEL exercises.

Methods.—Ten young men performed 3 exercises in random order, all using a pronated, closed grip: push-up (PU), a CKC/FEL activity; bench press with a load (BP-L), a MEL activity; and bench press with no load (BP-NL), an OKC/MNL activity. The investigators obtained EMG_{int} values from the pectoralis major and the long head of the triceps during each activity. For each muscle, a reference EMG value (EMG_{MVC}) was calculated from the mean integrated EMG values from 3 isometric maximal voluntary contractions. The EMG_{int} was divided by EMG_{MVC} to calculate a normalized EMG value for each muscle during the absorption and force phases.

Results.—The EMG values were similar for PU and BP, as equivalently load exercises with differing boundaries. However, there was a significant difference between BP and BP-NL, which were differently loaded but with equivalent boundaries, and between PU and BP-NL, which had different loads and different boundaries.

Conclusions.—Biomechanically similar exercises of similar loading have similar primary muscle EMG values, regardless of differences in boundary. The external load appears to be a better descriptor of human movement than the boundary condition. The type of articulations and their range of motion must also be considered in describing the movement.

▶ The terms CKC and OKC have been used extensively in recent years to describe 2 different types of rehabilitation exercises. In CKC exercises, the end segment is fixed and restricted from movement by a load, whereas in OKC exercises the end segment is free to move. However, there is blurring of these conditions, and some controversy, when the end segment is loaded and free to move. EMG and force plate analysis revealed that activities of similar biomechanical motions have similar muscle force requirements, regardless of the fixation of the end segment. The authors suggested elimination of the CKC and OKC classifications, and simply describing an exercise relative to the external load and to the articulations involved. This is an excellent suggestion that would eliminate the common use of 2 imprecise and unclear definitions.

M. J. L. Alexander, PhD

Relationship Between Muscle Fiber Pennation and Force Generation Capability in Olympic Athletes

Ichinose Y, Kanehisa H, Ito M, et al (Univ of Tokyo)
Int J Sports Med 19:541-546, 1998   8–13

Objective.—Previous studies have shown that muscle cross-sectional area (CSA) is closely related to force-generating ability. However, there is evidence that the hypertrophied muscle of athletes shows a negative correlation between CSA and force per unit of CSA (F/CSA), that is, athletes with large muscles cannot produce the same dynamic force for muscle size as untrained subjects or athletes with smaller muscles. One possible explanation is that the negative effect of muscle fiber pennation angles on force-generation capability may increase at greater CSA. The relationship between muscle fiber pennation and force-generating capability was studied in Olympic athletes representing various sports.

Methods.—The sample included Japanese male Olympic athletes from a wide range of sports, including wrestling, soccer, judo, running, rowing, and baseball. B-mode US was used to measure the thickness (TBmt) and fiber pennation angle (TBpen) of the triceps brachii muscle. In addition, the isokinetic force associated with elbow extension was assessed. The morphologic characteristics of the triceps brachii were compared with its functional performance, including the relationship between the fiber pennation angle and force-generating capability.

Results.—Participants in judo, wrestling, and gymnastics had larger values for TBmt and TBpen than other athletes did. The TBpen was

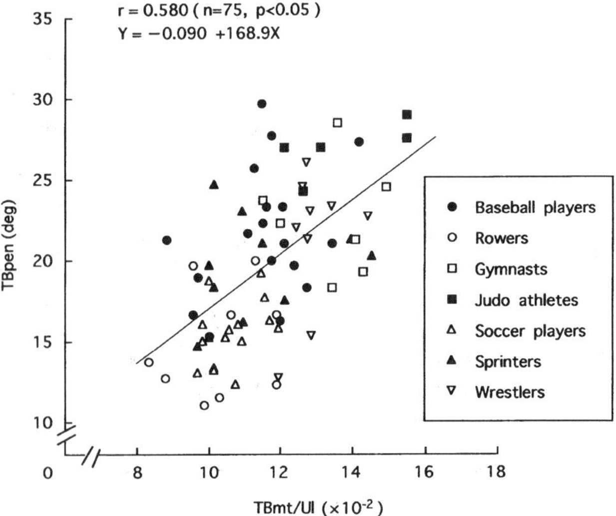

FIGURE 1.—Relationship between muscle thickness (TBmt) per unit of the upper arm length (TBmt/Ul) and muscle fiber pennation angle (TBpen). (Courtesy of Ichinose Y, Kanehisa H, Ito M, et al: Relationship between muscle fiber pennation and force generation capability in Olympic athletes. *Int J Sports Med* 19:541-546, 1998. Georg Thieme Verlag.)

significantly correlated with TBmt per unit of upper arm length; thus differences in TBpen reflected differences in TBmt (Fig 1). Measured at 2 different velocities, the isokinetic forces relative to the CSA, estimated from TBmt, were negatively correlated with CSA. The TBpen was also weakly but significantly and negatively correlated with the isokinetic forces per unit of CSA at both speeds. These negative correlations persisted even after normalizing for the effect of TBpen.

Conclusions.—A study of the triceps brachii muscles of elite athletes finds that the magnitude of pennation angles is related to muscle size. However, pennation angle cannot account for the lower F/CSA in athletes with larger muscles.

▶ It is generally accepted that athletes with larger muscle CSA have greater force output; however, some studies have reported that some athletes with large muscles cannot develop high levels of muscle force. This lack of force output could be caused by inefficient muscle pennation angles, which are the angles of the muscle fibers to the long axis of the muscle. A muscle with a greater pennation angle will have less contractile force directed along the tendon of attachment and more force directed perpendicular to the tendon. Imaging techniques now allow researchers to measure pennation angles in vivo to determine their relationship to force output. Previous studies have reported larger pennation angles for strength-trained athletes and lower force per unit of CSA in athletes with larger muscle size. Because the larger pennation angle is associated with a smaller rotational component of force, a larger CSA is not always associated with greater strength.

M. J. L. Alexander, PhD

Anthropometric Dimensions to Predict 1-RM Bench Press in Untrained Females
Scanlan JM, Ballmann KL, Mayhew JL, et al (Truman State Univ, Kirksville, Mo)
J Sports Med Phys Fitness 39:54-60, 1999   8–14

Background.—Studies in men have shown that anthropometric measurements can predict strength; however, the relationship between anthropometric dimensions and strength in women has received little attention. The ability of anthropometric dimensions to predict bench press performance in women was analyzed.

Methods.—A wide range of anthropometric measurements were obtained for 113 untrained female college students, and included skinfold thickness at 5 sites, circumference at 5 sites, and skeletal dimensions at 6 sites. These measurements were used to derive additional variables, including body mass index, percent body fat, fat-free mass, flexed arm cross-sectional area (CSA), ratio of shoulder to hip width, androgyny index, and somatotype. The ability of the anthropometric dimensions to predict the women's 1-repetition maximum (RM) bench press was calculated.

Results.—The dimensions with the greatest zero-order correlations with 1-RM bench press were arm CSA, flexed arm circumference, mesomorphic body type, and forearm circumference. Most correlations with bench press performed were decreased by first-order partial correlations, assuming a constant body mass or fat-free mass. Multiple regression analyses, using muscle, length, and fat factors identified by factor loading, were not highly predictive of 1-RM values. The equations had a mean coefficient of variation of 18.9% to 21.0%.

Conclusions.—Anthropometric measurements are not practical in estimating bench press performance among untrained women. The authors propose that women may be hesitant to achieve even modest levels of upper-body development because of social factors. Future studies might identify psychosocial factors that limit women from achieving physical performance consistent with their structural characteristics.

▶ Previous research examining male athletes has suggested that the CSA of the arm often has the highest correlation with 1-RM bench press. There is also some relationship between arm CSA and bench press in highly trained female athletes. This study attempted to examine whether several anthropometric variables were related to the 1-RM bench press in untrained women, and concluded that there were no significant correlations. Variables such as sum of skinfold thicknesses, percent fat, flexed arm CSA, shoulder and hip widths, and somatotype were all unrelated to bench press performance. This lack of correlation was likely caused by the wide range of strength and fitness levels in this group of untrained subjects, many of whom had not participated in any kind of strength or conditioning programs.

M. J. L. Alexander, PhD

Stoop or Squat: A Review of Biomechanical Studies on Lifting Technique

van Dieën JH, Hoozemans MJM, Toussaint HM (Vrije Universiteit, Amsterdam; Univ of Amsterdam)
Clin Biomech 14:685-696, 1999   8–15

Objective.—Studies have failed to show any benefits of lifting training and instruction on incidence of low back pain because individuals shift from the high-energy cost squat technique to the stoop technique. Evidence that lifting technique is an important risk factor for low back pain was reviewed.

Methods.—A search of multiple databases identified 27 biomechanical studies comparing the stoop and squat lifting techniques. The validity of indicators of compression and shear acting on the spine, tensile stresses in the posterior spine, and muscle force as indicators of back load were evaluated. Measurements of intradiscal pressure, intra-abdominal pressure, spinal shrinkage, and electromyography were compared.

Results.—Squat lifting, in terms of net moments and compression forces, provided a benefit only when lifting from a position between the feet, reducing the back load by about one third. When the load was not between the feet, net moment and compression were slightly lower with the stoop position. The squat lifting position provided no benefit or a slight disadvantage in other lifting tasks. Shear and bending moments were all higher in the stoop position. Parameters of back load must be weighted to determine the injury potential of the technique. Loss of balance was more likely to occur when using the squat technique. Other factors affecting mechanical load on the lower back include asymmetric lifting, speed of lift, horizontal and vertical position of the load, and load mass.

Conclusion.—There is no significant biomechanical evidence to support the squat over the stoop technique for lifting. Interventions for preventing low back pain associated with lifting should deal with asymmetry, speed, horizontal and vertical position of the load, and load mass.

▶ To prevent low back injuries when lifting, factors other than squatting or stooping should be stressed. The authors state the factors that should be stressed are asymmetry, speed, horizontal and vertical position of the load, and load mass.

F. J. George, ATC, PT

Abduction Moment Arm of Transposed Subscapularis Tendon

Nakajima T, Liu J, Hughes RE, et al (Mayo Clinic and Mayo Found, Rochester, Minn)
Clin Biomech 14:265-270, 1999   8–16

Background.—Superior transposition of the subscapularis tendon has been advocated for the surgical repair of massive rotator cuff tears. The effects of this procedure on shoulder biomechanics were investigated.

Methods.—Ten shoulders were harvested from fresh cadavers, aged 40 to 89 years at death. The moment arm about an instantaneous center of rotation was determined based on the slope of tendon excursion–glenohumeral angle curve. Pseudoinsertion sites were created to simulate insertion of the transposed subscapularis tendon (Fig 1).

Findings.—Superior transposition significantly increased the abduction moment arm of the subscapularis tendon. This effect was greatest when the simulated insertion site was lateral rather than medial and, to lesser degree, anterior rather than posterior.

Conclusions.—These data verify that superior transposition of the subscapularis tendon increases its abduction moment arm. Thus, the current analysis supports the use of subscapularis tendon transposition for restoring abduction strength to shoulders with a massive cuff tear.

▶ There is little agreement regarding the optimal surgical treatment of the massive rotator cuff tear involving the supraspinatus tendon. The use of the

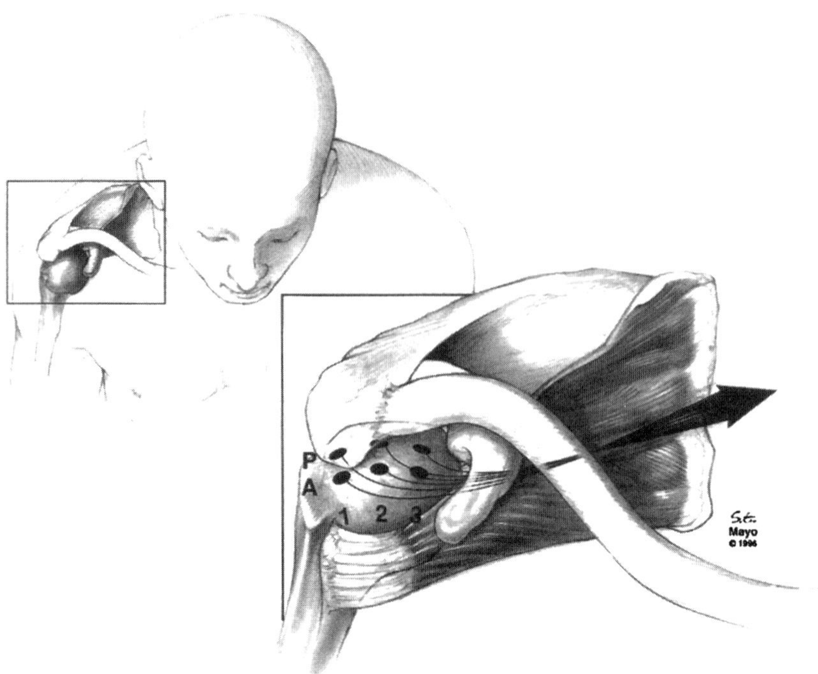

FIGURE 1.—Insertion sites on the humeral head simulating superior transposition of the subscapularis tendon. The pins and test nylon were arranged at the anterior and posterior pseudoinsertion sites (*row A and row P*) and at the lateral, intermediate, and medial sites (*pair 1, pair 2, and pair 3*). Row A corresponded to the midpoint of the greater tuberosity, row P to its posterior edge. Pair 1 was placed 3 mm medial to the insertion of the joint capsule. Pair 2 was 10 mm medial, and pair 3 was 17 mm medial to the insertion. (Reprinted from Nakajima T, Liu J, Hughes RE, et al: Abduction moment arm of transposed subscapularis tendon. *Clin Biomech* 14:265-270, 1999. Copyright 1999, with kind permission from Elsevier Science.)

subscapularis tendon as a replacement for the supraspinatus tendon in abduction was examined in this study. The subscapularis tendon is attached to the lesser tuberosity, and its line of action passes anterior to the center of rotation of the humeral head. The subscapularis tendon was transposed to a more superior location on 10 cadaver shoulders, and the resultant moment arms were measured. It was determined that moving the subscapularis tendon to a more superior location on the greater tuberosity increases the abduction moment arm significantly and helps to restore lost abduction strength.

M. J. L. Alexander, PhD

Older Adults Exhibit a Reduced Ability to Fully Activate Their Biceps Brachii Muscle

Yue GH, Ranganathan VK, Siemionow V, et al (Cleveland Clinic Found, Ohio)
J Gerontol 54A:M249-M253, 1999   8–17

Background.—Voluntary muscle strength decreases with age, partly as a result of muscle atrophy. However, aging may also affect the ability to maximally activate muscle. The effects of aging on biceps brachii muscle activation were studied.

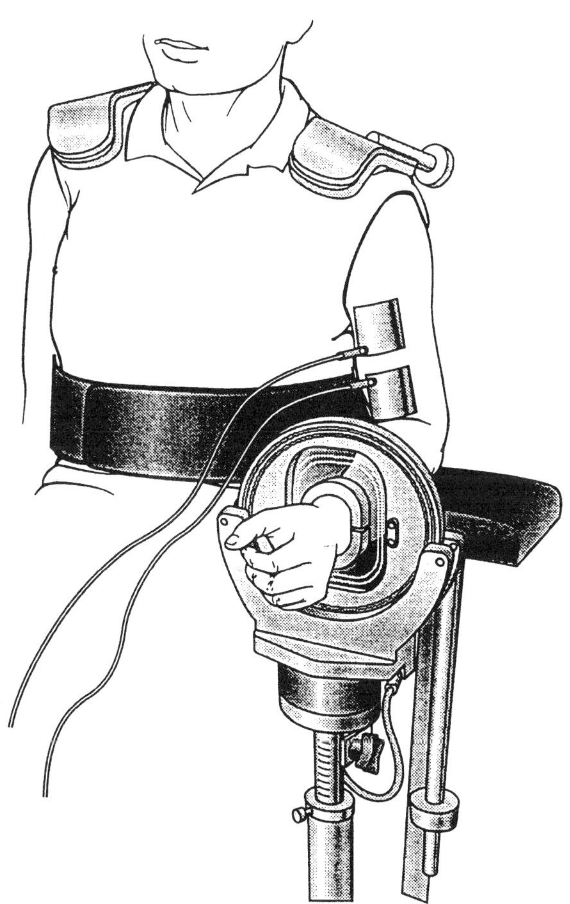

FIGURE 1.—Left arm of a subject in the apparatus used to measure the force exerted by the elbow-flexor muscles and evoked force by the biceps brachii muscle. The force transducer is the circular structure beneath the wrist. (Courtesy of Yue GH, Ranganathan VK, Siemionow V, et al: Older adults exhibit a reduced ability to fully activate their biceps brachii muscle. *J Gerontol* 54A:M249-M253, 1999. Copyright The Gerontological Society of America. Republished with permission of The Gerontological Society of America, 1030 15th Street, NW, Suite 250, Washington, DC 20005. Reproduced by permission of the publisher via copyright Clearance Center, Inc.)

Methods.—The study included 2 groups of volunteers: 14 young individuals (mean age, 31 years) and 14 older individuals (mean age, 71 years). In a special experimental setup connected to a force transducer, electrical stimulation was applied to the skin over the biceps brachii muscle as the subjects performed maximal voluntary elbow flexion contractions (Fig 1). Muscle activation level (AL) was assessed in terms of the magnitude of force evoked on the maximal voluntary force.

Results.—Expressed in percentage of complete activation, AL was 94% for the older group versus 97% for the younger group. The older group had a significantly lower AL than the younger group, although AL in both groups was significantly lower than 100%.

Conclusions.—The ability to activate the biceps brachii muscle is significantly reduced in elderly individuals compared with young adults. However, neither group can achieve full activation of this muscle. These findings suggest that aging-related loss of voluntary strength results from a combination of muscle atrophy and a reduced ability to activate muscle. Both of these factors should be addressed in programs to preserve or restore muscle strength in older adults.

▶ Aging is accompanied by a decrease in muscle strength of about 30% from age 60 to 90 years; some of this decrease is caused by muscle atrophy. However, loss of strength occurs at a faster rate than muscle atrophy, so other factors must affect these losses.

Electrical stimulation pulses were applied to the muscle during a maximal voluntary force output to determine activation levels, and older subjects had lower activation levels (94%) than younger subjects (97%). The decline in force output is partially caused by an impairment in the ability to fully activate the motor units; also, some motor units cannot be activated by voluntary effort because of aging in the brain. The aging brain suffers from a decrease in the number and size of axons, as well as a decrease in myelin and in excitability of spinal motor neurons. It is possible that strength training in older adults could improve CNS outflow to activate muscles more fully.

M. J. L. Alexander, PhD

The Effect of Wrist Guards on Bone Strain in the Distal Forearm

Staebler MP, Moore DC, Akelman E, et al (Brown Univ, Providence, RI)
Am J Sports Med 27:500-506, 1999   8–18

Objective.—Wrist injuries are common in snowboarders and in-line skaters. Although some individuals wear wrist guards to decrease their risk for injury, there are few epidemiologic and biomechanical studies of the effectiveness of such guards. To determine whether wrist guards reduce fracture risk by load sharing, bone strain was measured in the distal radius, distal ulna, and midshaft of the radius in cadaveric forearms with and without 2 types of commercially available wrist guards.

Methods.—Three pairs of fresh-frozen cadaveric upper extremities, without bone disease, from 3 men, ages 74, 78, and 88 years, were tested in a servohydraulic materials testing machine with and without 2 types of wrist guards (Fig 1). The forearms were potted at 75 degrees of dorsiflexion with no varus or volar tilt. The specimens were tested with a 5 newton preload, 20 preconditioning cycles to 50 newtons at 50 newtons/sec, and a single ramp load to 250 N at 100 newtons/sec. Bone strain was measured in the distal radius, distal ulna, and midshaft of the radius.

Results.—Guard A reduced distal and volar radius bone strain by 46% and 80%, respectively, and guard B by 23% and 30%. All reductions were significant except for the volar radius strain reduction by guard B. Guard A significantly reduced strains in the dorsal ulna and volar midshaft by

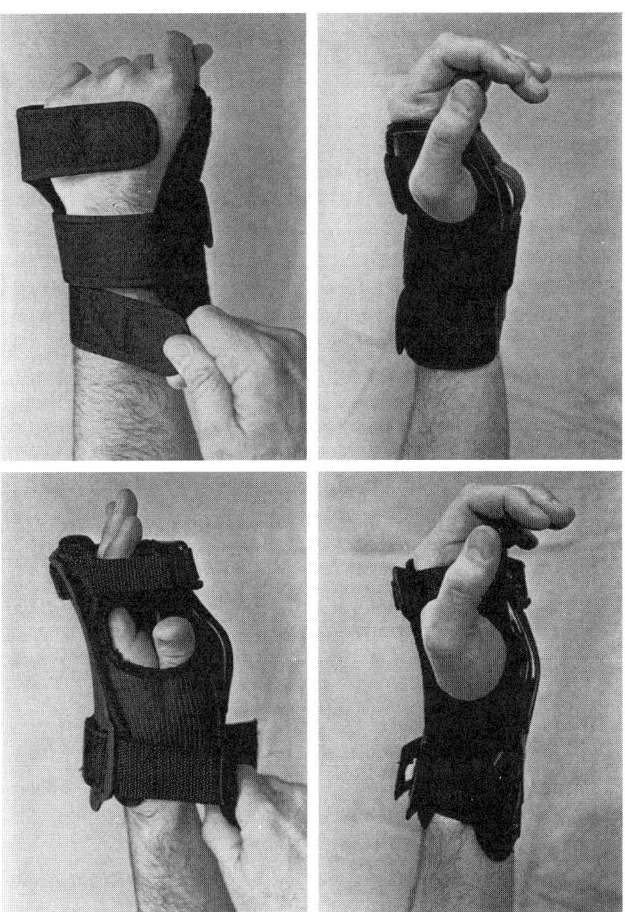

FIGURE 1.—The 2 types of wrist guards tested. **Top,** In the wrap-around guard A, the prominent volar plate was elevated off the heel of the hand. **Bottom,** In the slip-on guard B, the volar plate conformed closely to the heel of the hand. (Courtesy of Staebler MP, Moore DC, Akelman E, et al: The effect of wrist guards on bone strain in the distal forearm. *Am J Sports Med* 27:500-506, 1999.)

61% and 44%. The corresponding changes with guard B were −24% and 12%. Although both guards decreased wrist stiffness significantly at low loads, the reduction was not significant as the load increased.

Conclusion.—Both wrist guards lowered the risk for injury by load-sharing.

▶ The wrist guards described in this study can prevent injuries by absorbing impact energy and by dispersing the load, or, as the authors describe, load-sharing. Their results suggest that wrist guards with nonconforming volar plates may provide more protection than those with conforming volar plates.

F. J. George, ATC, PT

Biomechanical Risk Factors for Exercise-related Lower Limb Injuries
Neely FG (Defence Evaluation and Research Agency, Farnborough, England)
Sports Med 26:395-413, 1998   8–19

Objective.—The incidence of lower limb injuries during running is reported to be as high as 85%. Although biomechanical abnormalities of the lower limb have been implicated in many injuries, few studies have examined the reliability and reproducibility of the measurements of types of biomechanical abnormalities of the lower limb. The existing literature on this topic was reviewed and the likelihood of the various biomechanical abnormalities for being responsible for injury was evaluated.

Ankle Range of Motion.—Evidence that dorsiflexion or plantar flexion contributes to lower limb injuries is sketchy. Limitation of dorsiflexion may be a risk factor, but it is more probable that compensatory factors are the problem.

Femoral Anteversion/Hip Range of Motion.—Although limited range of hip eversion may contribute to lower limb injury, the relationship between hip range of movement and lower limb injuries has not been clearly established.

Genu Varum/Valgum.—The relationship between varus or valgus knee deformities and lower limb injuries is highly controversial.

Laxity, Flexibility, and Muscle Tightness.—There is little evidence that muscle tightness predisposes a runner to lower limb injuries. Excessive joint laxity may be an independent risk factor.

Leg Length Discrepancy.—It is not clear that leg length discrepancy is an independent risk factor for lower limb injury, but it does contribute to the development of low back pain.

Foot Type.—Excessive pronation or supination, excessively high arches, forefoot and rearfoot varus, and pes cavus increase the risk of lower limb injury.

Q angle.—An excessively large Q angle contributes to overuse knee pain.

▶ There is significant controversy regarding the biomechanical and structural risk factors for injuries that occur as a result of exercise. This extensive review of the literature noted that there is little evidence to suggest that abnormal range of ankle plantarflexion, genu varum or valgum, or undue muscle tightness are potential risk factors. Some likely risk factors for injury are: limited range of ankle dorsiflexion, limitation of range of hip lateral rotation, excessive joint laxity, leg length discrepancy, an excessively pronated or supinated foot, excessively high or low arches of the foot, and large Q angle. More prospective research studies are required to evaluate these risk factors for injury and to determine their value as screening tools for participants who may be at risk for lower extremity injury.

M. J. L. Alexander, PhD

Q-angle Influences on the Variability of Lower Extremity Coordination During Running

Heiderscheit BC, Hamill J, Van Emmerik REA (Univ of Massachusetts, Amherst)

Med Sci Sports Exerc 31:1313-1319, 1999   8–20

Background.—The quadriceps angle (Q-angle) may predict patellofemoral pain (PFP). An excessive Q-angle may change the patellofemoral

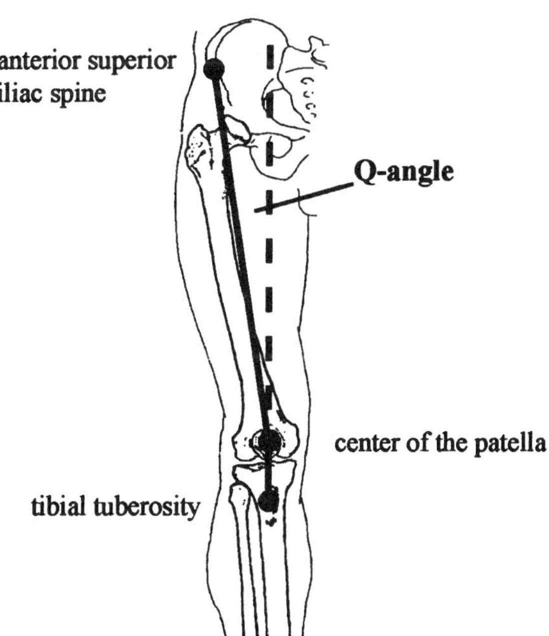

FIGURE 1.—Q-angle defined by the intersection of quadriceps vector and infrapatellar tendon at center of patella. (Courtesy of Heiderscheit BC, Hamill J, Van Emmerik REA: Q-angle influences on the variability of lower extremity coordination during running. *Med Sci Sports Exerc* 31:1313-1319, 1999.)

tracking, resulting in PFP. However, traditional methods for assessing changes in lower extremity angular kinematics have not confirmed this. A dynamic systems approach involving segment couplings was used to provide additional insight by addressing the variability of the intersegmental coordination.

Methods.—Thirty-two healthy persons with a variety of Q-angles were assessed and subgrouped based on sex and Q-angle (Fig 1). The participants ran overground for 10 trials, during which 3-dimensional kinematic data were collected on the thigh, leg, and foot. These data were used to calculate 3-dimensional segment angles and angular velocities. The variability of the continuous relative phase (CRP) of segment couplings was used to determine between-trial consistency at specific stance phase intervals.

Findings.—Participants with varying Q-angles did not have different CRP variability. The specific intervals of the couplings differed significantly, with the greatest variability noted during intial stance.

Conclusions.—Persons with and without abnormal Q-angles do not appear to have different CRP variability in the lower extremity. The significant differences among the stance phase intervals of running suggest that the coordination pattern variability is inherent. Increased pattern variability during initial stance may be important to the maintenance of external stability.

▶ Quadriceps angle is a measure of lower extremity alignment, as it measures the amount of valgus at the knee joint. A larger than normal Q-angle has often been suggested to produce knee injuries, notably patellofemoral problems, and excessive rearfoot pronation. Examination of running kinematics in this study revealed no relationship between abnormal running mechanics and increased Q-angle. However, all the runners tested in this study were injury free, and differences in running coordination patterns may be apparent in runners with running injuries and an increased Q-angle.

M. J. L. Alexander, PhD

Muscle Coordination and Function During Cutting Movements
Neptune RR, Wright IC, van den Bogert AJ (Univ of Calgary, Canada)
Med Sci Sports Exerc 31:294-302, 1999   8–21

Objective.—Ankle sprains represent 14% to 17% of sports injuries and occur often during cutting movements. Although coordination training has been shown to reduce the incidence of ankle sprains, the reason for the reduction is not understood because muscle activation and function measurements are lacking. Kinematic and electromyographic data of normal muscle function and coordination during cutting movements were collected and combined to describe normal muscle function and coordination during these movements and were used to identify potential muscle coordination deficiencies and mechanisms that may lead to injury.

Methods.—Kinematic, electromyographic, and ground reaction force data were collected from 10 recreationally active male volunteers, average age 23.4, who were fitted with retroreflective markers during side-shuffle and 45° forward v-cut movements (Fig 1). Lower extremity joint kinematics were measured with a video analysis system.

Results.—Muscle kinetics were similar during both the side shuffle and 45-degree forward v-cut movements. The primary function of the vasti muscle group and hamstrings was to decelerate the downward motion after impact and stabilize and extend the knee during the forward motion phase of both movements. The plantar flexor muscles absorb impact,

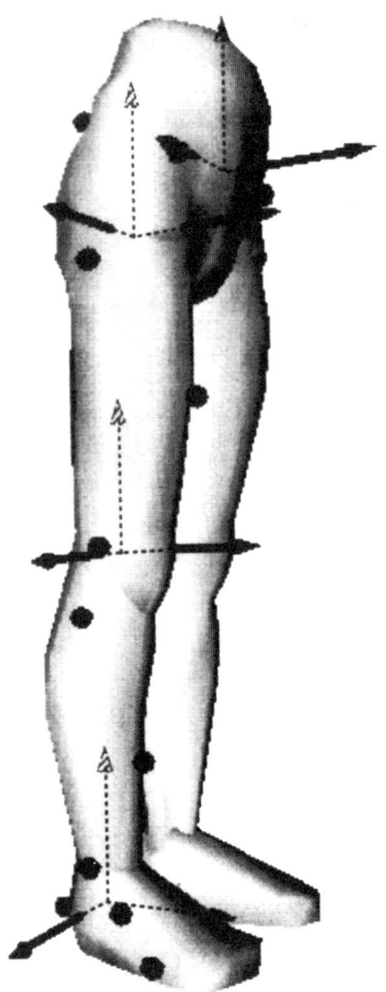

FIGURE 1.—Experimental retroreflective marker placement on the lower extremity. (Courtesy of Neptune RR, Wright IC, van den Bogert AJ: Muscle coordination and function during cutting movements. *Med Sci Sports Exerc* 31:294-302, 1999.)

reduce joint loading, and provide propulsion before toe-off during both movements. The tibialis anterior (TA) bends backward and turns the foot after toe-off during the side shuffle but maintains constant activity throughout the v-cut movement. The TA is the most important muscle in the prevention of ankle sprains. Because it has the highest rate of sustained muscle activity, fatigue that alters muscle timing may result in ankle sprain. Poor coordination between the TA and the peroneus longus may prevent adequate stabilization of the subtalar joint and contribute to excessive foot rotation, thus increasing the risk of sprain.

Conclusion.—Poor coordination or weakness of the TA and the peroneus longus may contribute to ankle sprain injuries. Coordination training may reduce the incidence of sprain. Rehabilitation programs including lower limb strengthening and coordination exercises may be beneficial.

▶ This study examined the role of 12 lower extremity muscles in stabilizing the ankle joint during cutting movements. Because ankle sprains are the most common injury in sport, knowledge of the muscle coordination patterns that protect the ankle during cutting movements may be important in prevention. They found significant activity in the muscles crossing the hip and knee joints that assist in deceleration and stabilization during cutting. The ankle joint muscles were strongly active during the movements, especially the gastrocnemius, which provides propulsion during toe-off as well as deceleration during touchdown. The TA and peroneus longus acted to stabilize the subtalar joint during push off to prevent excessive foot rotations. Ankle sprains may be caused by poor muscle coordination or to weakness in these important muscle groups, so rehabilitation should consist of both lower limb strengthening and overall coordination programs.

M. J. L. Alexander, PhD

Positive Versus Negative Foot Inclination for Maximum Height Two-Leg Vertical Jumps
Larkins C, Snabb TE (Ypsilanti, Mich; Univ of Michigan-Dearborn)
Clin Biomech 14:321-328, 1999   8–22

Objective.—It has been claimed that an athletic shoe with negative foot inclination, in which heel position is lower than forefoot position, can improve athletic performance. Various devices and shoe designs have been proposed to create negative foot inclination, although these have been untested to date. The effects of negative foot inclination on jump height, including the effects of a prototype shoe design incorporating the optimal degree of negative foot inclination, were examined.

Methods and Findings.—Thirteen collegiate track and field athletes participated in the study. The study used an adjustable platform to allow variations in foot inclination (Fig 1). The athletes performed standing 2-leg jumps at different levels of foot inclination: +4, 0, −2, −3, and −4 degrees. Analysis of repeated measures showed that a negative inclination

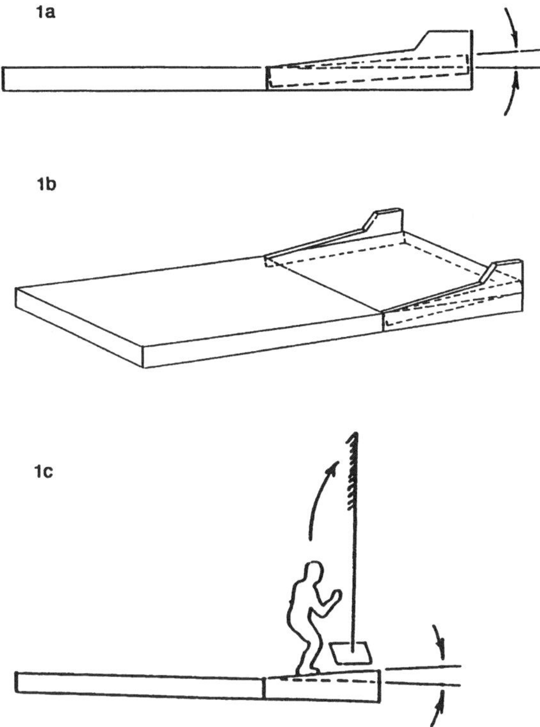

FIGURE 1.—Diagram of the jump platform constructed to allow for a continuous range of negative and positive degrees of foot inclination. (Reprinted from Larkins C, Snabb TE: Positive versus negative foot inclination for maximum height two-leg vertical jumps. *Clin Biomech* 14:321-328, 1999, with kind permission from Elsevier Science.)

of 3.5 degrees was associated with optimal performance on the standing jump: jumping height increased by an average of 4.8 cm, or 10%.

In the second phase of the study, 8 female volleyball players performed running vertical jumps at +4 degrees and −3.5-degrees of inclination. Negative foot inclination again improved jumping performance. Similar results were achieved in a third phase in which −3.5-degree prototype shoes were compared with standard +4-degree shoes.

Conclusions.—Negative foot inclination, with the heel lower than the forefoot, appears to improve jumping performance in athletes. The findings may be useful in athletic shoe design. However, questions remain as to how negative foot inclination improves performance, whether such a shoe might raise the risk of injury, and whether musculoskeletal adaptations would offset the performance benefit.

► Negative foot inclination is a foot position in which the heel is lowered in relation to the forefoot, producing dorsiflexion. It is possible to design shoes that place the foot into a permanent position of positive or negative foot inclination, which may affect jumping performance. A foot position in which the heel is lowered will place a stretch on the calf muscle complex, possibly enhancing jump performance by using stored elastic energy. This study examined the effect of different foot inclinations on jumping performance as measured by the Sargent Vertical Jump Testing Protocol and concluded that negative foot inclination significantly increased jump height. This finding suggests that negative-inclination shoes should be worn by jumping athletes, but the implications for muscle injury or Achilles tendon strain are unknown at this time.

M. J. L. Alexander, PhD

Three-dimensional Kinetic Analysis of Running: Significance of Secondary Planes of Motion
McClay I, Manal K (Univ of Delware, Newark; Joyner Sportsmedicine Inst, Harrisburg, Pa)
Med Sci Sports Exerc 31:1629-1637, 1999   8–23

Background.—Overuse injuries in runners are often caused by deviations in the secondary planes of motion. Little is known about the angular kinetics in these planes, so there is no reference for comparison.

Methods and Findings.—Three-dimensional kinematic and ground reaction force data were obtained on 20 recreational runners with normal rearfoot mechanics. Sagittal plane kinetic data were comparable to previously reported 2-dimensional studies. Sagittal plane data were least variable, comprising the largest percentage of positive or negative work done at the rearfoot and knee joints. Transverse plane kinetics were most variable, comprising the smallest percentage of work done at these joints.

Conclusions.—A substantial amount of positive work is done in the frontal plane at both joints, though relatively smaller than the sagittal plane component. These normative reference data will be useful when evaluating patients with abnormal mechanics.

▶ There are no other studies available in the literature that include a 3-dimensional kinetic analysis of running. The majority of the previous studies are sagittal planar studies and do not include the moments occurring in the frontal and transverse planes. Some interesting frontal plane findings reported were an inversion moment dominating during footstrike, controlled by tibialis posterior, and a knee abduction moment seen throughout footstrike controlled by the iliotibial band. The transverse plane moments were small and variable, with an initial external rotation moment at the ankle and knee during footstrike, followed by an internal rotation moment. It was concluded that the frontal plane moments are significant and should be considered in future kinetic analyses of running.

M. J. L. Alexander, PhD

Plantar Loading and Cadence Alterations With Fatigue
Willson JD, Kernozek TW (Univ of Wisconsin-La Crosse; Gundersen Lutheran Sports Medicine, La Crosse, Wis)
Med Sci Sports Exerc 31:1828-1833, 1999   8–24

Objective.—Although musculoskeletal injury is common among runners and walkers, the mechanism of such injuries is poorly understood. Repetitive loading of ligaments, cartilage, and bones has been shown to be a significant risk factor for running injuries. The effects of fatigue on loading variables of the feet while running were measured by with Pedar in-shoe measurement system.

Methods.—The Pedar in-shoe system was installed in the running shoes of 22 active, healthy volunteers. Pressure distribution measurements were performed at 7 anatomical regions while volunteers ran to fatigue on a treadmill with the Ohio State University protocol for exercise testing. Force-time integral (FTI), peak force (PF), peak pressure (PP), and pressure-time integral (PTI) were recorded under normal and fatigued conditions in a series of repeated measures. Multiple analysis of variance was performed.

Results.—Peak force was 70.0% of body mass under the heel and 37.2% of body weight under the second and third metatarsals. FTI values under the second and third metatarsals increased with longer contact time. Contact time, PF, PP, FTI, and PTI decreased significantly during fatigued running, and less force was distributed to the heel over a shorter period of time. PF values decreased from 70% of body mass during a rested condition to 62.5% of body mass in the fatigued condition. Simultaneously, contact time decreased from 179.3 to 163.3 msec. Contact times, PP, and PTI were also reduced during fatigue.

Conclusion.—Running when fatigued decreased stride length and increased cadence, resulting in decreased heel loading and increased midfoot loading.

▶ When fatigue sets in, a runner's step length decreases and the cadence increases. There is a significant shift in loading from the heel to the area under the first metatarsal. These factors may be a cause of the high incidence of stress fractures, tendonitis, and muscle strains in many runners. The authors did not suggest how to avoid these changes in the running gait other than not running when fatigued.

F. J. George, ATC, PT

Eccentric/Concentric Ratios at Selected Velocities for the Invertor and Evertor Muscles of the Chronically Unstable Ankle

Hartsell HD, Spaulding SJ (Univ of Iowa, Iowa City; Univ of Western Ontario, London, Canada)
Br J Sports Med 33:255-258, 1999   8–25

Background.—The use of muscle balancing to decide return to activity or discharge is not well understood. The eccentric-concentric (E/C) ratios for the invertor and evertor muscles at various velocities in normal and chronically unstable ankles were determined.

Methods and Findings.—Ten persons with normal ankles and 14 with chronically unstable ankles performed 5 maximal effort reciprocal E/C contractions on an isokinetic dynamometer at 4 velocities for each physiologic movement of inversion and eversion. Chronically unstable ankles were significantly weaker eccentrically and concentrically for inversion and eversion. However, the main effect of the E/C ratios for the ankle was not significant for either joint motion. The main effect of velocity was significant for each joint motion. There were no significant interaction effects. As velocity increased, the E/C ratio increased also, except at the highest velocities (180 and 240 degrees per second) for either ankle group (Fig 1).

Conclusions.—Chronic ankle instability and muscle weakness can occur together. In chronically unstable ankles, E/C ratios may be adequate when strength values are not normal.

▶ It is often the case that chronically injured joints also have weakened muscle groups surrounding them, caused either by underuse or by impaired neural feedback from the joint. This study reinforced this finding, in that the chronically unstable ankle was significantly weaker than the healthy ankle in both inversion and eversion. As well, the peroneal muscles of the unstable ankle were weaker in eccentric contractions at high-velocity movements,

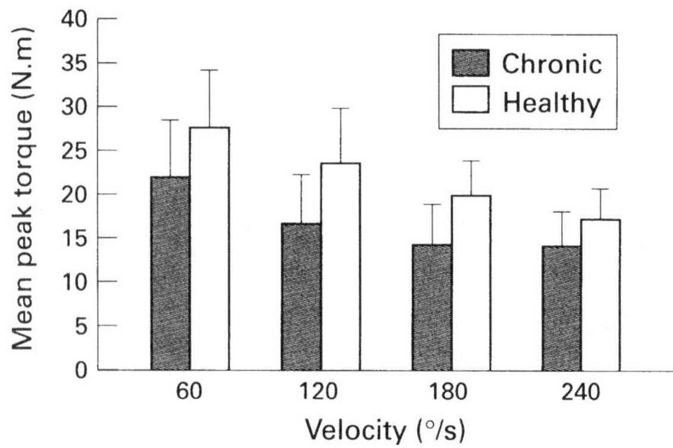

FIGURE 1.—Concentric peak torques for inversion by group. (Courtesy of Hartsell HD, Spaulding SJ: Eccentric/concentric ratios at selected velocities for the invertor and evertor muscles of the chronically unstable ankle. *Br J Sports Med* 33:255-258, 1999, with permission from the BMJ Publishing Group.)

such as those seen in sports activities. This finding suggests impaired muscle activity around the ankle during eccentric and high-velocity loads, which could lead to reinjury. This is an important consideration for clinicians when considering a return to normal activity for patients with chronic ankle injuries.

M. J. L. Alexander, PhD

Neuromuscular Properties and Functional Aspects of Taped Ankles
Lohrer H, Alt W, Gollhofer A (Inst of Sport Medicine Frankfurt am Main, Germany; Stuttgart Univ, Germany)
Am J Sports Med 27:69-75, 1999   8–26

Objective.—Studies on the effects of taping on an unstable ankle joint have investigated only neuromuscular pathways rather than the quantitative and qualitative effects of reflex muscle response. The sensitivity of functional joint stability to ankle taping and to athletic exercise was investigated by quantifying reflex-induced neuromuscular activation in relation to the maximum inversion amplitude of the ankle joint after controlled mechanical stimulus.

Methods.—A group of 40 volunteers (18 men) compared 2 tape materials. Group 1 (n = 20) used 3.75-cm wide Leukotape (made by Beiersdorf Medical), and group 2 used 3.8-cm wide 3M-tape (made by 3M Medica) on an inversion tilt platform with mechanical stimulus applied of 15° of plantar flexion and 30° of inversion with the right foot loaded with ≥90% body weight. Angular movement was measured with goniometers attached to the Achilles tendon and the calcaneus and with electrodes attached to the tibialis anterior, peroneus longus, gastrocnemius medialis, and vastus medialis muscles during 5 sprain simulations.

Results.—Active inversion was reduced to 11° in groups 1 and 2 from baseline values of 22° and 23°, respectively. Plantar flexion was similarly reduced to 33° for both groups from baseline values of 52° and 53°. After 20 minutes of exercise, inversion and plantar flexion mobilities increased to 14° (64% of baseline) and 50° (96%) in group 1 and to 15° (65% of baseline) and 46° (87%) degrees in group 2. After 24 hours, inversion and plantar flexion were 16° (73%) and 46° (88%) in group 1 and 18° (78%) and 49° (92%) in group 2. Mean maximum inversion decreased in both groups from 32° before wrapping to 18° after wrapping and to 21° in group 1 and to 23° in group 2 after 10 minutes of exercise. All differences were significant. After 20 minutes of exercise, inversion decreased to 21° and 23°, respectively. The difference was significant for group 2. The mean latency of the medial vastus muscle before Band after taping was a significant 4 msec shorter than for the other muscles. The proprioceptive amplification ratio increased significantly to 1.6 after taping from a baseline value of 1.0, decreased significantly to 1.2 after 20 minutes of exercise, and increased significantly to 1.5 after 24 hours.

Conclusion.—Taping protects the ankle joint from injury by reducing inversion amplitudes and tilting angular velocities.

▶ The results of this study are encouraging for those athletic trainers who routinely tape ankles to prevent and treat injuries. However, the type of tape used in this study is different from the conventional adhesive tape used in most athletic training rooms. The tape used in this study has a higher tensile strength.

F. J. George, ATC, PT

Chronic Eccentric Exercise: Improvements in Muscle Strength Can Occur With Little Demand for Oxygen

Lastayo PC, Reich TE, Urquhart M, et al (Northern Arizona Univ, Flagstaff; Univ of Bern, Switzerland)

Am J Physiol 276:R611-R615, 1999   8–27

Background.—The traditional view of skeletal muscle is shortening plus contraction to produce concentric (Con) work. However, eccentric (Ecc) work (force produced by muscle lengthening) is an important part of everyday movement. Because of the belief that Ecc contractions must cause muscle pain and injury, few studies have examined the effects of prolonged Ecc training on muscle injury and strength. This randomized study examined the effects of chronic Ecc training on locomotor muscle strength and injury, at energy intensities with no effect on concentrically trained muscles.

Methods.—The study included 9 healthy volunteers with a mean age of 21.5 years. They were assigned to 6 weeks of training on an Ecc or traditional Con cycle ergometer. In both groups, the frequency and duration of exercise increased progressively during training. The Ecc work rates were intended to increase leg strength, without producing muscle injury, at a level of oxygen consumption no greater than that produced by Con work. The 2 types of exercise were compared for their effects on lower extremity isometric muscle strength, oxygen consumption, and lower extremity soreness.

Results.—The Ecc exercise group had significant increases in isometric leg strength, whereas the Con group did not (Fig 2). Despite the fact that Ecc training began at a 3-fold higher work rate than Con training—increasing to a 7-fold difference by the end of the study—the oxygen requirement to perform Ecc work was less than or equal to that required for Con work. After the first 2 weeks, Ecc work caused little or no leg pain. There was no difference in ratings of perceived exertion between the 2 groups after the first week.

Conclusion.—Performing Ecc exercise at a progressively increasing work rate can yield significant gains in isometric strength. These increases are achieved with no muscle injury and with little or no increase in energy intensity, measured as oxygen uptake. The ability to improve strength

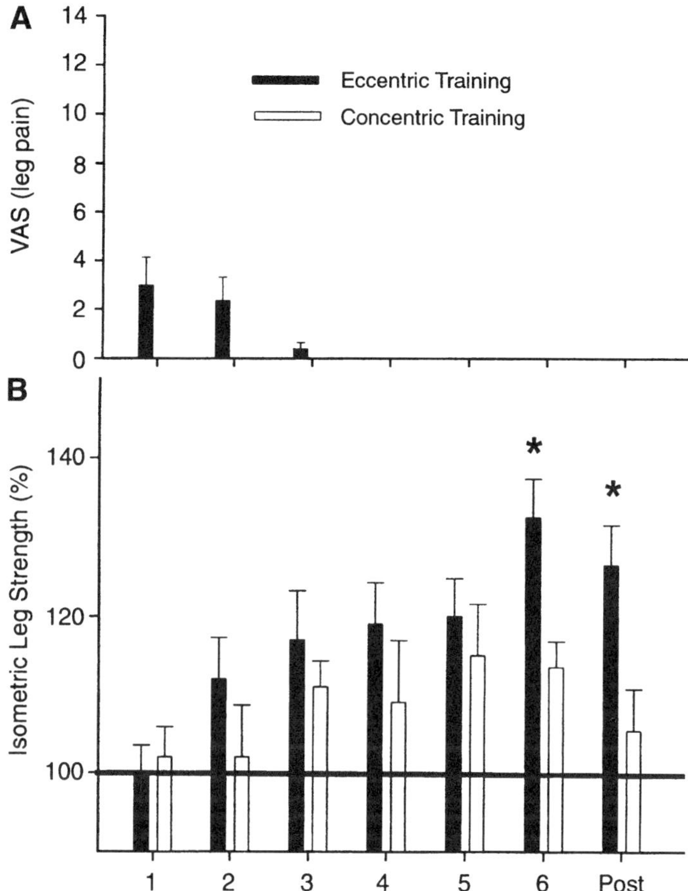

FIGURE 2.—Leg pain and isometric leg strength were measured weekly during training and before and after (2-3 days after) training. Mean values are shown with *error bars* equal to 1 SE. *Asterisk* indicates significant difference (*P* less than .05) from initial values. **A,** Leg pain was monitored with a 14-cm visual analogue scale (*VAS*). Very little leg/muscle soreness in the eccentric (Ecc) group was noted during the first 3 weeks and no leg pain thereafter. There was no leg pain in the concentric (Con) group at any time. **B,** Isometric leg extension strength for the Ecc and Con groups is shown as a relative percentage of their initial pretraining values. Overall, significant Ecc strength gains (*P* less than .05) were noted during the sixth week (33%) and at the 2- to 3-day posttraining measurement (27%). No significant increases in Con strength were noted at any time. (Courtesy of Lastayo PC, Reich TE, Urqhart M, et al: Chronic eccentric exercise: Improvements in muscle strength can occur with little demand for oxygen. *Am J Physiol* 276:R611-R615, 1999, copyright The American Physiological Society.)

through Ecc training, with minimal cardiac demand, could have important clinical applications, eg, for elderly patients with cardiovascular disease.

▶ This should be viewed as a preliminary study because of the small number of subjects (9). However, the study does have some promising indications. Ecc training intensity can be managed to minimize muscle injury and discomfort. Significant strength gains can be made by utilizing Ecc training, with less demands on the cardiovascular system.

F. J. George, ATC, PT

9 Women: Aging

Gender Comparisons of the Mechanomyographic Responses to Maximal Concentric and Eccentric Isokinetic Muscle Actions

Evetovich TK, Housh TJ, Johnson GO, et al (Univ of Nebraska-Lincoln)

Med Sci Sports Exerc 30:1697-1702, 1998

9–1

Background.—Mechanomyography (MMG) records the low-frequency sounds generated by the contraction of muscle. MMG can provide information about gross movements of muscle and dimensional changes in the fibers of active muscles and may be useful in examining muscle diseases and controlling external prostheses. However, differences in various factors, such as muscle mass, length, torque production, and velocity of muscle action, affect the amplitude of the MMG signal. The MMG signal is also influenced by differences in the thickness of the adipose tissue layer. Differences between men and women in these factors and in the thickness of the adipose tissue layer may cause gender-related differences in MMG amplitude during muscular activity. With one exception, previous studies of MMG responses to dynamic muscle actions have not included female subjects. Gender-related differences in velocity-related patterns of MMG response to isokinetic muscle actions were examined in this study.

Methods.—The study group comprised 15 men and 16 women. A Cybex 6000 dynamometer was used to test all subjects at 3 randomly ordered muscle action velocities for maximal concentric (CON) and eccentric (ECC) isokinetic peak torque (PT) using the dominant leg. The MMG signal was detected with a Hewlett-Packard 21050A sensor. MMG analysis was done for the trial, resulting in the highest PT for CON and ECC isokinetic muscle actions. A standardized range of motion of 90 degrees was used for comparison among the muscle action velocities.

Results.—There were declines in concentric peak torque for both men and women at all three different mucle action velocities tested; however, this decline was greater in women (Fig 2). The MMG amplitude for men was greater than that for women at all concentric velocities. There was no gender-related difference in eccentric peak torque, which remained constant at all velocities in both men and women. In both men and women, the MMG amplitude for eccentric velocities was consistently lower than the amplitude for concentric velocities.

Conclusions.—Muscle mass and adipose tissue layer thickness, among other factors relating to muscle structure, influence MMG amplitude. The

"

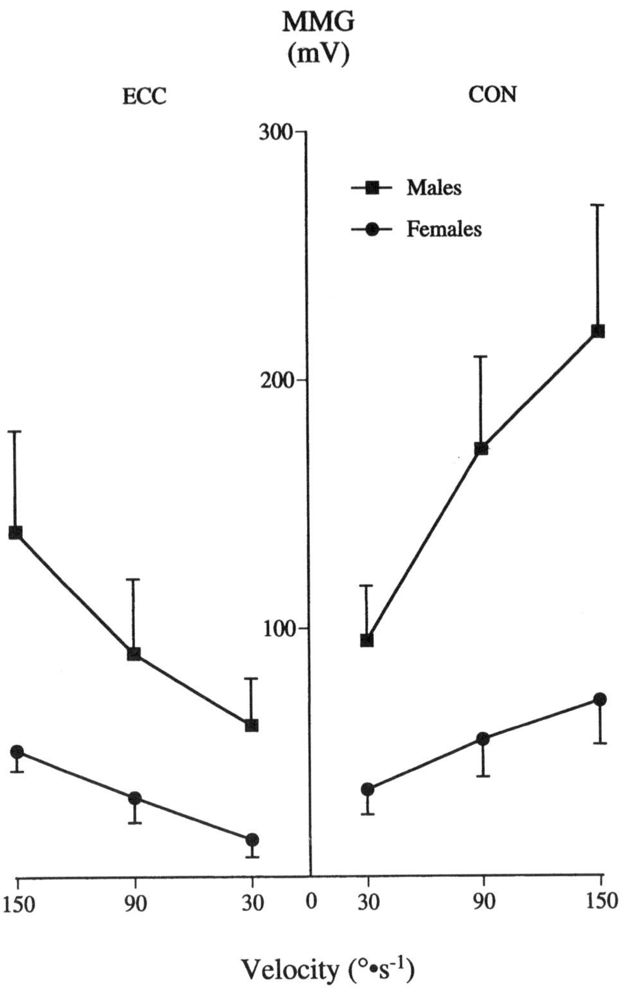

Velocity ($°•s^{-1}$)

FIGURE 2.—The relationship ($\overline{X}$ ± SEM) between CON and ECC MMG amplitude (mV) and muscle action velocity (degrees per second) for men and women. (Courtesy of Evetovich TK, Housh TJ, Johnson GO, et al: Gender comparisons of the mechanomyographic responses to maximal concentric and eccentric isokinetic muscle actions. *Med Sci Sports Exerc* 30:1697-1702, 1998.)

tendency toward greater muscle mass in men and the difference between men and women in thickness of the adipose tissue layer may account for the greater MMG amplitude at concentric velocities in men. Thus, the increase in MMG amplitude in men may relate more to the structure rather than to the function of muscle.

▶ Mechanomyography (MMG) records the low-frequency sounds generated by muscle during contraction; it can be used to determine the gross movement of the muscle and to determine the dimensional changes of active muscle fibers. MMG amplitude increased with velocity for both the men and the women. Maximal isokinetic testing at three different velocities produced declines in concentric peak torque for both men and women, with a greater decline in concentric peak torque in women. At all concentric velocities, men exhibited greater MMG amplitude than women. Eccentric peak torque remained constant with increasing velocity for both men and women, the MMG amplitude was consistently lower for eccentric than for concentric torque, and there was no gender difference in MMG amplitude across eccentric velocities. Since MMG is related to muscle mass and adipose layer thickness, increased MMG in male subjects may be related to structure rather than to muscle function. The value of MMG in analysis of muscle performance during maximal contractions remains unproven by this article.

M. J. L. Alexander, PhD

Gender Differences in Musculoskeletal Injury Rates: A Function of Symptom Reporting?

Almeida SA, Trone DW, Leone DM (Naval Health Research Ctr, San Diego, Calif)
Med Sci Sports Exerc 31:1807-1812, 1999

9–2

Background.—Exercise-related musculoskeletal injuries are associated with significant morbidity, lost work time, increased use of medical resources, and attrition from exercise programs. In military trainees, such injuries are associated with lost training time, medical attrition, and increased training costs. Sex differences in the voluntary reporting of lower extremity musculoskeletal injuries among US Marine Corps recruits were investigated.

Methods.—Two hundred forty-one women and 176 men were followed up prospectively through weeks 12 and 11, respectively, of boot camp training. Medical records were reviewed for reported injuries. To determine the occurrence of unreported injuries, recruits were given a questionnaire and a medical examination on completion of training.

Findings.—Among women, the most commonly reported injuries were patellofemoral syndrome (20%), ankle sprain (9.1%), and iliotibial band syndrome (5.8%). The most common unreported injuries were patellofemoral syndrome in 2.1%, metatarsalgia in 1.7%, and unspecified knee pain in 1.7%. Among men, the most commonly reported injuries were iliotibial band syndrome in 4%, ankle sprain in 2.8%, and Achilles tendinitis/bursitis in 2.8%. The most common unreported injuries in men were shin splints (4.6%), iliotibial band syndrome (4%), and ankle sprain (2.8%). Women were more likely to have reported injuries than men and were less likely to have an unreported injury. Overall, injury rates were high in both women and men, at 53.5% and 45.5%, respectively. These rates were not significantly different.

Conclusions.—The higher injury rates previously reported for female military trainees may be explained by women's greater tendency to report injuries. In this study, when both reported and unreported injuries were considered, injury rates did not differ significantly between the sexes.

▶ This politically correct document confuses injury and injury rates with subjective complaints of "knee pain," "foot pain," "metatarsalgia," etc.

J. S. Torg, MD

Anterior Cruciate Ligament Injury Patterns Among Collegiate Men and Women
Arendt EA, Agel J, Dick R (Univ of Minnesota, Minneapolis; Natl Collegiate Athletic Assoc, Overland Park, Kan)
J Athletic Train 34:86-92, 1999   9–3

Objective.—There are differences in anterior cruciate ligament (ACL) injury rates in male and female athletes. Basketball and soccer injury pattern data for the last 10 years were collected from the National Collegiate Athletic Association database and reviewed.

Methods.—Data on sex-specific knee injuries were collected and expressed as injuries per 1000 athletic exposures for 1989 to 1993 and for 1994 to 1998.

Results.—The 1989-1993 ACL injury rates for soccer were 0.31 for women and 0.13 for men. The primary mechanism for injury in women was no contact (63%) and player contact (37%), whereas for men it was player contact (52%) and no contact (48%). Women were twice as likely as men to have an ACL injury after player contact. The ACL injury rates for basketball were 0.29 for women and 0.07 for men. The cause for men and women was no apparent contact (80%) and player contact (20%). During the 1994-1998 period, women continued to have a higher injury rate than men in soccer and basketball. Female volleyball players had a significantly lower incidence of ACL injury than female soccer and basketball players. The profile of the ACL-injured athlete revealed that the mechanism of injury was pivoting or landing from a jump.

Conclusion.—The ACL injury rate in female athletes is significantly higher than in male athletes playing the same sports. The mechanism of ACL injury to female athletes appears to be multifactorial and requires further study.

▶ The conclusion of the authors is that the increased incidence of ACL disruption in women compared with men is "not clearly attributable to any physical or historical measurements that were monitored." That is, comparative and relative hormone levels were not determined.

J. S. Torg, MD

Knee Joint Laxity and Neuromuscular Characteristics of Male and Female Soccer and Basketball Players
Rozzi SL, Lephart SM, Gear WS, et al (College of Charleston, SC; Univ of Pittsburgh, Pa)
Am J Sports Med 27:312-319, 1999
9–4

Background.—Injuries to the anterior cruciate ligament (ACL) are among the most common injuries of athletes. As the participation of women in intercollegiate sports has increased, the incidence of ACL injuries among women has also increased and is significantly higher than among their male counterparts. Various explanations for this disproportionate incidence of ACL injuries among women in intercollegiate sports have been advanced, including knee joint laxity, muscle strength, balance, proprioception, distal femur dimensions, shoe-surface interface, and muscle fatigue. However, recent research has focused on the role of proprioception and muscle activity in stabilizing the knee joint.

It is thought that proprioceptive deficits—possibly resulting from excessive laxity in the knee joint—may leave the joint unable to sense and respond to stress. This, in turn, could lead to injury to the ligament and connective tissue. The possible role of knee joint laxity in ACL injuries was investigated, and the neuromuscular characteristics of the joint in a group of male and female intercollegiate soccer and basketball players were examined.

Methods.—A group of 34 collegiate athletes, evenly divided as to male and female athletes, participated in the study. All of the participants were healthy soccer or basketball players without a history of significant ligament injury to either knee joint, and all had functionally stable ankle joints. The participants were tested for knee joint laxity, joint kinesthesia, lower extremity balance, time required to generate peak torque of the knee flexor and extensor muscles, and electromyographic muscle activity. Significant gender differences were determined by means of independent *t*-tests.

Results.—There was a significant difference in joint laxity values between the male and female participants, with the women having much higher values. Time required to peak torque was also significantly different between the 2 groups, with the women having a much longer time in detecting the movement of the joint into extension. The women scored better than men in single-leg balance and demonstrated much greater electromyographic peak amplitude and area of the lateral hamstring on landing from a jump.

Conclusion.—It appears from the data produced that the women had excessive joint laxity, which would seem to contribute to diminished proprioception. This increases the risk of injury to the knee by leaving it less sensitive to potentially damaging stresses. The electromyographic results indicate that in healthy female athletes, functional stabilization of the joint is accomplished through compensatory mechanisms of increased hamstring activity.

▶ "Why can't a woman be more like a man?" Interestingly, the authors do not entertain the possibility of a correlation between testosterone and androgenic hormone levels and the propensity for ACL disruption.

J. S. Torg, MD

The Relative Incidence of Anterior Cruciate Ligament Injury in Men and Women at the United States Naval Academy
Gwinn DE, Wilckens JH, McDevitt ER, et al (US Naval Academy, Annapolis, Md; Uniformed Services Univ of Health Sciences, Bethesda, Md)
Am J Sports Med 28:98-102, 2000   9–5

Introduction.—Recent investigations have reported significant increases in knee injuries, particularly of the anterior cruciate ligament (ACL), in female athletes. Most of these trials have evaluated only National Collegiate Athletic Association Division I collegiate athletes. This health issue is also a concern in the US military, which has an increasing number of females in a physically rigorous training environment. The incidence of ACL injuries between 1991 and 1997 was compared among male and female intercollegiate athletics, intramural athletics, and US Naval midshipmen participating in the obstacle course and instructional wrestling.

Methods.—Data were collected at the time of injury. Teach coaches and athletic trainers completed questionnaires to determine the total number of athletic exposures, which included any practice or game. Data concerning the midshipman population was collected from records at the Registrar's office.

Results.—Intercollegiate soccer, basketball, and rugby female athletes had a relative injury risk of 3.96, compared with male athletes. For coed soccer, basketball, softball, and rugby, female athletes had a relative risk of injury of 1.40, compared with male athletes. Compared with men in the military, their female counterparts had a relative injury risk of 9.74. The overall annual ACL relative risk of injury among female midshipmen was 2.24, compared with male midshipmen.

Conclusion.—Female midshipmen, particularly athletes, are at increased relative risk of ACL injury, compared with male midshipmen. The increase in risk was not significant at the intramural level of athletics.

▶ As Professor Henry Higgins (*My Fair Lady*) asked: "Why can't a woman be more like a man?" The politicalization of today's military, attempting to establish gender physical equality by subjecting male and female cadets to "regimented training programs at identical facilities," is one of the absurdities of our times. Clearly, today's military is "not the military of our fathers." However, to this observer, gender differences should be recognized and physical demands be in keeping with the physical capabilities of the gender.

J. S. Torg, MD

The Relationship Between Body Composition and Physical Performance in Older Women

Zamboni M, Turcato E, Santana H, et al (Università di Verona, Italy; CNR Program on Aging, Padua, Italy; Natl Inst of Aging, Bethesda, Md; et al)
J Am Geriatr Soc 47:1403-1408, 1999   9–6

Purpose.—Disability becomes more prevalent with age, particularly among women. Older adults with higher body mass index (BMI) are more likely to become disabled, but the important component in this relationship may be loss of skeletal muscle mass. The association between body composition and physical disability was investigated in a group of elderly women.

Methods.—The study included a random population sample of 144 Italian women aged 68 to 75 years. All subjects were able to walk at least one-half mile without difficulty and had a Mini-Mental Status Examination score of higher than 24. All underwent dual-energy x-ray absorptiometry and bioimpedance studies to assess body composition. Based on a combination of physical function scales, 63 women were classified as having limitations of physical functioning and 81 as being nondisabled.

Results.—The women with disability had a greater body weight, BMI, waist and hip circumference, sagittal diameter, total body and leg fat mass, and fat percent, compared with the nondisabled women. The ratio of body cell mass to fat-free mass was lower in the disabled group. Body cell mass was significantly lower for women in the lowest tertile of muscle strength, compared with those in the highest tertile.

Conclusions.—Older women with physical disability have higher BMI, higher body fat, and higher percent body fat than nondisabled women. Lower extremity muscle strength is significantly related to fat-free mass. Although larger studies including both sexes are needed, the ratio of body cell mass to fat-free mass may be a useful indicator of muscle quality as related to function.

▶ Physical frailty and disability in old age traditionally have been associated with being underweight, rather than overweight. However, it seems likely that with improved health care, overweight individuals are now living longer, and disability in this population is becoming more apparent. Indeed, in this study of women aged 68 to 75 years, disability was associated with a high body fat content. Even more surprising was the finding that muscle strength was reduced in disabled women, despite the fact that lean body mass tended to be higher than in normal, age-matched women. Physical activity habits were not assessed in this study, but it seems likely that sedentary behavior could lead to both increased adiposity and reduced muscle function, leading to premature disability.

W. M. Kohrt, PhD

Reliability and Validity of Body Composition Measures in Female Athletes

Fornetti WC, Pivarnik JM, Foley JM, et al (Michigan State Univ, East Lansing)
J Appl Physiol 87:1114-1122, 1999
9–7

Introduction.—Although a high ratio of fat-free mass (FFM) to fat mass (FM) is generally regarded as favorable in athletes, a body fat level that is too low can adversely affect health and performance. For professionals working with athletes, a radical change in body composition should trigger concern about potential health problems. For female athletes, the triad of disordered eating, amenorrhea, and osteoporosis is a common and potentially devastating problem. Percentage body fat (%BF) has traditionally been measured by means of dual-energy x-ray absorptiometry (DEXA). In recent years, new electronic measurement tools have became available, including bioelectric impedance (BIA) and near-infrared interactance (NIR). The reliability and validity of BIA and NIR for assessing body composition in female athletes were assessed and compared with the standard of DEXA.

Methods.—The study included a total of 132 women (mean age, 20 years) participating in collegiate varsity sports. All underwent DEXA to establish the criterion measure of FFM. Body composition was also estimated by BIA and NIR, and stepwise multiple regression was carried out to derive an equation for BIA and NIR estimates of FFM.

Results.—All 3 measures yielded very high reliability coefficients for multiple and single trials, with a low standard error of the mean for all variables. The mean DEXA measurement of FFM was 49.5 kg, corresponding to a %BF of 20.4%. Predicted FFM values of the other techniques were 49.4 kg for BIA and 49.5 kg for NIR. An equation that was developed using only height and weight predicted an FFM of 49.4 kg.

Conclusions.—In a sample of female collegiate athletes, the electronic BIA and NIR techniques are highly valid and reliable in estimating body composition. Their performance in predicting %BF, based on DEXA measurements of FFM, is slightly better than predictions based on height and weight alone. With careful attention to measurement technique, BIA and NIR can provide highly accurate results with only a single trial.

Anthropometry and Bioelectrical Impedance Inconsistently Predicts Fatness in Women With Regional Adiposity

Swan PD, McConnell KE (Arizona State Univ, Tempe)
Med Sci Sports Exerc 31:1068-1075, 1999
9–8

Objective.—Dual-energy x-ray absorptiometry and other advanced techniques are highly accurate in assessing body composition and body fat distribution. Field methods such as anthropometric measurements and bioelectrical impedance (BIA) are more practical for use in diverse settings, although they are associated with greater error. Field methods have frequently been used with regression equations, which may be population specific or generalizable. This study assessed the accuracy of generalizable anthropometric and BIA regression equations for use in estimating body fat in women with differing patterns of body fat distribution.

Methods.—The study included a community sample of 36 premenopausal women. On the basis of waist-to-hip circumference ratio (WHR), they were classified as having a lower body (LB) fat distribution with a WHR of 0.73 or less or an upper body (UB) fat distribution with a WHR of 0.80 or more. The 2 groups consisted of 18 women each, matched for age and percentage body fat on hydrostatic weighing. Anthropometric measurements and BIA were performed as well. Five published equations to estimate percentage body fat based on anthropometric data and three equations based on BIA were evaluated in the 2 groups.

Results.—Compared with hydrostatic weighing, the 5 equations based on anthropometric data significantly overestimated percentage body fat in women with a UB distribution. Of the 3 BIA equations, 1 overestimated percentage body fat in UB women, 1 overestimated in both groups, and 1 underestimated in LB women.

Conclusions.—Some regression equations based on anthropometric or BIA data can accurately predict percentage body fat in women with a LB pattern of fat distribution. However, these equations are not reliable in women with a primarily abdominal fat pattern. Pending the development of appropriate equations, anthropometric estimates of percentage body fat should be derived cautiously in women with a UB fat distribution pattern. The regional pattern of fat distribution has less effect on estimates produced by equations in which BIA data are used.

▶ Body composition is a determinant of successful performance in many athletic events, particularly those that require carrying (eg, distance running) or lifting (eg, gymnastics) of body mass. Although reduction of body weight does not necessarily result in improved performance and may, in fact, lead to amenorrhea and increased risk of osteoporosis, many athletes are nevertheless driven to lose weight in the hope of gaining success. Evaluating the effects of weight loss on performance poses a significant challenge to the sports medicine community. One aspect of this challenge involves identifying methods that accurately assess body composition, particularly in field or office settings. Hydrodensitometry and DEXA are usually the methods of choice, but both are laboratory-based procedures that require relatively expensive equipment. Essentially all other methods provide indirect estimates of body composition and are evaluated for accuracy by comparison with established methods. This typically involves establishing a mathematical relationship between the reference method and the experimental method, so that it is possible to convert what is actually measured by the experimental method (such as skinfold thicknesses in anthropometry or resistance in BIA) to meaningful measures of body composition (such as fat-free mass or body fat content). These 2 articles emphasize the caution that must be exercised in using indirect methods of assessing body composition. Although equations to predict body composition accurately can be developed, as in the study by Fornetti et al, the equation may be accurate only in the population in which it was developed. As illustrated in the article by Swan and McConnell, large errors in estimation of body composition can occur, even when equations thought to be appropriate for the population are used. Parents, coaches, and health care professionals should be strongly discouraged from using indirect methods of assessing body composition to judge whether an athlete should be encouraged to lose weight to enhance performance.

W. M. Kohrt, PhD

Reduced Resting Metabolic Rate in Athletes with Menstrual Disorders

Lebenstedt M, Platte P, Pirke K-M (Ctr for Psychobiology and Psychosomatic Research, Trier, Germany)
Med Sci Sports Exerc 31:1250-1256, 1999   9–9

Background.—An increased incidence of menstrual disturbances as a result of endurance exercise has been described in a number of previous studies. Dieting with minor or moderate weight loss has been associated with menstrual cycle disturbances and may contribute to the development of reproductive dysfunctions in healthy women of normal weight. Athletes participate in a variety of dietary and weight control practices to lower their weight or maintain a low weight. This is particularly true among endurance athletes. Metabolic and nutritional determinants that are associated with menstrual disorders in athletes were investigated.

Methods.—The study group comprised 21 athletes with normal menstrual function and 12 athletes with menstrual disorders. Assessment of salivary progesterone concentrations were used to determine the quality of the menstrual cycle. Researchers measured the resting metabolic rate and diet-induced thermogenesis with indirect calorimetry. Researchers also assessed body composition, energy intake, and restrained eating scores. One-factor ANCOVA was used on the statistical analysis.

Results.—After adjusting for body composition in the statistical analysis, the resting metabolic rate was significantly lower in athletes with menstrual disorders than in those without menstrual disorders. There were no differences between the 2 groups in daily energy intake and diet-induced thermogenesis. Scores on the Restraint Eating Scale were significantly higher among athletes with menstrual disorders than among those without menstrual disorders. When researchers analyzed thyroid hormones using a competitive chemiluminescent immunoassay, they found that levels were within the normal range and did not differ between groups.

Conclusions.—The results of this study support the hypothesis that restrained eating and low resting metabolic rate are associated with disturbances of menstrual cycle in athletes.

▶ The incidence of the female athlete triad is growing among young women who participate in sports or activities in which a benefit is conferred from having low fat mass, either for esthetic purposes or because body weight must be carried or lifted (eg, gymnastics, distance running, ballet). The triad, which has been recognized as such only in the past decade, consists of disordered eating, amenorrhea, and high risk for osteoporosis. The mechanisms for the hormonal dysfunction are not fully understood, nor are the potential physiologic consequences. The findings of Lebenstedt and colleagues suggest that even subtle disturbances in endocrine function in eumenorrheic athletes can have a significant impact on metabolism. It remains to be determined whether disordered eating is truly the trigger for these events.

W. M. Kohrt, MD

Effects of Short-term Strenuous Endurance Exercise Upon Corpus Luteum Function

Williams NI, Bullen BA, McArthur JW, et al (Boston Univ; Med and Technical Research Associates, Wellesley, Mass; Penn State Univ, Univ Park, Pa)
Med Sci Sports Exerc 31:949-958, 1999   9–10

Introduction.—The long-term reduction in estrogen levels associated with athletic amenorrhea has known adverse effects, such as delayed puberty, bone demineralization, and a possible increase in risk of heart disease. However, few studies have assessed the consequences of corpus luteum dysfunction occurring in athletes who maintain normal menstrual cycles. It is not known whether the corpus luteum is more vulnerable to exercise stimuli occurring during different phases of the menstrual cycle (ie, follicular vs luteal phase). The effects of short-term strenuous exercise limited to the follicular or luteal phase on corpus luteum function were prospectively studied.

Methods.—The analysis included a total of 19 menstrual cycles in 9 untrained women: 5 who performed a high volume of exercise during the follicular phase only and 4 during the luteal phase. Six control women were studied as well: 3 were progressively conditioned to a low level of exercise and 3 remained sedentary. Women assigned to the follicular or luteal phase group performed intense exercises 5 days per week only during the assigned phase, which was based on temperature and serum progesterone levels. In between phases, they refrained from all exercise and moderate activity. Exercise volume increased progressively until the occurrence of ovulation in the follicular group or menses in the luteal group. The women were monitored closely to ensure maintenance of body weight. The study definition of a luteal defect was a short luteal phase (ie, less than 9 days) or an inadequate luteal phase, based on reduced progesterone excretion.

Results.—None of the control women had any disturbances in luteal phase. In contrast, the rate of luteal phase disturbances was 40% in the follicular group and 50% in the luteal group. Fifty percent of menstrual cycles were disrupted in the follicular group and 30% in the luteal group. This difference was not significant, but both groups had a higher proportion of cycles disrupted than the control group.

Conclusions.—Abrupt exercise can have an impact on luteal function, whether it occurs during the follicular or luteal phase of the menstrual cycle. Mild luteal disturbances can occur at relatively low volumes of exercise. No characteristics that can identify women who are and are not susceptible to luteal disturbances are identified. A larger study would help to clarify whether there is a true difference in susceptibility of the corpus luteum to follicular versus luteal phase exercise.

▶ The increasing popularity of sports participation among girls and young women has raised the level of interest in studies of the effects of vigorous exercise on reproductive function. The vast majority of studies have been descriptive in nature, providing characterizations of athletes who have either normal or disturbed menstrual function. The study by Williams and colleagues employed a novel approach to study prospectively the effects on luteal function of performing vigorous exercise during either the follicular or the luteal menstrual phase. A limitation of this study was that it involved small numbers of women and may not have been sufficiently powered to detect changes in hormone disturbances; negative results must therefore be interpreted with caution.

W. M. Kohrt, PhD

Prospective Decrease in Progesterone Concentrations in Female Lightweight Rowers During the Competition Season Compared With the Off season: A Controlled Study Examining Weight Loss and Intensive Exercise
Morris FL, Payne WR, Wark JD (Univ of Melbourne, Australia)
Br J Sports Med 33:417-422, 1999   9–11

Background.—More and more women are being seen with alterations in reproductive function related to intense exercise, particularly during competition seasons. Although the range of exercise-related changes in ovarian function has been well defined, there are few data on the patterns of change in response to changes in seasonal intensity of exercise training. The sport of lightweight rowing poses 2 risk factors for altered ovarian function: not only intensive training in season but also body weight reduction. Ovarian hormone levels were monitored in female lightweight rowers during the competition season and during the off-season.

Methods.—The study included 12 women who were members of the Australian national lightweight rowing program, excluding those who were using oral contraceptives. Also studied were 10 sedentary control women, matched for age, height, and off-season body weight. During the competitive season and the subsequent off-season, the women's ovarian hormone function was monitored by measurement of urinary estrone glucuronide (E_1G) and pregnanediol glucuronide (PdG) excretion. The findings were analyzed to assess the effects of intensive training and weight reduction on ovarian hormone levels.

Results.—The rowers' menstrual cycles were significantly longer than those of the control women during the competition season (mean, 48 days) but not during the off-season (mean, 28 days). The in-season prolongation of menstrual cycles was associated with a significant increase in follicular phase duration and a decrease in the luteal phase. The athletes showed significantly reduced peak and average progesterone metabolite excretion in season but not in the off-season. The peak level of PdG excretion was 13.0 µmol/24 hr for controls versus 6.4 µmol/24 hr for rowers in season. During the competition season, the rowers lost a mean of 5.8 kg, or 9.3% of their preseason body weight. Regression analysis showed that weight loss was the main determinant of the in-season change in progesterone metabolite excretion.

Conclusions.—Female lightweight rowers show significant reductions in ovarian hormone function in association with in-season training and seasonal weight loss. Progesterone metabolite excretion is significantly reduced, whereas estrogen metabolite excretion decreases nonsignificantly. These changes are most pronounced in women who lose the greatest amounts of body weight to achieve competition weight. These athletes have the lowest body fat levels, train the longest, and have a history of previous menstrual cycle irregularity.

▶ The mechanisms of the oligomenorrhea and amenorrhea that occur among young female athletes are only partially understood. There is growing evidence that it is negative energy balance, rather than exercise *per se*, that is a predictor of menstrual disturbances. This has been challenging to study, as most of the young sportswomen who have been evaluated (ie, distance runners, gymnasts) maintain high levels of training and relatively stable body weights year round. In this respect, the study by Morris and colleagues makes a unique contribution to the literature, in that they studied a group of athletes who were required to meet weight restrictions for competition. The rowers who participated in this study had to reduce body weight by nearly 10%, which was a fairly drastic reduction since the women were not over-weight before weight loss. The magnitude of weight loss accounted for nearly 50% of the variance in progesterone levels. It will be important to determine whether certain factors, such as method of achieving weight loss (ie, increasing energy expenditure or decreasing energy intake) or the rate of weight loss, can be manipulated so as to maintain normal sex hormone levels in young athletes who must lose weight for competition.

W. M. Kohrt, PhD

Randomized Trial of the Short-term Effects of Dieting Compared With Dieting Plus Aerobic Exercise on Lactation Performance

McCrory MA, Nommsen-Rivers LA, Molé PA, et al (Univ of California, Davis)
Am J Clin Nutr 69:959-967, 1999   9–12

Background.—The importance of weight loss during lactation is emphasized by evidence that excessive weight retention postpartum is a contributing factor in the development of obesity. However, there has been little evaluation of the effects of weight loss on lactation. The possible adverse effects on lactation of weight loss by dieting alone and in conjunction with aerobic exercise were examined.

Methods.—Women who were breast-feeding exclusively were randomly assigned to 1 of 3 groups: 22 women in a diet-only group; 22 women in a diet-plus-exercise group; and 23 women in a control group. Duration of the intervention was 11 days. The exercise group used a treadmill daily. Dietary intake, energy expenditure, and anthropometry and body composition, as well as plasma prolactin concentration and infant weight before and after the study, were assessed for all groups. Volume and composition of the breast milk, as well as feeding frequency and total breast-feeding time, were assessed for 4 consecutive days and again on days 5, 6, 9, and 10 of the study.

Results.—There were no significant changes in milk volume, milk lipid concentration, and energy density among the 3 groups. There was a significant and similar decrease in milk protein concentration in all the groups, but no significant changes in milk nonprotein nitrogen. Weight loss in the diet-only group averaged 1.9 kg, compared with 1.6 kg in the diet-plus-exercise group and 0.2 kg in the control group. The weight loss in the diet group consisted of 67% fat, compared with 100% fat in the diet-plus-exercise group. A significant interaction was noted between group and baseline percentage body fat in the diet-only group; milk energy output decreased in leaner women and increased in fatter women.

Conclusions.—Short-term weight loss through a combination of dieting and aerobic exercise appears to be safe for lactating women, and is preferable to weight loss by dieting only, which reduces lean body mass. However, more research should be done to determine whether these conclusions apply to women undergoing moderate long-term weight loss during lactation, especially those women with a lean body build.

▶ The prevalence of overweight and obesity in the United States has been increasing steadily, with more than 50% of Americans now falling in these categories. Pregnancy increases the risk for becoming obese because of the retention of excess body weight postpartum. Recommendations for safe weight loss for overweight lactating women are in place (0.5 kg/week), but these guidelines may be overly cautious considering the long-term health risks of excess weight retention. This study represents an initial attempt to evaluate the effects of short-term rapid weight loss, induced by either diet alone or diet plus exercise, on lactation. The finding that lactation performance was not negatively affected by a rate of weight loss 2 to 3 times more rapid than the recommended rate suggests that a more aggressive approach in the postpartum period to ensure return to normal body weight may be warranted. Further studies evaluating the effect on lactation of varying duration and degree of negative energy balance are necessary before standards of care can be revised.

W. M. Kohrt, PhD

Knee Joint Kinematics During the Sidestep Cutting Maneuver: Potential for Injury in Women
McLean SG, Neal RJ, Myers PT, et al (Univ of Queens, Brisbane, Australia; Holy Spirit Hosp, Brisbane, Australia)
Med Sci Sports Exerc 31:959-968, 1999

9–13

Objective.—With the increase in women's participation in sports, it has become apparent that noncontact anterior cruciate ligament (ACL) injuries are 3 to 5 times more frequent in female athletes than in male athletes. These injuries have a significant impact on athletic performance and morbidity. Few studies have examined the biomechanics of the lower limb in women performing movements associated with high risk of noncontact ACL injury, such as the sidestep cutting maneuver. The kinematics of this maneuver were compared between women and men.

Methods.—The study included highly competitive athletes deemed proficient in the sidestep cutting maneuver. A high-speed video analysis system was used to record bilateral knee joint kinematic data while the subjects performed the sidestep maneuver. A custom software package was then used to provide clinically relevant knee kinematic data during both sidestepping and running.

Methods.—Few clinically significant differences were noted between the sexes; for all clinical knee joint rotations, maximum values were well within the limits of safe knee motion. The coefficient of variation for external/internal rotation during the stance phase of the sidestep maneuver was significantly larger in women than in men. However, this difference was significantly correlated with level of experience and was unrelated to gender or the interaction between gender and experience.

Conclusions.—The observed gender differences in knee motion between female and male athletes during the sidestep cutting maneuver do not explain the increased risk of noncontact ACL injuries in women. Experience appears to be a better determinant of variability in knee joint kinematics, although any potential effect on risk of ACL injury remains speculative. More study is needed to examine the gender effects of other factors that affect ACL risk, including joint geometry, ligament morphology, and physical conditioning.

▶ Female athletes experience significantly higher rates of ACL injury (3-5 times) than do men. Many reasons for this discrepancy have been proposed, including levels of muscle strength, lower limb alignment, joint geometry, ligament laxity, skill and experience level, and others. This study examined the performance of the sidestepping maneuver between male and female athletes, to determine whether there were technique differences that may lead to increased risk of injury in women. They found that there were no significant differences in technique that could account for the greater injury incidence in women, but women had greater variability in the joint angles attained during the movement. It may be that one of the contributing factors to increased ACL injury is the previous experience level of the participants, which tends to favor male athletes.

M. J. L. Alexander, PhD

A Prospective Study of Walking as Compared With Vigorous Exercise in the Prevention of Coronary Heart Disease in Women

Manson JE, Hu FB, Rich-Edwards JW, et al (Harvard Med School, Boston)
N Engl J Med 341:650-658, 1999   9–14

Background.—The benefits of moderate-intensity exercise for preventing coronary heart disease is controversial. The benefits of walking versus vigorous exercise for preventing coronary events were prospectively compared in a large cohort of women.

Methods.—In 1986, 72,488 female nurses, aged 40 to 65 years, without cardiovascular disease or cancer, reported information on their walking, hiking, jogging, running, bicycling, sports, and aerobic activity, number of flights of stairs climbed per day, and walking pace. Information was updated in 1988 and 1992. A weekly metabolic-equivalent (MET) score for physical activity was calculated. Outcome measures were coronary events before 1994. The relative risk of a coronary event was calculated for each MET quintile.

Results.—During the follow-up period, 475 nonfatal myocardial infarctions and 170 coronary deaths occurred. Total physical activity score was significantly and inversely related to the risk of coronary events and was a significant predictor of coronary event risk, according to multivariate analysis, even after controlling for age, smoking status, body mass index, and other covariates (Table 2). To control for a change in activity level during the follow-up period, physical activity status was assessed in 1980. Women who were sedentary in 1980 and remained sedentary in 1986 had significantly higher rates of coronary events compared with women who became active in 1986. Among women who walked, those in the 2 highest quintiles for walking scores had a significantly lower risk of coronary events than women in the lowest quintile. Multivariate analysis showed walking pace to be an independent predictor of the risk of coronary events. Although women who walked and engaged in vigorous exercise had larger reductions in risk of coronary events, the magnitude of reduction for women who exercised vigorously was similar to that for women who walked when MET-hours per week were comparable. The role of vigorous

TABLE 2.—Relative Risk of Coronary Events According to Quintile Group for Total Physical-Activity Score*

Variable	Quintile Group for Total Physical Activity					P for Trend
	1	2	3	4	5	
MET-hr/wk						
Median	0.8	3.2	7.7	15.4	35.4	
Range	0-2.0	2.1-4.6	4.7-10.4	10.5-21.7	>21.7	
No. of coronary events	178	153	124	101	89	
Person-yr of follow-up	106,252	116,175	112,703	110,886	113,419	
			Relative Risk (95% CI)			
Type of analysis						
Age-adjusted	1.0	0.77 (0.62-0.96)	0.65 (0.52-0.82)	0.54 (0.42-0.69)	0.46 (0.36-0.60)	<0.001
Multivariate†	1.0	0.88 (0.71-1.10)	0.81 (0.64-1.02)	0.74 (0.58-0.95)	0.66 (0.51-0.86)	0.002
Multivariate, excluding first 2 yr†‡	1.0	0.91 (0.71-1.16)	0.79 (0.61-1.03)	0.69 (0.52-0.92)	0.66 (0.49-0.88)	0.004
Multivariate, excluding biologic intermediates†§	1.0	0.85 (0.69-1.06)	0.78 (0.62-0.99)	0.69 (0.54-0.88)	0.60 (0.46-0.77)	<0.001

*The total physical-activity score was computed as the cumulative updated average number of MET-hours per week for 1986, 1988, and 1992. The primary end point, events caused by coronary heart disease, included nonfatal myocardial infarction and death due to coronary causes. In each type of analysis, the women in the lowest quintile group served as the reference group. *CI* denotes confidence interval.

†The model included variables for age (in 5-year categories), period during the study (four two-year periods), smoking status (never smoked, previously smoked, or currently smokes 1 to 14, 15 to 24, or ≥25 cigarettes per day), body-mass index (in five categories), menopausal status (premenopausal, postmenopausal without hormone-replacement therapy, postmenopausal with previous hormone-replacement therapy, or postmenopausal with current hormone-replacement therapy), parental history with respect to myocardial infarction before the age of 60 years, multivitamin-supplement use, vitamin E supplement use, alcohol consumption (0, 1 to 4, 5 to 14, or ≥15 g per day), history of hypertension, history of diabetes, history of hypercholesterolemia, and aspirin use (none, 1-6 doses per week, or 7 or more doses per week).

‡In this analysis, data from the first 2 years of follow-up after the completion of the physical-activity questionnaire were excluded in order to minimize potential bias due to subclinical disease.

§In this analysis, biologic intermediary covariates that may have had a role in mediating the effect of exercise (body-mass index, hypertension, high cholesterol level, and diabetes) were excluded from the model.

(Reprinted by permission of the New England Journal of Medicine, from Manson JE, Hu FB, Rich-Edwards JW, et al: A prospective study of walking as compared with vigorous exercise in the prevention of coronary heart disease in women. *N Engl J Med* 341:650-658. Copyright 1999, Massachusetts Medical Society. All rights reserved.)

exercise alone could not be assessed because of the small number of women involved.

Conclusion.—Women who increased their activity level had a lower risk of coronary events than women who were sedentary. The benefits of activity showed a dose-response relationship.

▶ Although it is well documented that habitual exercise is associated with reduced risk for heart disease, whether exercise intensity is an important determinant of the extent of the risk reduction remains controversial. In this evaluation of data from the Nurses' Health Study, the investigators sought to determine whether moderate intensity exercise was as effective as vigorous exercise in preventing coronary heart disease in women, aged 40 to 65 years. Two very important findings emerged from the study. First, total physical activity level was associated with a reduced incidence of coronary events in a dose-dependent fashion. Second, sedentary women who became physically active during the follow-up period of the study had fewer coronary events than women who remained sedentary. Thus, in a broad sense, these findings indicate that more exercise leads to more cardioprotection, even in previously sedentary women.

The investigators also reported that vigorous exercise was no more effective than brisk walking in reducing coronary events, but this finding must be interpreted cautiously. Vigorous exercise was defined as an activity that required a rate of energy expenditure of at least 6 metabolic-equivalents, or METS. However, it is conventional to express exercise intensity in relative terms (ie, as a percentage of an individual's maximal aerobic power, maximal heart rate, or heart rate reserve), rather than in absolute terms (ie, METS). A physical activity that requires a rate of energy expenditure equivalent to 6 METS may represent a relative exercise intensity of 90% (vigorous intensity) for a fit 65 year-old women, but only 50% (moderate intensity) for a fit 40 year-old woman. Brisk walking may indeed be vigorous exercise for older women, although it would not have been classified as such for the purposes of this study. Because the method used in this study to categorize exercise intensity is problematic, the results should not be used to endorse walking as being as cardioprotective as more vigorous exercise.

W. M. Kohrt, PhD

Physical Activity and Cardiovascular Disease Risk in Middle-aged and Older Women
Sesso HD, Paffenbarger RS, Ha T, et al (Harvard School of Public Health, Boston; Harvard Med School, Boston; Stanford Univ, Calif)
Am J Epidemiol 150:408-416, 1999   9–15

Background.—For men, low physical activity is associated with high cardiovascular disease (CVD) risk. Although the same is assumed to be true for women, available data on this question have been inconsistent. The findings suggest possible sex differences in the way physical activity and coronary risk factors affect CVD risk. Data from a large follow-up study of women were used to assess the relationship between physical activity and CVD risk.

Methods.—The study included 1564 women who were participants in the College Alumni Health Study. All had graduated from the University of Pennsylvania between 1928 and 1940. At initiation of the cohort in 1962, the women's mean age was 46 years, and all were free of CVD. At that time, the women provided information on the number of flights of stairs they climbed and the number of city blocks they walked per day, as well as the sports in which they participated. These data were used to classify the women into approximate thirds of physical activity: less than 2093, 2093 to 4181, or 4186 or more kJ/week. During 35,021 person-years of follow-up, 181 CVD events were reported. The effects of physical activity level on CVD risk were calculated.

Results.—The higher levels of physical activity were not associated with significantly lower risk for CVD, after adjustment for coronary risk factors. The one exception was walking: for women who walked 10 or more blocks per day, CVD risk was reduced by one third. There was a significant interaction between body mass index and physical activity: CVD risk was reduced with exercise only for women with a BMI of less than 23 kg/m^2. The relationship between physical activity and CVD was unaffected by menopausal status, whether defined as a cutoff age of 55 years or at other ages. Analysis of a subset of women who provided repeated data on physical activity found a marginally significant reduction in CVD risk among more active women: relative risk was 0.94 for each 2093 kJ/week increase in physical activity.

Conclusions.—These long-term follow-up data do not support the assumption that physical activity reduces CVD risk in women. Walking does appear to have a significant protective effect; however, this finding may be related to more precise reporting of walking, compared with other types of activity. Further studies of this issue are needed, including data on changes in physical activity level over time.

▶ It has become axiomatic among health care professionals and the lay community that regular physical activity reduces the risk for CVD. What is not appreciated is that while this appears to be true for men, convincing evidence that this is also the case for women is lacking. The study by Sesso and colleagues adds to the uncertainty, as high levels of total physical activity were not cardioprotective, but walking 10 or more blocks per day was. A serious limitation of the study was that physical activity level was evaluated on only 1 occasion, 14 to 29 years before the self-reports of cardiovascular events, and included only number of city blocks walked, number of flights of stairs climbed, and participation in sports. Answering the question of whether physical activity prevents CVD in women requires a gender-sensitive approach. For example, the tool used to assess physical activity level must include activities in which women are likely to engage. It must also be recognized that some of the benefits of exercise on disease risk may be secondary to the maintenance of appropriate body weight. In this regard, because of their lower exercise capacity and lean mass, the rate of energy expenditure is typically lower in women than in men. Such factors must be considered when evaluating the sex specificity of the cardioprotective benefits of physical activity.

W. M. Kohrt, PhD

Effects of Cardiac Rehabilitation and Exercise Training Programs in Women With Depression

Lavie CJ, Milani RV, Cassidy MM, et al (Ochsner Heart and Vascular Inst, New Orleans, La)

Am J Cardiol 83:1480-1483, 1999

9–16

Background.—Cardiac rehabilitation and exercise training programs have been found to be beneficial for modifying coronary artery disease (CAD) risk factors; reducing psychologic stress, especially depression; and improving quality of life after CAD events. However, women, especially older women, are often not referred to or encouraged to participate in outpatient cardiac rehabilitation programs. The effects of depression and of cardiac rehabilitation and exercise training programs in a large series of women with CAD were reported.

TABLE 2.—Benefits of Cardiac Rehabilitation and Exercise Training Program in Depressed Women With Coronary Artery Disease (n = 23)

Parameter	Before Rehabilitation	After Rehabilitation	% Change	p Value
Exercise capacity (estimated METs)	3.7 ± 1.7	5.3 ± 3.1	+33%	<0.01
Body mass indexes (kg/m^2)	27.0 ± 5.6	25.6 ± 7.0	−5%	0.19
Body fat (%)	33.9 ± 6.1	32.3 ± 8.1	−5%	0.05
Total cholesterol (mg/dl)	222 ± 44	224 ± 33	+1%	0.78
Triglycerides (mg/dl)	234 ± 137	198 ± 96	−15%	0.11
HDL cholesterol (mg/dl)	41 ± 13	47 ± 13	+14%	0.02
LDL cholesterol (mg/dl)	135 ± 33	138 ± 28	+2%	0.37
LDL/HDL	3.54 ± 1.3	3.27 ± 1.4	−8%	0.38
Behavioral characteristics (U*)				
Depression	10.7 ± 3.7	4.8 ± 6.0	−55%	<0.0001
Anxiety	13 ± 5	6 ± 6	−54%	<0.0001
Somatization	11 ± 4	5 ± 6	−55%	<0.0001
Hostility	6 ± 5	3 ± 4	−50%	<0.01
Quality of life (U†)				
Total	79 ± 19	103 ± 21	+30%	<0.0001
Mental health	16 ± 6	22 ± 5	+38%	<0.01
Energy	10 ± 5	14 ± 5	+40%	0.01
General health	19 ± 4	21 ± 5	+11%	0.02
Pain	6 ± 3	8 ± 2	+33%	0.05
Function	27 ± 8	37 ± 8	+37%	<0.0001
Well-being	33 ± 11	44 ± 11	+33%	<0.01

*A lower score indicates a more favorable behavioral trait.
†A higher score indicates a favorable quality of life parameter.
(Reprinted by permission of the publisher from Lavie CJ, Milani RV, Cassidy MM, et al: Effects of cardiac rehabilitation and exercise training programs in women with depression. *Am J Cardiol* 83:1480-1483, 1999. Copyright 1999 by Excerpta Medica, Inc.)

Methods and Findings.—One hundred two consecutive women with CAD were referred to and completed a phase II cardiac rehabilitation and exercise training program. At baseline, 23% met criteria for depression. The depressed and nondepressed groups were comparable in age, body mass index, total cholesterol, and low-density lipoprotein cholesterol. However, compared with women without depression, depressed women had lower exercise capacity, high-density lipoprotein (HDL) cholesterol, and quality of life scores. They also had higher triglyceride levels and scores for anxiety, somatization, and hostility. After cardiac rehabilitation, the depressed women showed significant improvements in exercise capacity, percent body fat, HDL cholesterol, and scores on depression, anxiety, somatization, and hostility. They also had better total quality of life. Compared with the nondepressed group, the depressed group had greater relative improvements in body mass index; HDL cholesterol; total quality of life; and the quality of life components of well-being, pain, and mental health (Table 2). After cardiac rehabilitation, the prevalence of depression declined to 12%. Only 7 of the women with depression at baseline were still depressed after the program.

Conclusions.—Depression is prevalent among women with CAD. In this study, depressed women had markedly abnormal overall cardiovascular risk profiles. An outpatient phase II cardiac rehabilitation program resulted in significant benefits in exercise capacity, obesity indexes, behavioral characteristics, depression, and quality of life.

▶ When we first demonstrated depression in many of our patients following myocardial infarction,[1] one reviewer suggested that we were merely looking at the side effects of antihypertensive medication. Nevertheless, our study demonstrated that a substantial proportion of our patients had sufficient depression to be of clinical concern. Further, the exercise program progressively relieved this depression without any change in medication. As in the study of Lavie et al, we did not have any control group who did not perform exercise. Thus, purists might argue that the decrease in depression score seen in that subsample who were initially depressed was no more than a reversion to the mean. However, the changes were very large, and given also the positive effect of exercise on other types of depression,[2] I, at least, am persuaded that we were dealing with a real phenomenon. Although the present authors argue that the problem of coronary-induced depression is more prevalent in women,[3] this seems unlikely; the percentage of patients meeting the criteria for depression (23%) was actually somewhat smaller than what we found in our original male sample (35%).

R. J. Shephard, MD, PhD, DPE

References

1. Kavanagh T, Shephard RJ, Tuck JA: Depression after myocardial infarction. *Can Med Assoc J* 113:23-27, 1975.
2. North TC, McCullagh P, Tran ZV: Effect of exercise on depression. *Exerc Sports Sci Rev* 18:379-416, 1990.

3. Lavie CJ, Milani RV: Benefits of cardiac rehabilitation and exercise training in elderly women. *Am J Cardiol* 79:664-666, 1997.

Influence of Age and Gender on Exercise Training–induced Blood Pressure Reduction in Systemic Hypertension

Ishikawa K, Ohta T, Zhang J, et al (Natl Inst of Health and Nutrition, Tokyo; Univ of Tokyo; Univ of Colorado, Boulder)
Am J Cardiol 84:192-196, 1999   9–17

Background.—Previous studies have shown that regular exercise can reduce blood pressure (BP) in young and older adults with essential hypertension. However, the effects of age and gender on this relationship remain unclear. Patients with stage 1 or 2 essential hypertension participating in an aerobic exercise program were studied to analyze the effects of age and gender on the BP-reducing effects of exercise.

Methods.—The analysis included 109 previous sedentary subjects with stage 1 or 2 essential hypertension who participated in the Japanese Multiple Risk Factor Intervention Trial. In this study, the subjects performed 8 weeks of mild-intensity exercise training at 22 fitness clubs. The exercise group consisted of 74 men and 35 women, with exercise durations of 60 to 240 min/wk. They were compared with 42 nonexercising controls. The effects of exercise on BP were analyzed in sex and age subgroups; the age subgroups were 30 to 49 years and 50 to 69 years.

Results.—All 4 subgroups achieved significant reductions in BP with exercise. Mean reductions were $-15/-11$ mm Hg for men aged 30 to 49 years, $-10/-5$ mm Hg for men aged 50 to 69 years, $-16/-14$ mm Hg for women aged 30 to 49 years, and $-10/-6$ mm Hg for women aged 50 to 69 years. Although a significant age $\times$ time interaction was noted for both systolic and diastolic BP, there was no significant sex $\times$ time interaction. Age significantly affected BP reduction from week 4 to 8 of exercise, with adjustment for baseline BP, exercise duration, and changes in body mass and salt intake (Fig 1). Age and sex showed no significant interaction on changes in BP.

Conclusion.—This study confirms clinically significant reductions in BP with exercise among subjects with essential hypertension. In an 8-week exercise program performed at fitness clubs, older subjects have lesser reductions in BP at weeks 4 and 8 compared with younger subjects. The mechanism of this effect remains to be defined. Gender did not significantly influence the effect of exercise on BP.

▶ It is now generally agreed that exercise is an effective method of treating moderate hypertension. Pitfalls in such an analysis are bias in those recording BP and the initial fears of patients undergoing clinical examination.[1] The present study was careful to avoid these problems and used an automatic oscillometric system to measure BP and conducting duplicate determinations at fitness centers rather than in a normal medical office. The magnitude

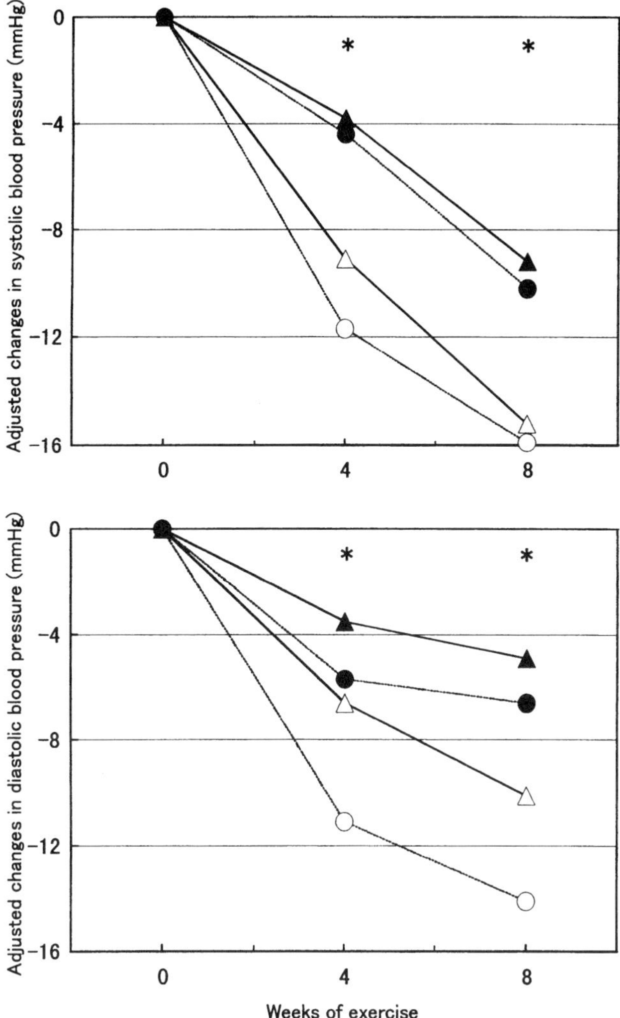

FIGURE 1.—Time courses of systolic and diastolic blood pressure reduction with exercise training. Changes were adjusted for baseline blood pressure, exercise duration, and changes in body mass and salt intake. *Open triangles*, 30- to 49-year-old men; *closed triangles*, 50- to 69-year-old men; *open circles*, 30- to 49-year-old women; *closed circles*, 50- to 69-year-old women. *Asterisks* indicate significant age difference (*P* less than .01). (Reprinted by permission of the publisher from Ishikawa K, Ohta T, Zhang J, et al: Influence of age and gender on exercise training–induced blood pressure reduction in systematic hypertension. *Am J Cardiol* 84:192-196, 1999, copyright 1999 by Excerpts Medica, Inc.)

and speed of response of both systolic and diastolic BP to quite moderate exercise compare very favorably with what could be achieved with many pharmacologic forms of treatment. The age-related difference in response could not be explained by a greater intensity of training or a larger reduction in body fat in younger participants; presumably, it reflects a structural rather than a functional component to the hypertension of the elderly.[2]

R. J. Shephard, MD, PhD, DPE

References

1. Young MA, Rowlands DB, Stallard TJ, et al: Effect of environment on blood pressure; Home versus hospital. *Br Med J* 286:1235-1236, 1983.
2. Vaitkevicious PV, Fleg JL, Engel JH, et al: Effects of age and aerobic capacity on arterial stiffness in healthy adults. *Circulation* 88:1456-1462, 1993.

Physical Activity and Weight Gain and Fat Distribution Changes With Menopause: Current Evidence and Research Issues
Astrup A (Royal Veterinary and Agricultural Univ, Frederiksberg, Denmark)
Med Sci Sports Exerc 31(suppl):S564-S567, 1999   9–18

Background.—Only a handful of studies have addressed the changes in body fat and distribution of body fat in menopausal women. In light of the relationship between obesity and a host of diseases, including cardiovascular disease and certain cancers, notably breast cancer, in postmenopausal women, the changes in fat distribution that occur with menopause are an important issue. Typically, a woman's body weight reaches its maximum at the onset of menopause, and at any given weight there is an increase in relative body fat and abdominal fatness with advancing age. In this study, researchers analyzed the role of physical activity in weight gain and changes in fat distribution that accompany menopause.

Methods.—For this investigation, a search of the Medline database was conducted.

Results.—Cross-sectional observational studies have shown that postmenopausal women who engage in a high level of physical activity have less abdominal fat and a lower percent body fat. In addition, longitudinal studies show that women who are physically active are less likely than sedentary women to gain body fat and abdominal fat after menopause. The investigators found few randomized controlled trials that compared exercise with no intervention or diet versus diet plus exercise. The results of these studies offer no substantive conclusions regarding whether physical activity might prevent or minimize total fat gain and abdominal fat gain after menopause, or whether physical activity may play an effective role in an obesity treatment program.

Conclusion.—Randomized controlled trials are needed to evaluate the role and effectiveness of increased physical activity and physical fitness in the prevention of body fat and abdominal fat gain that are associated with menopause and aging in women of normal weight. Researchers should also investigate the effectiveness of various exercise training programs in treating existing overweight and obesity in postmenopausal women.

▶ Excess accumulation of fat in the abdominal region confers greater risk for cardiovascular and metabolic disease than does total degree of obesity. Although men have a propensity for abdominal adiposity at any age, women do not tend to deposit fat in the abdominal region until after menopause. Studies of older male athletes over a 20-year span indicate that habitual exercise markedly attenuates the increase in fat mass, particularly in the abdominal region, that occurs with aging in sedentary men.[1] Whether habitual exercise is similarly effective in women, in whom abdominal fat deposition is apparently triggered by sex hormone deficiency, is unknown.

This article summarizes the limited published data in this area and highlights the need for further randomized clinical trials. It is important to determine the extent to which exercise, in the absence of hormone replacement therapy, can prevent abdominal adiposity and the related risk for cardiovascular and metabolic disease in postmenopausal women.

W. M. Kohrt, PhD

Reference

1. Pollock ML, Mengelkoch LJ, Graves JE, et al: Twenty-year follow-up of aerobic power and body composition of older track athletes. *J Appl Physiol* 82:1508-1516, 1997.

Lean Body Mass and Leg Power Best Predict Bone Mineral Density in Adolescent Girls
Witzke KA, Snow CM (Oregon State Univ, Corvallis)
Med Sci Sports Exerc 31:1558-1563, 1999   9–19

Background.—Increasing peak bone mass by increasing bone mass during youth has been suggested as a way to prevent osteoporosis in later years. Although peak bone mass is reached soon after the end of girls' longitudinal growth, research has suggested that loading activities can continue to increase peak bone mass through the third decade of life. It has also been reported that there is a relationship between muscle strength and power and adult bone mass. There are indications that this relationship also exists in children, so that children with higher lean body mass with higher levels of both growth and physical activity would also have increased bone mass. Although body weight has long been established as a strong predictor of bone mineral density (BMD), there is disagreement as to whether fat mass or lean mass is more closely related to body mass. Most researchers have reported that lean mass seems more predictive of bone mass, but research by Reid et al has demonstrated repeatedly that fat mass rather than lean mass is more predictive of bone mass. Better awareness of the relationships between fat and lean mass and BMD would help in elucidating effective exercise regimens for building bone. In addition, health implications are involved if fat mass is shown to be more protective against osteoporosis than lean mass. The relationships between bone mineral content (BMC) and BMD as specific indicators of muscular fitness, such as lean mass, leg power, and leg strength, were examined, and the hypothesis that leg strength and power and bone-free lean mass would be independent predictors of bone mass was tested.

Methods.—The study group comprised 54 healthy girls age 14 years (22.7 ± 14.0 months past menarche). After completion of detailed health and menstrual histories, the subjects and their parents were interviewed. Height, weight, and level of physical activity were assessed. Type and frequency of activity were scored. BMC and BMD were assessed for the whole body and for the right proximal femur, femoral neck, greater trochanter, lumbar spine L2-L4, and right midfemoral shaft using dual-energy x-ray absorptiometry (Hologic QDR-1000/W). Investigators then assessed knee extensor strength and leg power using the Kin-Com 500H and the Wingate Anaerobic Power Test. Data were then analyzed statistically.

Results.—The closest correlates to BMD measures were bone-free lean mass and leg power. The best predictor of BMD at the hips was leg power, and lean mass was the best predictor of BMD in the whole body, femoral midshaft, and lumbar spine. In regression analyses, fat mass was not found to be a significant contributor.

Conclusions.—According to these results, bone-free lean mass strongly predicts BMD and BMC in the whole body, lumbar spine, and femoral shaft in adolescent girls, and leg power is the strongest predictor of bone mass in the hip. Taken together, these results indicate the importance of developing muscle mass during growth to maximize peak bone density.

▶ During puberty, rapid increases in bone growth and density occur, with peak bone density achieved between the ages of 20 and 30 years. About 90% of the adult bone mineral content is deposited by the end of adolescence, and this process is affected by both genetic and lifestyle factors. The period between ages 9 and 20 years is critical in building up an optimal bone density as a safeguard against losses later in life. Osteoporosis is thus now viewed as a pediatric health problem.

This cross-sectional study confirms that adolescents who have stronger muscles through vigorous exercise also have denser bones, which should translate to a reduced risk of osteoporosis later in life.[1]

D. C. Nieman, DrPH

Reference

1. Snow CM: Exercise and bone mass in young and premenopausal women. *Bone* 18(suppl):51S-55S, 1996.

A Cross-sectional Study of Smoking and Bone Mineral Density in Premenopausal Parous Women: Effect of Body Mass Index, Breastfeeding, and Sports Participation

Jones G, Scott FS (Menzies Centre for Population Health, Hobart, Tasmania, Australia)
J Bone Miner Res 14:1628-1633, 1999   9–20

Background.—Although cigarette smoking is a known risk factor for osteoporosis in men and postmenopausal women, few studies have examined such risk factors in premenopausal women. The relationship of smoking and body composition, lactation, and physical activity to osteoporosis was investigated in premenopausal parous women in Southern Tasmania.

Methods.—Questionnaires were mailed to 278 women in 1997 who had undergone bone mineral density (BMD) determinations in 1996. Maternal weight, smoking during pregnancy in 1988, breastfeeding habits with that child, and diet during the third trimester were assessed at baseline. The questionnaire requested information about the number of children, lactation history, contraceptive use, calcium intake, physical activity, and change in physical activity. Multivariate analysis was used to examine the association between these variables and smoking to assess the effect on BMD.

Results.—Questionnaires were returned by 263 (95%) women including 118 current smokers. Smokers with a body mass index (BMI) of less than 25 kg/m² had a 4% to 5% decrease in bone mass at all sites. Smokers with a BMI of more than 25 kg/m² experienced no detrimental effect (Fig 1). There was an inverse dose-response relationship between smoking and

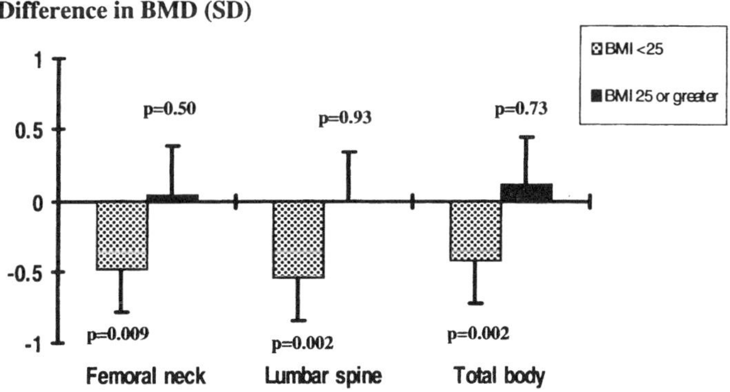

FIGURE 1.—Smoking and bone mass in premenopausal women: interaction with BMI. In women with a BMI below 25 kg/m², current smoking is associated with deficits in bone mass at all sites as compared with nonsmokers. In contrast, current smoking is not associated with deficits in bone mass at any site in overweight or obese women (BMI > 25 kg/m²). Results are presented as Z scores ± 95% CI. (Reproduced from Jones G, Scott FS: A cross-sectional study of smoking and bone mineral density in premenopausal parous women: Effect of body mass index, breastfeeding, and sports participation. *J Bone Miner Res* 14:1628-1633, 1999, with permission of the American Society for Bone & Mineral Research.)

BMD loss in women with a BMI of less than 25 kg/m^2 but not in overweight or obese women. Multivariate analysis confirmed a significant negative relationship between smoking and BMD at all sites as BMD decreased. Current smoking was more strongly associated than other variables with bone mass for all women. Multivariate analysis revealed that BMD was decreased in smokers who had breastfed at least 1 child, but it was increased in smokers who participated in competitive sports. There were no similar associations for nonsmokers.

Conclusion.—Bone loss was increased in smokers with a BMI of more than 25 kg/m^2. Smokers who had breastfed at least 1 child had an even greater BMD deficit. Smokers who participated in competitive sports had a significant increase in BMD at all sites.

▶ Cigarette smoking is regarded as a risk factor for osteoporosis, yet studies of premenopausal women do not uniformly find reduced BMD, the best predictor of osteoporosis in smokers as compared with nonsmokers. Although it is possible that the risk to skeletal integrity conferred by smoking becomes apparent only later in life, this study sheds new insight into the potential interactions of smoking with other factors that may have an impact on BMD of young women. For example, the investigators found a robust interaction between smoking and BMI, with deleterious effects of smoking on BMD apparent only in those women with a BMI of less than 25 kg/m^2. It should be noted, however, that BMD of the overweight women (BMI >25 kg/m^2) who were smokers was only normal, when, in fact, BMD is typically above normal in overweight individuals. The results of this study suggest that the negative impact of smoking on bone health of young women may have been underestimated in previous studies because of the failure to consider confounding factors. It will be important to confirm these findings in a larger prospective trial.

W. M. Kohrt, PhD

Running and Ovulation Positively Change Cancellous Bone in Premenopausal Women

Petit MA, Prior JC, Barr SI (Univ of British Columbia, Vancouver, Canada)
Med Sci Sports Exerc 31:780-787, 1999   9–21

Background.—Other studies have demonstrated that exercise decreases the loss of cancellous bone in premenopausal women, and it has been previously reported that there is a positive relationship between progesterone and cancellous bone changes. In healthy premenopausal women with normal levels of estrogen, these effects may be related to ovulatory characteristics. Whether changes in spinal cancellous bone mineral density (BMD) in premenopausal women who exercise regularly are related to their ovulatory characteristics was determined.

Methods.—Comparisons over 1 year were made in 3 separate analyses among a group of 66 women: nonrunners, consistent runners, and runners

TABLE 2.—Changes in Bone Mineral Density by Quantitative CT (mg·cm^{-3}) in Runners and Nonrunners by Tertile of Mean Luteal Length

Tertile	Luteal Length (d)	N*	QCT Change	N	QCT Change
			Runners		Nonrunners
1	<9.9	15	−5.9 ± 4.2	6	−7.1 ± 3.7
2	9.9-10.9	16	−2.4 ± 4.5	7	−4.5 ± 3.5
3	>10.9	11	0.72 ± 4.6	10	−2.6 ± 3.6

*Chi square = 7.65, P = .177.

(Courtesy of Petit MA, Prior JC, Barr SI: Running and ovulation positively change cancellous bone in premenopausal women. *Med Sci Sports Exerc* 31(6):780-787, 1999.)

training for a marathon. First, the luteal lengths of the consistent and marathon groups combined were compared with the nonrunning group. To determine the possible link between exercise and changes in BMD, the women were divided into tertiles based on their average luteal length. In the second analysis, runners and nonrunners with normal ovulatory cycles were compared to determine a possible relationship between exercise and changes in BMD. A third analysis investigated possible contributing factors to BMD changes in runners by contrasting the cancellous bone characteristics of runners in the upper tertile of luteal phase length with those in the lower tertile. CT was used to measure cancellous bone density from the twelfth thoracic to the third lumbar vertebrae. All 66 women completed daily records of activity, resting heart rate, exercise heart rate, basal temperature, and menstrual cycle. Statistical analysis of the data was performed with both parametric and nonparametric tests.

Results.—Table 2 shows the changes in BMD by tertile as determined by quantitative CT. Among the runners, those with shorter average luteal lengths had a 3.6% loss of BMD versus an insignificant 0.5% loss among runners with longer average luteal lengths. However, there was a negative correlation between distance run per week and changes in BMD.

Conclusions.—Statistical analyses of the data indicated that both luteal length and activity had independent positive effects on BMD. The results of this study indicate that, in healthy women with regular menstrual cycles and normal levels of estrogen, exercise and luteal length have positive, but independent, effects on changes in cancellous bone.

▶ Prior et al[1] reported previously that cancellous BMD was positively related to luteal phase length and that exercise, in the form of running, had no significant effect on bone mineral status. The data from that study were reanalyzed and the investigators now report independent, positive effects of running and luteal phase length on cancellous BMD. Although the practice of retrospectively reanalyzing previously published data should not be encouraged, this article exemplifies the importance of considering the potential interaction of mechanical loading with other factors that influence bone metabolism, including hormonal status and nutritional environment.

W. M. Kohrt, PhD

Reference

1. Prior JC, Vigna YM, Schechter MT, et al: Spinal bone loss and ovulatory disturbances. *N Engl J Med* 323:1221-1227, 1990.

Hormone Replacement Therapy and Hip Fracture Risk: Effect Modification by Tobacco Smoking, Alcohol Intake, Physical Activity, and Body Mass Index
Høidrup S, Grønbæk M, Pedersen AT, et al (Copenhagen Univ; Bispebjerg Hosp, Copenhagen; Copenhagen Municipal Hosp)
Am J Epidemiol 150:1085-1093, 1999   9–22

Background.—There is a substantial amount of evidence to indicate that hormone replacement therapy (HRT), when begun soon after spontaneous menopause or oophorectomy, prevents the loss of bone and lessens the risk for postmenopausal fractures. The effectiveness of HRT apparently increases with longer use, but decreases quickly when HRT is discontinued. This would suggest that HRT should be used indefinitely after menopause to protect against fracture. Thus far, there is little knowledge concerning the effects of behavioral and physiologic factors on the effectiveness of HRT, particularly the effects of smoking. The overall effect of HRT on the risk of hip fracture and whether tobacco smoking, alcohol intake, physical activity, and body mass index modify these effects was investigated.

Methods.—The study population comprised 6159 postmenopausal women from the Copenhagen Center for Prospective Population Studies in Denmark. The women were first examined in the years from 1976 to 1978 and were followed until 1993. Women were surveyed regarding their current use of HRT, which in this study included all forms of systemically administered hormones for postmenopausal replacement therapy. Other covariates included in the study were age at menopause, parity, alcohol intake, smoking habits, leisure time physical activity, educational level, cohabitation, marital status, and body mass index. End point for this study was the first occurrence of hip fracture.

Results.—Three hundred and sixty-three hip fractures were identified during follow-up. Women who were current users of HRT had a lower risk of hip fracture than those who were not using HRT, and the use of HRT was associated with a lower risk in former and current smokers, but not among those women who never smoked. HRT was also associated with a lower risk for hip fracture in sedentary women and those who consumed alcohol, but was not associated with a lower risk among women who were nondrinkers or among women who were physically active. No evidence was found of an interaction between body mass index and the use of HRT.

Conclusions.—Women who are smokers, who consume alcohol, and who are sedentary appear to gain the greatest protective effect from HRT in decreasing the risk of hip fracture. The results of this study suggest that behavioral history provides important information regarding the probable degree of protection HRT provides against hip fracture.

▶ The osteoprotective effects of HRT in older women are well established. An important question that has not been addressed is whether appropriate lifestyle habits, such as regular exercise and appropriate nutrition, can effectively counteract the deleterious effects of sex hormone deficiency on bone. This prospective population-based study found that the incidence of hip fracture was reduced in women who never used tobacco or alcohol and who were physically active, but not further reduced by HRT. Although these findings are certainly encouraging, they must be confirmed in appropriate, well-controlled, clinical trials. The fact that young female athletes who are amenorrheic are often at high risk for osteoporosis suggests that mechanical loading is not an effective substitute for hormones in maintaining bone mass.

W. M. Kohrt, PhD

One-Mile Run Performance and Cardiovascular Fitness in Children
Rowland T, Kline G, Goff D, et al (Baystate Med Ctr, Springfield, Mass; Univ of Massachusetts, Amherst; Agawan Public Schools, Mass)
Arch Pediatr Adolesc Med 153:845-849, 1999   9–23

Objective.—School physical fitness tests include an endurance component that determines cardiovascular fitness by measuring maximum oxygen consumption (VO_{2max}). Maximum oxygen consumption, which is correlated with body weight and 1-mile run time, is affected by body fat content. The influence of body fat and maximum values of oxygen consumption per unit time, stroke volume, heart rate, and arteriovenous oxygen differences on 1-mile run time were evaluated in healthy 6th-grade boys.

Methods.—The relative contributions of body fat and oxygen consumption per unit time per kilogram to 1-mile run time was assessed in 36 boys who performed cycle testing to exhaustion and ran 1 mile.

Results.—VO_{2max} per kilogram of body mass and 1-mile run velocity were significantly correlated (0.77). Percent body fat and VO_{2max}/kg were significantly and negatively correlated (−0.73). According to multiple regression analysis, percent body fat and VO_{2max}/kg together accounted for 60% of the variance in 1-mile run time, with fat content responsible for 31% and VO_{2max}/kg for 28%. Forty percent of the variance could not be explained by body fat or cardiovascular fitness. Cardiovascular fitness can explain only 28% of the variance in 1-mile run velocity, supporting the role of anaerobic factors in endurance performance. Although a 15-year-old boy can run a mile in little more than half the time it takes a 7-year-old boy, both have similar VO_{2max}/kg values.

Conclusion.—VO_{2max}/kg is responsible for about 25% of the variance in 1-mile run times for boys aged 12. Only stroke volume is related to run performance. Body fat content and cardiovascular fitness both influence endurance performance to a similar extent, with anaerobic factors contributing significantly.

▶ Maximal endurance runs on the track (typically 1 or 1.5 miles) are practical, inexpensive, less time-consuming than laboratory tests, and easy to administer to large groups. Although VO_{2max} and 1-mile run time were correlated in this study ($r = 0.77$), closer examination showed that cardiovascular fitness and body fat content together accounted for only 60% of the variance in run time. The 1.5 mile run may provide a better indication of cardiorespiratory fitness in older children and youth.

D. C. Nieman, DrPH

Adolescent Physical Activity and Inactivity Vary by Ethnicity: The National Longitudinal Study of Adolescent Health
Gordon-Larsen P, McMurray RG, Popkin BM (Univ of North Carolina, Chapel Hill)
J Pediatr 135:301-306, 1999   9–24

Introduction.—Being overweight is a major health problem for American children and adolescents, and inactivity is a key contributing factor. There is some evidence that minority adolescents have lower levels of physical activity than their non-Hispanic white peers. Data from a nationwide sample of adolescents were used to analyze in detail the relationship between physical activity level and ethnicity.

Methods.—The analysis, drawn from the nationally representative sample of the 1996 National Longitudinal Study of Adolescent Health, included 13,157 US adolescents in grades 7 to 12. Blacks, Hispanics, and Asians were well represented. Questionnaire responses were used to assess hours per week in physical inactivity, including time spent watching television and playing video games, and times per week spent in moderate to vigorous physical activity. Logistic regression was used to assess levels of physical activity and inactivity, and adjustment was made for sociodemographic factors.

Results.—Rates of overweight (Fig) were highest for non-Hispanic black girls and Hispanic boys and girls and lowest for Asian girls. Among specific ethnic subpopulations, Cuban females and Puerto Rican males had particularly high levels of overweight. Boys overall and non-Hispanic blacks of both sexes watched more television per week than other groups. The mean hours of television viewing per week were 20 for non-Hispanic blacks versus 13 for non-Hispanic whites. Male adolescents also had higher composite levels of inactivity. One third of study participants reported engaging in moderate to vigorous physical activity at least 5 times per week. Girls and minority study participants had the lowest levels of physical activity. The racial/ethnic differences in inactivity were far greater than those for moderate to vigorous physical activity.

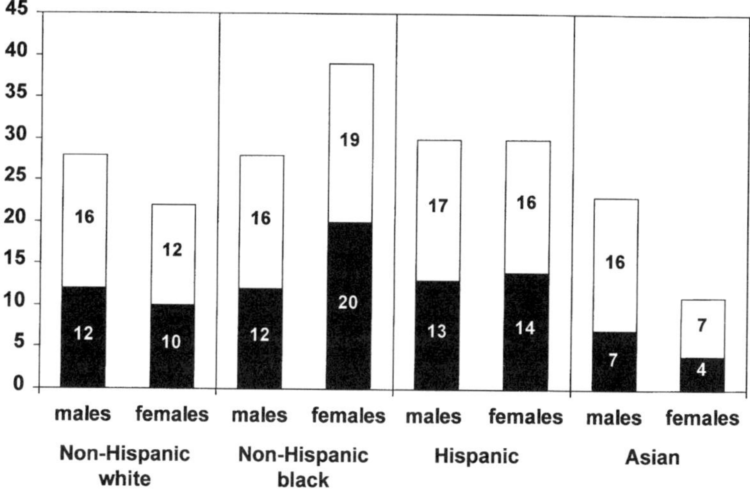

FIGURE.—Percent of adolescents with BMI greater than or equal to 85th and 95th percentiles NHANES I by sex and ethnic group, weighted to be nationally representative with the error terms corrected for design effects. *Abbreviations*: *BMI*, body mass index; *NHANES I*, National Health and Nutrition Examination Survey I. (Courtesy of Gordon-Larsen P, McMurray RG, Popkin BM: Adolescent physical activity and inactivity vary by ethnicity: The National Longitudinal Study of Adolescent Health. *J Pediatr* 135:301-306, 1999.)

Conclusions.—This study documents high rates of physical inactivity among adolescents of most racial/ethnic groups. Specifically, the results suggest that Hispanics and non-Hispanic blacks are less physically active and spend more time watching television than non-Hispanic whites. Efforts to address the problem of adolescent overweight should target female, older, and minority adolescents.

▶ There is increasing evidence of a secular trend toward increased obesity and reduced physical fitness in US children and adolescents, and government officials are worried that health gains achieved during the later half of the 20th century may be reversed.[1] Data from the 1996 National Longitudinal Study of Adolescent Health indicate that there is, indeed, cause for concern, especially among minority youth.

D. C. Nieman, DrPH

Reference

1. Morrison JA, James FW, Sprecher DL, et al: Sex and race differences in cardiovascular disease risk factor changes in schoolchildren, 1975-1990: The Princeton School Study. *Am J Public Health* 89:1708-1714, 1999.

Predictors of Five-Year Mortality in Older Canadians: The Canadian Study of Health and Aging

Østbye T, Steenhuis R, Wolfson C, et al (Univ of Western Ontario, London, Canada; McGill Univ, Montreal; Sisters of Charity of Ottawa Health Service, Ont, Canada)
J Am Geriatr Soc 47:1249-1254, 1999

9–25

Introduction.—Dementia is a major risk factor for death—along with age, sex, major disease, and physical impairment. Data from the population-based Canadian Study of Health and Aging were analyzed to assess the importance of cognitive function and other factors as predictors of 5-year mortality in older adults.

Methods.—The analysis included a random sample of 10,263 Canadians, aged 65 years or older, living in the community or in long-term care institutions. Subjects aged 75 and older were oversampled. Screening data only were available for 8949 community-dwelling subjects. The remaining 2914 subjects—including all of the long-term care residents, all community subjects who screened positive for cognitive impairment, and a subsample of community subjects with normal cognitive function—underwent a clinical examination. Predictor variables of death within 5 years after the initial survey were evaluated.

Results.—Overall, the 5-year mortality rate was 30%. The 5-year mortality rate doubled with each 10-year increase in age and was about 50% higher in men than in women. In the community sample, cognitive impairment was associated with a significantly increased risk of death, similar to that associated with impairment in activities of daily living. In the clinical sample, functional ability was more strongly related to mortality than was cognitive impairment. Institutionalization was associated with an increased risk of death, although this relationship was weakened after adjustment for cognitive and physical status and specific disease factors.

Conclusions.—Sex, age, functional status, cognitive status, and health variables are all significant predictors of 5-year mortality in older adults. Cognitive and physical impairment are powerful predictors, which may tend to obscure the effects of weaker predictors. Information about risk factors and prognosis in older adults can be useful for care planning as well as clinical decision making.

▶ Although not emphasized in this article, the investigators found that physical disability, as assessed by dependence in activities of daily living, was a strong determinant of mortality and that it was largely independent of disease state. Moreover, physical disability was a stronger predictor of death for women than for men. The increasing life expectancy in Western societies has heightened the awareness that age-related loss of bone and muscle mass leads to a decline in functional abilities and loss of independence in individuals, particularly women, who are otherwise healthy. Such preventive measures as exercise training—alone or in combination with nutritional, hormonal, or pharmacologic therapies—may be effective in enhancing physical abilities and sustaining functional independence in the elderly.

W. M. Kohrt, PhD

Declining Physical Abilities With Age: A Cross-sectional Study of Older Twins and Centenarians in Denmark

Andersen-Ranberg K, Christensen K, Jeune B, et al (Odense Univ, Denmark)
Age Ageing 28:373-377, 1999

9–26

Purpose.—Physical disability is more frequent in women over the age of 75 years than in men of the same age. Disabled elderly individuals need additional care, which could pose major social and economic issues as the population ages. A cross-sectional study was performed to assess whether physical ability plateaus or continues to decline with age.

Methods.—Two groups of elderly Danish subjects were studied: 276 who turned 100 years old during a 1-year period from 1995-96 and 3075 twins aged 75 to 94 years. Physical ability was assessed in terms of the basic activities of daily living as well as the ability to walk outdoors.

Results.—For each of the selected activities, the proportion of subjects who could perform the activity independently decreased with advancing age. Women were less likely to be able to perform the activities than men, and this difference became more pronounced with advancing age. By the age of 100, only 20% of the women and 44% of the men were able to perform all of the selected ADLs, compared with 84% of the women and 83% of the men aged 75 to 79 years.

Conclusions.—Among the very old—up to and including 100 years of age—physical ability gradually declines in both men and women. Even though mortality is lower in women, rates of physical disability are higher, and this difference becomes more marked at the oldest ages. The reasons for this paradox—and their amenability to intervention, as through exercise training—are unclear.

▶ This population-based study described the ability of women and men 75 to 100 years of age to perform activities of daily living. Although the findings that disability increased with advancing age and was higher in women than in men may intuitively seem obvious, it is the prevalence of disability and the magnitude of the sex differences that should be noted. By the age of 85, more than 50% of the women reported being disabled; however, this prevalence of disability was not apparent in men until the age of 100. The extent to which lower muscle mass and strength of women contributes to the sex dimorphism in disability must be better described, as these are potentially modifiable factors.

W. M. Kohrt, PhD

Smoking, Physical Activity, and Active Life Expectancy

Ferrucci L, Izmirlian G, Leveille S, et al (Natl Research Inst, Florence, Italy; Natl Inst on Aging, Bethesda, Md; Univ of Padova, Italy)
Am J Epidemiol 149:645-653, 1999   9–27

Objective.—Smoking and sedentary lifestyle are associated with disability and shorter life expectancy. The relative magnitude of these 2 effects on total survival and time of disability onset have not been thoroughly studied. Data from a large longitudinal study of a population-based sample of older individuals examined the joint effect of smoking and physical activity on active life expectancy and disabled life expectancy.

Methods.—Baseline data between 1981 and 1983 and follow-up data on autonomy, disability, death, demographics, smoking, and physical exercise from the Established Populations for Epidemiologic Studies of the Elderly (EPESE) were analyzed. Baseline interviews were conducted with 10,294 individuals, aged 65 or older. Those with disability or with disability status unknown and those who died or were lost to follow-up were excluded from the study. Outcome measures were mortality and disability over the next 6 follow-ups.

TABLE 3.—Disabled Life Expectancy (DLE) and Expected Age at Death (Age T) Estimated for Men and Women Aged 65 Years, According to Smoking Status and Level of Physical Activity, Established Populations for Epidemiologic Studies of the Elderly (EPESE), 1981-1989

Sex	Smoked	Physical Activity	DLE At Age 65 (Years)	Expected Age (Years) At Death for the Group (Age T)	Expected Length of Disabled Life (Years) for Average Men and Women Dying at Exactly Age T*
Men	Never	High	2.5	83.7	3.0
		Moderate	2.6	82.0	2.4
		Low	2.6	78.7	1.4
	Ever†	High	1.3	79.2	1.9
		Moderate	1.3	76.8	1.5
		Low	2.0	76.5	1.4
Women	Never	High	3.8	87.2	4.6
		Moderate	3.9	85.1	3.9
		Low	3.8	81.5	2.8
	Ever†	High	2.2	82.5	3.4
		Moderate	2.2	79.8	2.6
		Low	3.1	79.2	2.4

*The last column reports, for comparison, the expected number of years spent in a state of disability by men and women in the whole study population (regardless of physical activity and smoking status) who are assumed to die exactly at age T.
†Includes both past and present smokers.
(Courtesy of Ferrucci L, Izmirlian G, Leveille S, et al: Smoking, physical activity, and active life expectancy. *Am J Epidemiol*, 1999, 149:645-653. 1999, by permission of Oxford University Press.)

Results.—The 8604 individuals without disability at baseline were divided by gender and classified as "ever" or "never" smokers and participators in low, moderate, or high levels of physical activity. Women had significantly lower smoking and physical activity levels than men did. Smoking was significantly associated with a higher risk of dying, and each increment in physical activity was associated with a lower risk of dying, a much lower risk of new disability, and a higher probability of functional recovery for both disabled and nondisabled individuals. Never smokers who engaged in high levels of physical activity spent less time disabled than did the other groups (Table 3).

Conclusion.—Elderly never smokers who engage in physical activity, particularly high levels of physical activity, live longer and spend less time disabled than smokers and those who do not exercise.

▶ Jack Guralnik and his associates have completed some important studies of habitual physical activity and quality-adjusted life expectancy in populations from the eastern seaboard of the United States. In the present report, data are broken down by smoking habits; however, whether subjects smoke or not, there is good evidence that an active lifestyle not only extends overall life expectancy, but also very substantially reduces the number of years of disabled survival. It is also worth comment that although the activity questionnaire was relatively simple, the difference in expected age at death between high and low levels of activity for nonsmokers (about 6 years) was substantially greater than what has been promised to us in the studies of Paffenbarger and associates.[1] This tends to reinforce my personal hunch that a better classification of habitual physical activity is sometimes obtained by a simple rather than a complex questionnaire, although the sample is demographically more representative than Paffenbarger's, and an alternative explanation could be that covariates other than smoking contribute to the advantage of the active group.

R. J. Shephard, MD, PhD, DPE

Reference

1. Paffenbarger R, Hyde RT, Wing AL, et al: Physical activity, all-cause mortality and longevity of college alumni. *N Engl J Med* 314:605-613, 1986.

Aging Successfully: The Importance of Physical Activity in Maintaining Health and Function
Galloway MT, Jokl P (Yale Univ, New Haven, Conn)
J Am Acad Orthop Surg 8:37-44, 2000   9–28

Introduction.—By the year 2010, more than half of all Americans will be older than 35 years and 25% will be 55 years or older. It is widely believed that increasing age means progressive decline in physical function and loss of independence. Recent evidence shows that deterioration of physical function and resultant frailty are not inevitable aspects of aging.

The importance of physical activity in maintaining health and function is discussed.

Physical Activity.—Declines in musculoskeletal function can be markedly decreased by participation in some form of regular exercise. Record review of masters athletic competitions has been used to ascertain the true rate of age-related functional decreases in healthy individuals in excellent physical shape. Reductions in physical abilities for masters athletes are gradual, indicating that for many, the potential for participation in competitive sports may continue well into the seventh decade of life. Recent trials show that health gains may be realized with low volumes of exercise. Significant health benefits may be gained with a cumulative total of 30 to 50 minutes of aerobic exercise performed 3 to 5 times weekly and 1 set of resistance exercises targeting the major muscle groups performed twice weekly. The aerobic conditioning component does not need to be a formal or structured activity. It may be achieved through regular participation in several common physical activities, including walking, gardening, and housekeeping. Musculoskeletal injuries are an important cause of noncompliance with any exercise program and are particularly debilitating for older adults. Prompt recognition and treatment of injuries and alternative conditioning exercises that minimize "downtime" can help older adults maintain physical activity.

Conclusion.—An active lifestyle is important in preserving health and function in older adults. Many reductions in musculoskeletal function commonly attributed to aging may be minimized with regular exercise. The physician's role is to encourage appropriate physical activity in older adults and prompt recognition and treatment of musculoskeletal injuries.

Exercise, Mobility and Aging

Daley MJ, Spinks WL (Australian Inst of Sport, Canberra, Australian Capital Territory, Australia; Univ of Technology, Sydney, New South Wales, Australia)
Sports Med 29:1-12, 2000   9–29

Objective.—The number and percentage of elderly is increasing and so are the costs of treating those who are in poor health. Preventive measures need to be instituted to forestall projected increases in health services costs.

Exercise.—Although many of the functional limitations that many of the elderly experience may be improved or delayed by exercise, only 4% to 16% of males and females between 60 and 78 are vigorously active. Exercise improves fatigue levels, increases energy levels, speeds recovery from illness, minimizes future health problems, and promotes a sense of well-being. Aging progressively decreases work capacity and level of physical conditioning and increases cardiac hypertrophy.

Age-related Effects.—Anthropometric and morphometric changes occur, along with postural hypotension and a decreased capacity to undertake aerobic activity. The immune, respiratory, and central nervous systems undergo adverse changes, and the senses of sight, hearing, and taste diminish. Muscle strength and mass decline and resorption and redeposition of bone is slowed. Flexibility and range of motion of joints decrease, while joint stiffness increases. With increasing frailty, individuals are less able to perform activities of daily living. Postural sway increases and gait slows, leading to falls.

Exercise-related Effects.—The decline in exercise capacity is not inevitable and can be reversed with exercise. Exercise improves endurance, reduces the incidence of hypertension, hyperlipidemia, obesity, type 2 diabetes mellitus, and impaired glucose metabolism. Exercise can strengthen muscles and improve mobility, balance, and gait, decreasing the risk of falls.

Acute Exercise.—Most of the studies in the elderly have examined the effects of long-term exercise. Acute exercise may have additional benefits in terms of increased coping and relaxation and improved gait economy.

Conclusion.—Most of the physiologic changes that accompany the aging process can be forestalled or reversed by exercise, improving the lives of the elderly and decreasing the cost of health services.

▶ Both articles (Abstracts 9–28 and 9–29) are a comprehensive review of the subject matter. Of note, the Daley article has an extensive bibliography consisting of 135 citations. As a certifiable member of the "over-the-hill gang," it is encouraging to know that "exercise is known to slow the decline."

J. S. Torg, MD

Are Aerobically Fit Older Individuals More Physically Active in Their Free-living Time? A Doubly Labeled Water Approach

Brochu M, Starling RD, Ades PA, et al (Univ of Vermont, Burlington)
J Clin Endocrinol Metab 84:3872-3876, 1999   9–30

Background.—The most variable component of daily energy expenditure is free-living daily physical activity energy expenditure (PAEE). PAEE is a significant predictor of age-related change in body composition, mortality, and morbidity, and consists of volitional movements (such as purposeful physical activity) and nonvolitional movements (such as fidgeting). Experimental overfeeding studies have shown that nonvolitional movements are an important buffer against fat gain. There is a great deal of controversy regarding the factors that regulate free-living PAEE. The authors of this study suggest that free-living PAEE is under regulatory control because individuals increase their nonvolitional activity during caloric surplus to offset weight gain, and decrease their nonvolitional activity during intense exercise to preserve energy. Recent studies have suggested that maximal aerobic fitness is a potential modulator of free-living PAEE. Some studies have found a positive relationship between these 2 variables, but others have not found an association. The relationship between maximal aerobic capacity (VO_{2max}) and PAEE in older individuals was examined.

Methods.—Peak VO_2 max and PAEE were directly assessed using the largest sample size to date in a doubly labeled study. Total energy expenditure was measured from doubly labeled water in 180 healthy individuals from 45 to 90 years old. PAEE was determined by calculating the difference between total energy expenditure, resting metabolic rate, and estimated thermic effect of a meal, assuming that the thermic effect of feeding is 10% of total daily energy expenditure in elderly individuals. Total daily energy expenditure was calculated with the doubly labeled water technique over 10 days. Resting metabolic rate was determined by 45 minutes of indirect calorimetry by means of the ventilated hood technique. Leisure time activities (LTA) were measured using the Minnesota LTA questionnaire. The energy cost of nonvolitional activity was estimated by the equation: nonvolitional activity = PAEE (cal/day) – volitional activity (LTA, cal/day). Regression-based analysis was used to compensate for variables of age, fat mass, and fat-free mass on peak VO_2 and PAEE.

Results.—Significant correlations were found, after correcting for variables, between peak VO_2 and PAEE in both older men and older women (Fig 2), although there was significant variation among the participants. Division of the group by tertiles based on peak VO_2 revealed that men with

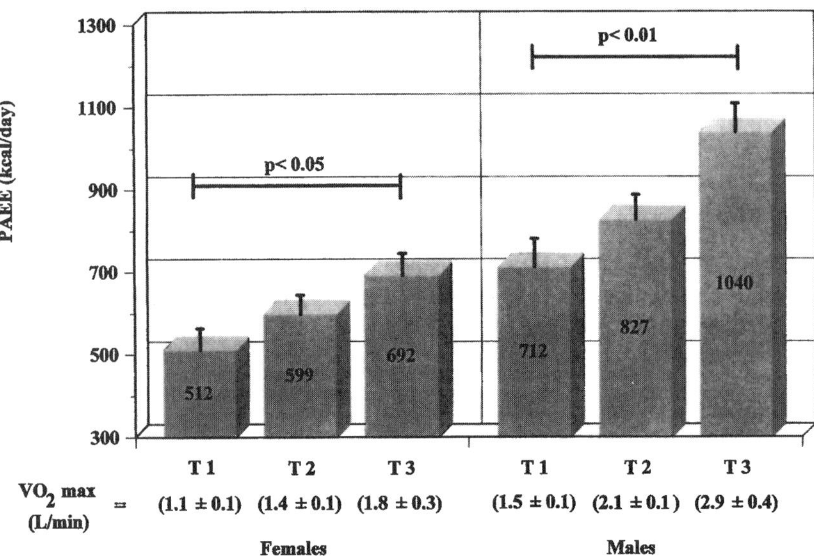

FIGURE 2.—Average PAEE in sedentary male and female subjects when characterized on the basis of low (T1), average (T2), and high (T3) peak VO_2 (liters per min.) Values are the mean ± SE. Analysis of covariance was used to remove the potential linear effect of age, fat-free mass, and fat mass on peak VO_2 and PAEE. ANOVA was used for the comparison between groups, and the Tukey–Kramer highest significance test was used for *a posteriori* comparisons among the 3 groups. A level of significance of $p <$ .05 was used for hypotheses testing. (Courtesy of Brochu M, Starling RD, Ades PA, et al: Are aerobically fit older individuals more physically active in their free-living time? A doubly labeled water approach. *J Clin Endocrinol Metab* 84:3872-3876, 1999. Copyright The Endocrine Society.)

the highest peak VO_2 showed greater free-living PAEE than those with low peak VO_2. Results were similar among women. It is likely that the high intensity of the exercise program fatigued those participants who had not adapted to the short exercise program. PAEE comprises mainly the energy expenditure resulting from physical activity, both volitional and nonvolitional, other than regularly performed exercises. In this study, nonvolitional activity accounted for 65% to 70% of PAEE.

Conclusions.—Results of this study indicate a positive correlation between higher peak VO_2 and greater free-living PAEE in older individuals, with the relationship being stronger among men than in women. The greater free-living PAEE may help these individuals to preserve leanness and buffer fat gain as they age.

▶ Humans expend energy in 3 ways: through the resting metabolic rate, physical activity, and the thermic effect of food.[1] For most people, resting metabolic rate represents about two thirds of daily energy expenditure, and thermic effect of food about 10%. The greatest variability in energy expenditure from 1 person to another is through physical activity, which can be volitional (eg, swimming laps) or nonvolitional (eg, fidgeting). Nonvolitional physical activity typically accounts for two thirds of all energy expended through muscular movement and is an important determinant of obesity.

Are aerobically fit older individuals more physically active in their free-living time? This has been a difficult question to answer, in part because of methodological shortcomings. In this large study of 180 middle-aged and elderly men and women, energy expended through all forms of physical activity (estimated with the doubly labeled water technique) was positively related to peak VO_2, but significant variation was measured that decreased the strength of the correlation. The authors hypothesized that the increased energy expended through physical activity (primarily nonvolitional) may in part be caused by increased levels of sympathetic nervous system activity in the aerobically fit subjects.

D. C. Nieman, DrPH

Reference

1. Ravussin E, Bogardus C: A brief overview of human energy metabolism and its relationship to essential obesity. *Am J Clin Nutr* 55:242S-245S, 1992.

Exercise—It's Never Too Late: The Strong-for-Life Program
Jette AM, Lachman M, Giorgetti MM, et al (Boston Univ; Brandeis Univ, Waltham, Mass; New England Research Insts, Watertown, Mass; et al)
Am J Public Health 89:66-72, 1999   9–31

Objective.—Even though elderly individuals benefit from exercise, 70% or more do not exercise regularly. Whether the Strong-for-Life Program, a course of home resistance exercises designed for older adults with some

TABLE 2.—Comparison of Treatment Groups With Respect to Baseline Values and 3- and 6-Month Change

	Baseline Value		Adjusted Mean (SE) 3-Month Change		6-Month Change	
	Exercise	Control	Exercise	Control	Exercise	Control
Strength*, kg						
Hip extension	10.41 (0.40)	10.48 (0.40)	0.69 (0.52)	−0.16 (0.52)	1.66† (0.51)	0.35 (0.49)
Hip abduction	8.36 (0.26)	8.01 (0.26)	0.38 (0.34)	0.38 (0.34)	1.15† (0.33)	0.22 (0.31)
Knee extension	13.79 (0.48)	13.63 (0.47)	0.06 (0.54)	−0.22 (0.54)	1.12‡ (0.53)	0.17 (0.51)
Shoulder flexion	9.62 (0.33)	9.54 (0.33)	−0.28 (0.38)	−0.10 (0.38)	0.24 (0.37)	0.25 (0.35)
Shoulder abduction	9.27 (0.29)	9.38 (0.28)	−0.92 (0.35)	−1.05 (0.35)	−0.20† (0.35)	−1.07 (0.33)
Elbow extension	8.58 (0.25)	8.59 (0.24)	−0.79 (0.32)	−0.58 (0.32)	−0.15 (0.32)	−0.50 (0.30)
Balance and function§						
Tandem gait (0-10 steps)	3.59 (0.33)	3.54 (0.33)	1.24‡ (0.41)	0.43 (0.41)	1.22‡ (0.40)	0.48 (0.38)
Unilateral stand (0-30 s)	6.55 (0.74)	4.96 (0.74)	1.68 (0.77)	1.83 (0.77)	1.22 (0.75)	1.53 (0.72)
Up-and-go, s	13.39 (0.46)	13.68 (0.46)	−1.00‡ (0.36)	−0.32 (0.36)	−1.02 (0.35)	−0.74 (0.33)
Functional reach, in	9.76 (0.28)	9.15 (0.28)	−0.42 (0.31)	−0.09 (0.31)	−0.04 (0.31)	−0.18 (0.29)
Mood state‖						
Depression	1.49 (0.06)	1.51 (0.06)	−0.06 (0.06)	−0.01 (0.06)	−0.06 (0.06)	−0.01 (0.06)
Anger	1.38 (0.06)	1.41 (0.06)	0.04 (0.05)	0.01 (0.05)	−0.04 (0.05)	0.01 (0.05)
Tension	1.50 (0.06)	1.59 (0.06)	0.05 (0.06)	0.04 (0.06)	0.01 (0.06)	−0.02 (0.06)

Confusion	‾.65 (0.05)	1.70 (0.05)	0.01 (0.05)	0.00 (0.05)	0.01 (0.05)	0.02 (0.05)
Vigor	2.88† (0.09)	2.56 (0.09)	−0.10† (0.08)	0.17 (0.08)	−0.11 (0.09)	0.04 (0.08)
Fatigue	‾.83 (0.08)	2.01 (0.07)	0.05 (0.08)	−0.04 (0.08)	0.13 (0.08)	−0.03 (0.08)
Disability¶						
ln(overall disability)	1.52 (0.15)	1.66 (0.15)	−0.43 (0.10)	−0.24 (0.10)	−0.55† (0.10)	−0.27 (0.10)
(range: −1.04 to 4.10)						
ln(physical disability)	1.53 (0.14)	1.62 (0.14)	−0.47† (0.09)	−0.19 (0.09)	−0.45‡ (0.09)	−0.21 (0.09)
(range: −0.60 to 4.03)						
ln(psychological disability)	1.50 (0.13)	1.67 (0.13)	−0.09 (0.11)	−0.15 (0.11)	−0.31 (0.11)	−0.15 (0.10)
(range: −0.08 to 4.43)						

Note: Strength models are adjusted for gender, age, height, weight, and assessor. Balance models are adjusted for age and assessor. Mood state models are adjusted for gender. Disability models are adjusted for gender and age.

*Higher values better.

†*P* < .05.

‡Borderline statistical significance.

§Higher values better except for up-and-go.

‖1-5 scale; lower numbers better except for vigor.

¶Lower numbers better.

(Courtesy of Jetter AM, Lachman M, Giorgetti MM, et al: Exercise - It's never too late: The strong-for-life program. *Am J Public Health* 89:66-72, 1999, copyright by American Public Health Association.)

degree of physical disability, improved their health was tested in a randomized controlled trial.

Methods.—Strength (dynamometer manual muscle testing), balance (functional reach, one foot balance, and heel-toe walk), mobility (up-and-go test), mood (Profile of Mood States Short Form), and degree of disability (Sickness Impact Profile 68) were assessed in 215 older individuals who performed a 6-month home-based resistance exercise training program (n=107) and in a control group (n=108). The program consisted of a 35-minute videotaped program of 11 exercise routines led by a trainer, to be performed three times weekly, and using color-coded elastic bands of varying thickness to individualize resistance. Individuals received two home visits from a physical therapist and six or seven telephone calls. Outcome measures were assessed at baseline and at 3 and 6 months.

Results.—On average, individuals performed 89% of exercises. Compared with the control group, the exercise group had improvements in almost all variables measured at 6 months (Table 2).

Conclusion.—The Strong-for-Life Program is an effective and inexpensive home intervention for improving the exercise level of older individuals with disability.

▶ This report describes an intervention that seems quite attractive from a public health point of view. Muscle strengthening exercises were performed faithfully at home over a 6-month period, with use of a minimum of equipment (color-coded elastic bands) and supervision (a motivational videotape which presupposes a clientele wealthy enough to own a videoplayer), 2 home visits, and 6-7 phone calls). Good compliance was attributed to use of cognitive and behavioral strategies. Over the 6-month period, participants showed modest gains in strength (6-12%) and a reduction in physical disability as measured by the Sickness Impact Profile.[1] However, in contrast to some supervised programs, there were no significant gains in scores on tests of balance or mobility, and mood state did not change. One practical problem that may have limited the magnitude of response was that the rubber bands stretched over the 6-month interval, so that the applied resistance decreased rather than increased. Possibly, the rate of deterioration of the rubber in a given environment could be estimated, and prescriptions adjusted to take account of this change.

R. J. Shephard, MD, PhD, DPE

Reference

1. DeBruin AF, Buys M, DeWitte P, et al: The Sickness Impact Profile: SIP68, a short generic version, and first evaluation of the reliability and reproducibility. *J Clin Epidemiol.* 1994;8:863-871.

Lack of Age-associated Elevations in 24-h Systolic and Pulse Pressures in Women Who Exercise Regularly
Seals DR, Stevenson ET, Jones PP, et al (Univ of Colorado, Boulder; Univ of Colorado, Denver)
Am J Physiol 277:H947-H955, 1999   9–32

Background.—As people age, their arterial blood pressure increases. The greatest elevations occur in systolic blood pressure, and the increases in systolic pressure and subsequent pulse pressure in women from their premenopausal years to their postmenopausal years are roughly 2 times greater than increases seen in men over the same years. The hypothesis that these age-associated changes in 24-hour systolic and pulse pressures did not occur or occurred to a lesser degree in women who exercise regularly compared with sedentary women was tested.

Methods.—Investigators studied 4 groups of healthy, normotensive women. Group 1 consisted of 12 sedentary premenopausal women, and group 2 consisted of 29 postmenopausal sedentary women. Group 3 comprised 14 premenopausal endurance-trained distance runners, and group 4 comprised 12 postmenopausal endurance-trained distance runners. Seven of the 12 endurance-trained postmenopausal women used estrogen-based hormone supplementation for at least 1 year before the study, as did 11 of the 20 sedentary postmenopausal women. None of the women were smokers, and none took medication that could affect blood pressure. A noninvasive ambulatory monitor (Spacelabs model 90207) was used to record blood pressure over 24 hours of normal daily activity. The carotid augmentation index (AI) was obtained with the subjects in a supine position. The pressure waveform and amplitude were recorded from the right common carotid artery.

Results.—Figure 1 shows the mean daytime and nighttime systolic arterial pressure in the 4 groups. Both systolic pressure and pulse pressure were about 10 mm Hg higher in the sedentary postmenopausal women than in the sedentary premenopausal women. However, there were no significant differences in systolic pressure and pulse pressure between the endurance-trained premenopausal and postmenopausal women. Load and variability of systolic blood pressure were, in general, greater with increasing age among the sedentary women but not among the endurance-trained women. In the whole test group, there was a correlation between 24-hour systolic blood pressure and pulse pressure and waist-to-hip ratio and carotid augmentation index. Taking the influence of either of these factors into account in the sedentary women eliminated the age-associated differences in 24-hour systolic blood pressure and pulse pressure.

Conclusions.—The results if this study seem to support the hypothesis that age-related elevations in 24-hour systolic blood pressure and pulse pressure that occur with age in sedentary women may not occur in women who regularly engage in endurance exercise. This appears to be related to the lack of age-associated abdominal adiposity and arterial stiffness in women who exercise regularly.

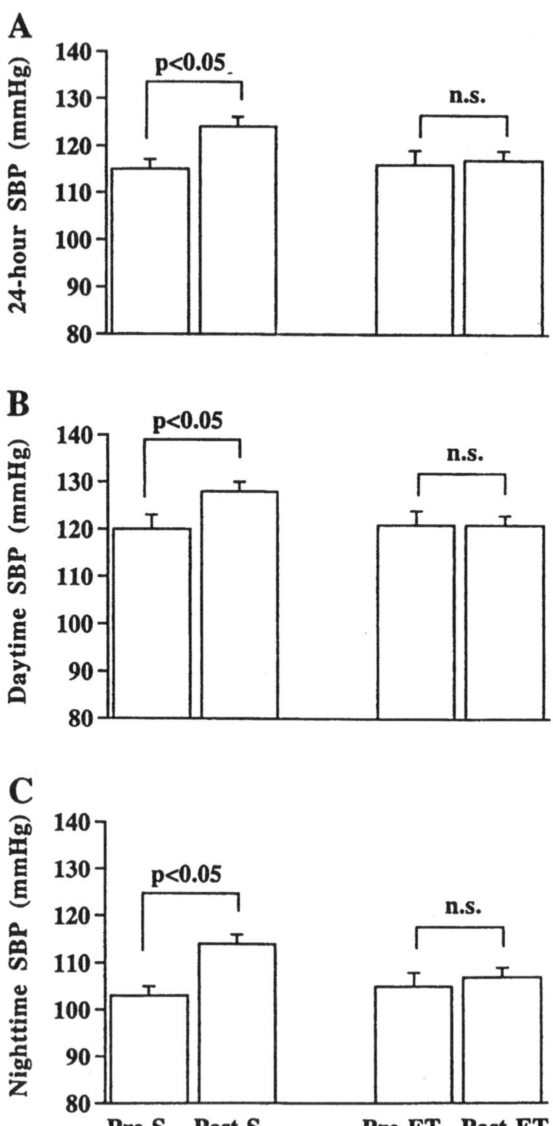

FIGURE 1.—24-hour (**A**), daytime (**B**), and nighttime (**C**) systolic arterial blood pressure (*SBP*) in premenopausal and postmenopausal sedentary (*S*) and endurance exercise-trained (*ET*) women. Data are means ± SE. *Abbreviation: NS*, not significant. (Courtesy of Seals DR, Stevenson ET, Jones PP, et al: Lack of age-associated elevations in 24-h systolic and pulse pressures in women who exercise regularly. *Am J Physiol* 277:H947-H955, 1999. Copyright The American Physidogical Society.)

▶ Increased diastolic blood pressure is commonly viewed as the principal indicator of clinical hypertension. However, with aging, it is systolic pressure that is typically elevated, often in the presence of normal diastolic pressure. This is likely caused by increased stiffness (ie, reduced compliance or elasticity) of the central arteries. It is not known whether arterial stiffness is a normal consequence of the aging process, or whether it is related to such secondary factors of aging as reduced physical activity or increased adiposity. Although the results of this study must be interpreted cautiously, because of its cross-sectional design, they suggest that systolic pressure is not elevated in older women who exercise regularly. An indirect measure of arterial stiffness was also normal in exercisers, but was elevated in sedentary older women. Regular exercise may confer benefits on both vascular structure and function that protect against the development of cardiovascular disease. This study contributes to the growing awareness that many physiological changes traditionally associated with aging are more likely related to life style than to the aging process.

W. M. Kohrt, PhD

Effects of Walking on Coronary Heart Disease in Elderly Men: The Honolulu Heart Program

Hakim AA, Curb JD, Petrovitch H, et al (Univ of Virginia, Charlottesville; Univ of Hawaii, Honolulu; Kuakini Med Ctr, Honolulu, Hawaii; et al)
Circulation 100:9-13, 1999   9–33

Introduction.—Previous results from the Honolulu Heart Program suggest that walking may reduce mortality from coronary heart disease in elderly men. However, these reports included follow-up data on too few men to assess associations with total coronary heart disease. Longer follow-up of a larger sample was used to assess the effects of walking on risk of coronary heart disease in older men.

Methods.—The analysis included 2678 physically capable men of Japanese ancestry living in Hawaii, aged 71 to 93 years. Baseline information on distance walked per day was collected between 1991 and 1993. During 2 to 4 years' follow-up, information on incident coronary heart disease from all causes was collected. The effects of distance walked on coronary heart disease morbidity and mortality were analyzed.

Results.—Coronary heart disease occurred in 109 men during follow-up. The incidence of coronary heart disease was 2.5% for research subjects who walked more than 2.4 km/d compared with 5.1% for those who walked less than 0.4 km/d. The reduction in risk remained significant when distance walked was considered as a continuous variable. Coronary heart disease risk for men who walked between 0.4 to 2.4 km/d was 4.5%. The beneficial effects of walking were maintained after adjustment for age and other risk factors (Table 3).

Conclusions.—Among physically capable elderly men, coronary heart disease risk decreases as walking distance increases. As in younger age

TABLE 3.—Estimated Age-adjusted and Risk Factor–adjusted Relative Risks of Coronary Heart Disease Comparing Ranges of Distance Walked Per Day

Comparison Between Ranges of Distance Walked, Mile/d	Age-Adjusted Relative Risk	Risk Factor-Adjusted Relative Risk (95% CI)*
<0.25 vs >1.5	2.2‡ (1.3-3.7)	2.3‡ (1.3-4.1)
0.25 to 1.5 vs >1.5	1.8† (1.1-3.0)	2.1† (1.2-3.6)
<0.25 vs 0.25 to 1.5	1.2 (0.8-1.8)	1.1 (0.7-1.7)
Test for trend	$P=0.002$	$P=0.002$

*Relative risks are adjusted for age, total and high-density lipoprotein cholesterol, hypertension, diabetes, alcohol use, performed physical function score, and number of years lived in Japan during childhood.
†Significant excess of coronary heart disease ($P < .05$).
‡ Significant excess of coronary heart disease ($P < .01$).
(Courtesy of Hakim AA, Curb JD, Petrovitch H, et al: Effects of walking on coronary heart disease in elderly men: The Honolulu Heart Program. *Circulation* 100:9-13, 1999.)

groups, an active lifestyle appears to reduce cardiovascular disease significantly risk for elderly people. Encouraging elderly people to walk could have important health benefits.

▶ The capability of a walking program to protect against coronary heart disease continues to be debated vigorously. A study from the Honolulu Heart Program[1] reported only 1 year previously failed to find a benefit in men aged 61 to 81 years in terms of a reduced risk of death from coronary heart disease and stroke. The authors now recognize that this may have been because their sample, and thus the number of coronary events, was insufficient to yield a significant effect. In the present study, the sample size was increased approximately fourfold, and the likelihood of a cardiac event was increased by looking at subjects aged 71 to 93 years; the events counted were also expanded to include not only sudden death and fatal myocardial infarction but also clearly diagnosed incidents of nonfatal myocardial infarction. It is a pity that the earlier publication was not held in a drawer until this statistically more powerful trial had been completed! The present report suggests that, in the middle-old, much of the benefit is associated with walking as little as 0.4 km/d. This is not to suggest that a benefit will be derived from such a mild volume of exercise in younger adults. For example, in the Harvard Alumni study,[2] the benefit from walking an estimated 2.1 km/d is only a 20% reduction in the risk of death as compared with the 52% reduction in adjusted risk seen here with a walk of only 0.4 km/d. The benefit in the Honolulu sample persisted and, indeed, was marginally increased after adjustment of the data for age, total and HDL cholesterol, hypertension, diabetes, alcohol use, physical function score, and number of years lived in Japan. It must thus be presumed that exercise is either serving as a marker of an overall healthy lifestyle or is acting through some other unmeasured cardiac risk factor.

R. J. Shephard, MD, PhD, DPE

References

1. Hakim AA, Petrovich H, Burchfiel CM, et al: Effects of walking on mortality among nonsmoking retired men. *N Engl J Med* 338:94-99, 1998.
2. Paffenbarger RS, Hyde RT, Wing AL, et al: Physical activity, all-cause mortality, and longevity of college alumni. *N Engl J Med* 314:605-613, 1986.

Muscle Quality and Age: Cross-sectional and Longitudinal Comparisons
Metter EJ, Lynch N, Conwit R, et al (Natl Inst on Aging, Baltimore, Md; Johns Hopkins School of Medicine, Baltimore, Md; Univ of Maryland, College Park)
J Gerontol 54A:B207-B218, 1999   9–34

Background.—This study investigated whether changes in muscle quality, expressed in terms of force per unit of muscle mass, accompany the aging process, in an effort to better understand the declines in strength associated with aging. Some studies have found that muscle quality changes are not associated with aging, whereas other studies have demonstrated consistent declines. However, unlike most other studies, this one was conducted as both a longitudinal and a cross-sectional study.

Methods.—Three groups were used. The first group comprised 617 men and women in whom the isometric arm strength was examined cross-sectionally by estimation of muscle mass by means of arm circumference and 24-hour urinary creatinine excretion (CREAT). The second group consisted of 412 men in whom the measures used in the first group were studied longitudinally for 10 to 25 years. The third group consisted of 675 men and women in whom isometric knee extensor strength was studied cross-sectionally. In this third group, muscle mass was estimated by CREAT, cross-sectional area (CSA) was taken from thigh circumference, and leg nonosseous fat free mass was determined by dual energy x-ray absorptiometry. Statistical and cross-sectional analysis of the data were performed.

Results.—On cross-sectional analysis, declines in muscle quality were seen in both the arm and leg using CSA and fat free mass, but not with CREAT measurements. However, CREAT and CSA did not indicate any decline in muscle quality associated with age in longitudinal analysis.

Conclusion.—This is the first study to combine cross-sectional and longitudinal analyses of muscle quality in upper and lower extremities across the entire age span of adults. Analysis of the data obtained in this study suggest that there may be a decline in muscle quality with increasing age. However, this relationship is dependent on how the muscle mass is estimated, as well as whether the study is conducted cross-sectionally or longitudinally. It is also possible that CREAT measures a property of muscle that is not measured by the CSA or fat free mass methodologies.

▶ Unfortunately, the authors did not concern themselves with activity levels, testosterone or lack thereof, and other factors relating to muscle quality.

It appears to this observer that the study dealt more with research design than with real-life phenomena.

J. S. Torg, MD

Effects of Resistance Training on Selected Indexes of Immune Function in Elderly Women
Flynn MG, Fahlman M, Braun WA, et al (Purdue Univ, West Lafayette, Ind; Wayne State Univ, Detroit; Univ of Toledo, Ohio; et al)
J Appl Physiol 86:1905-1913, 1999   9–35

Objective.—Loss of strength in the elderly has important implications for functional status, risk of falls, and independence. There is evidence that resistance training can improve strength and functional capacity in older adults. However, there is some concern that the stress of a rigorous resistance training program could cause impairment of immune function. The effects of resistance exercise on immune indices in older women were examined.

Methods.—The randomized trial included 29 67- to 84-year-old women. One group completed a 10-week resistance training program, and a control group maintained normal activity. Blood samples were taken for analysis both after acute resistance training and at the end of the 10-week program. Immune parameters measured included mononuclear cell number, lymphocyte proliferative response to mitogen, natural cell-mediated cytotoxicity (NCMC), and serum cortisol level.

Results.—Women assigned to resistance training had a significant increase in strength. Exercise had no effect on lymphocyte phenotypes CD3+, CD3+CD4+, or CD3+CD8+. However, exercise had a significant time effect on the CD3−CD16+CD56+ phenotype. There was no significant difference between groups in lymphoproliferative response to mitogen. The resistance training group showed a significantly increased NCMC response after acute exercise at the beginning of the study, whereas both groups had an increased NCMC response at week 10. In both groups at both times, NCMC values were elevated above baseline when measured 2 hours after exercise.

Conclusions.—Resistance exercise does not cause impairment of immune function in elderly women, either acutely or over the course of a 10-week resistance training program. Resistance exercise can safely be prescribed to increase muscle strength in women aged 67 to 84 years without affecting immune function negatively or positively.

▶ The effects of exercise on immune function in young healthy individuals are not well understood, as both beneficial and detrimental effects have been reported. Numerous factors contribute to this discordance in the literature, but it is generally thought that deleterious changes in immunity may occur in response to high-intensity exercise in individuals who are unaccustomed to performing such exercise. This raises concern that vigorous exercise may have undesirable effects in the elderly, in whom immunity may be compromised. To study this, these investigators challenged the immune system of sedentary older women before and after 10 weeks of high-intensity resistance exercise training. Although they did not find any beneficial effects of the exercise program on the immunity outcomes that were measured, neither did they find negative effects. However, the volunteers for the study were quite healthy for their age, so whether the findings are generalizable to the elderly population is not known.

W. M. Kohrt, PhD

Diving
  dermatitis associated with, allergic
      contact, 184
  recreational, circulating venous bubbles
      in, 275
DonJoy ROM-Walker brace
  photograph of, 119
Doping, 251
  blood, in athletes, 282
Drugs
  anti-inflammatory, nonsteroidal, for
      chronic patellofemoral pain
      syndrome, outcome study, 79

E

Eating
  disorders
      college coaches' knowledge of, 215
      in wrestling, 221
Eccentric
  /concentric ratios for invertor and
      evertor muscles of chronically
      unstable ankle, 322
  exercise
      chronic, 324
      protocols, adverse events associated
          with, 206
  isokinetic muscle actions, maximal,
      gender comparisons of
      mechanomyographic responses to,
      327
Economic
  costs of obesity and inactivity, 216
Edema
  cerebral, high-altitude, and high-altitude
      retinopathy, 257
  pulmonary
      after exercise at altitude, radiographic
          evidence of, 254
      high-altitude, exaggerated endothelin
          release in, 256
Ejection
  fractions in athletes participating in
      Hawaii Ironman Triathlon, 203
Elbow
  ulnar collateral ligament injuries of,
      operative treatment, 64
Elderly
  adipose tissue lipoprotein lipase in, in
      men, 233
  adoption of active lifestyle by, effect of
      medical clearance on (*see* Medical
      clearance)
  biceps brachii muscle activation
      reduction in, 311
  body composition in

effect of resistance training on, in
    men *vs.* women, 235
  physical performance related to, in
    women, 333
cardiac catastrophe in, exercise-induced,
    avoidance of, xix
exercise in, 367
  cardiovascular risks associated with,
      xviii
  contraindications to, permanent, xxiv
  contraindications to, relative, xxiv
  contraindications to, temporary, xxiv
  life span and, quality-adjusted, xxii
  longevity and, xxii
  maximal, effects on natural killer cell
      cytotoxicity and responsiveness to
      interferon-α, 210
  risks of, xxiv
heart disease in, coronary, walking
    effects on, in men, 373
lipoprotein-lipid profile in, effect of
    resistance training on, in men *vs.*
    women, 235
mortality in, 5-year, predictors of, 360
osteoarthritis of knee in, radiographic
    and symptomatic, level of physical
    activity and risk of, 174
physical abilities in, declining, 361
physical activity in
  assessment of, 190
  free-living time, and aerobic fitness,
      365
resistance training in, effects on indexes
    of immune function, in women,
    376
Electrical
  stimulation
    leg cycling in paraplegics,
        cardiorespiratory responses to, 179
    neuromuscular, after anterior cruciate
        ligament surgery, 95
Electrocardiogram
  stress, fallibility in medical clearance for
      adoption of active lifestyle by
      elderly, xviii
  wall motion analyses in athletes
      participating in Hawaii Ironman
      Triathlon, 203
Electrolyte
  -carbohydrate ingestion during
      intermittent high-intensity running,
      240
Electromyographic
  analysis, use in challenging kinetic chain
      terminology, 304
  measurements, comparison of two
      abdominal training devices with
      abdominal crunch using, 290

Author Index

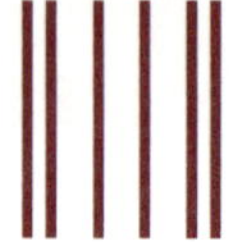

BUSINESS REPLY MAIL
FIRST-CLASS MAIL   PERMIT NO 135   ST LOUIS MO

POSTAGE WILL BE PAID BY ADDRESSEE

SUBSCRIPTION SERVICES
MOSBY
A HARCOURT HEALTH SCIENCES COMPANY
11830 WESTLINE INDUSTRIAL DRIVE
ST. LOUIS   MO 63146-9988

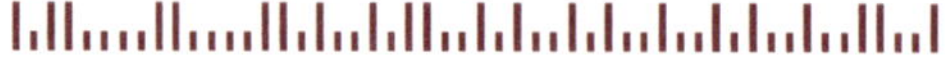

BUSINESS REPLY MAIL
FIRST-CLASS MAIL   PERMIT NO 135   ST LOUIS MO

POSTAGE WILL BE PAID BY ADDRESSEE

SUBSCRIPTION SERVICES
MOSBY
A HARCOURT HEALTH SCIENCES COMPANY
11830 WESTLINE INDUSTRIAL DRIVE
ST. LOUIS   MO 63146-9988

NO POSTAGE
NECESSARY
IF MAILED
IN THE
UNITED STATES

Want to speed up the process?

To order a *Year Book* or *Advances*,
or to subscribe to a journal today,
call toll-free in the U.S.:
1-800-453-4351
Or fax 314-432-1158
Outside the U.S., call: 314-453-4351
Visit us at: *www.mosby.com/periodicals*

Mosby
Subscription Services
11830 Westline Industrial Drive
St. Louis, MO   63146 U.S.A.

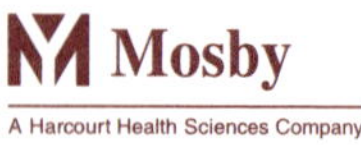

RC